RUNNING REDS

CHRIS DARBY

Copyright © 2021 Chris Darby

All rights reserved.

ISBN: 9798546277574

DEDICATION

Lauren, you will always be my Doodlebugs

All rights reserved. No part of this publication may be reproduced, stored, distributed or transmitted in any form or by any means, including photocopy, recording or other electronic or mechanical methods, without the prior written permission of the author, except in the case of brief quotations for critical reviews and specific other non-commercial uses permitted by copyright law. Chris Darby retains any and all rights to the contents of this book.

For permission requests, contact the author: info@runningreds.ca

Available at Amazon.com in Kindle format or softcover book.

RUNNING REDS – Author Chris Darby, Copyright © 2021 by Chris Darby

Every effort has been taken to protect confidential information following Provincial legislation in PHIPA. Specific addresses, patients, coworkers, allied responders, and hospital staff names where used have been changed to maintain privacy.

Views and opinions expressed in this book are solely that of the author and are not endorsed by the Ministry of Health, past or present employers. Any medical procedures or opinions in this writing should not be taken as medical advice. For medical aid, call 911 or consult a physician.

CONTENTS

	Introduction	1
1	In the beginning	4
2	Are We Happy Today?	20
3	Poor Fido	39
4	You Know, Stuff Just Happens	55
5	A B C	82
6	Strictly Crashes Act I	139
7	Oh Babies Cute Babies	188
8	Regulars I have Known and Loved	212
9	Vignettes From Richmond Street	248
10	Triple Tragedy	285
11	Strictly Crashes Act II	308
12	Guns and Knives Good Grief	352
13	A Strange But True Collection	389
14	Postmortem	441

ACKNOWLEDGMENTS

Lauren, you are the reason this book project was created and has come to fruition. Your encouragement and professional insight are priceless. I am delighted that dad's "war stories" didn't drive you away after all. Thanks, I love you.

Peggy and Pam, your patience with my endless talk of the project used up all my family get out of jail free credits. I owe you both.

To my nephew Matt, thanks for your contribution and opinion. Your advice was invaluable. – Uncle Wonderful

Bones, your insatiable pursuit of humour and the artistic talent you shared over the years carried countless paramedics, hospital staff and friends when we needed it the most. Thanks for granting me permission to convey your messages in this book. R.I.P. brother.

Chris Slabon, your sense of humour and technical authority in pre-hospital care are awe-inspiring. Your students reap the true rewards of your experience and spirit, leading them to their careers. Thanks for your time reviewing and evaluating the manuscript.

Introduction

Nearly two years following retirement, I find myself driving down the highway with family returning from a mission. Amid a global pandemic, it was our turn to be vaccinated. The earliest opportunity popped up at an out-of-town clinic weeks before the chance to seek protection locally.

Familiar with the route, I settled into the drive as the conversation reduced itself to small talk, leaving me to daydream. Passing mostly trucks delivering the essentials, there were gaps in the traffic. The view was a repetition of decades of highway travel ranging from open fields about to spring into action yielding crops to wooded areas with bare trees showing the earliest signs of their leaves.

Ask anyone what they daydream about; the response will range from past experiences or interests to recent activities or future plans. For me, a current project or problem often draws on my subconscious, drafting a solution or plan to fix the self-imposed dilemma. Just ask my family. I drive them silly when they bring up a topic, and I offer unsolicited advice. I am often directed to mind my own business, clarifying that their statement was purely rhetorical.

For those readers that know nothing of the author, some would label me a catastrophist. Although some tragic circumstances are described in my book, the parallel theme to the mayhem is helping. Responders often have their skills and powers usurped by overwhelming odds and the reality that some things just cannot be reversed. When patient care is not enough, the opportunity to support others surrounding the incident or the patient who has succumbed to the odds may be the only chance to effect change in a terrible situation.

Cruising along at 110 kilometres an hour (sorry, Ontario Provincial Police, no stunt driving here), something drew my attention into a wooded lot. A plume of smoke rose beyond the trees, reminding me of a recent conversation with an old emergency management acquaintance. I recalled a poster in our city's emergency operations centre illustrating an event from 1973. So much for thoughts of designing a shelf for my sister's place.

It was early into the 2nd of my 17 years as a volunteer firefighter in Lambeth when the wail of the station's siren interrupted the morning. Called into the City of London to assist their fire service, this incident became a life-changer for so many.

During some construction on Riverside Drive, a pressure regulator on a natural gas line was damaged, sending vapour clouds through gas lines into basements. This touched off a series of residential structure fires unequalled in local history. The sheer quantity of alarms overwhelmed local resources. On route, cresting "Winery Hill" at Wharncliffe Road and Commissioners Road, distinct columns of smoke rose in the distance.

Arriving on scene, houses on several streets in Oxford Park burned uncontrollably after the gas exploded, igniting the shattered structures. A city fire captain turned to our pump crew, shouting, "pick one!" That day 10 families lost their homes, and 40 more were damaged. Fortunately, no one was injured from the explosions or fires. Surrounded by firefighters, police officers and paramedics, it was a true "baptism by fire" for this nineteen-year-old, inspiring my commitment to a career of answering calls for help.

Rejoining the conversation in the car, I handed a notepad to my wife and dictated a few lines to remind me of the daydream. This story is one of my earliest recollections from a life of public service. I am over the work, miss friends and coworkers and continue to foster the desire to serve.

There were stars in my eyes as an impressionable young lad, protected by an unimaginable innocence. Occasionally startled by reactions from friends and coworkers, it was impossible at times to accurately tell whether they were laughing at me or with me relating and sharing the circumstances serving the public. I understand now, more than ever, wanting to help is as much a weakness as a driving force.

For forty-seven years, I was a first responder; this is my story.

1

In the Beginning - Can I help?

In my youth, mom and dad would say it was your badge of honour to declare you had been employed in the same place for however many years. Dad spent his best twenty-five years with the same company in sales. Before she was married, mom was very successful in her brief career as an interior decorator. Mom was happy and satisfied that she realized her goal, though it was short-lived.

Mom lost the argument, and in keeping with the times, dad whisked her away to the east coast when they married. My father was the same as many other dads in the day: he was the breadwinner, and that was that. It was a decision mom, and I discussed on occasion over the years. I disagreed but deferred to her judgement. In her words, "Honey, times were different."

Thankfully those days changed decades ago. Coworkers will laugh at the statement that they think they are about to read here. There have been three jobs in my life; part-time at a milk store while in high school, a labourer - truck driver in a lumber yard following school, and finally, EMS.

Every kid grew up wanting to do something. Remember the adage, "when I grow up, I want to be a firefighter"? That one never crossed my mind until I worked across from the fire station in our village. Martin, a neighbour serving with the volunteer department, invited me to join. We met at the door one evening; he was canvassing for Muscular Dystrophy. In my case, it was an adventure that lasted seventeen years in volunteer service. It was a simple desire driven by the heart: I loved the excitement and wanted to help.

A career in EMS? Now there was an introduction that spanned years. There was no foreshadowing, just a fascination. It started at age seven or eight.

There was a commotion outside grandma's house one summer day. I ran to see what the siren was all about. Parked outside was an old white panel van. A driver and an attendant in white uniforms picked up a fellow having what I later realized was a seizure. Off they went, lights blinking, the old grinder siren wailing away. Cool!

Several years later, some high school friends and I walked to the variety store after school to get a snack. We looked up to see a blue and white SUV ambulance arrive in front of us, lights and sirens. Two attendants jumped out. They cared for a fellow who was knocked off his motorcycle after colliding with a car. My schoolmates walked on. I stood, mesmerized by the action.

Shortly after signing on as a volunteer firefighter, there was an accident just outside the village. We responded on the pumper to find the first of two ambulances at the scene; it was a nasty crash. Standing beside a badly smashed car was a man I was later introduced to as Howard. Our first meeting did not go well. The spray from my hose line soaked him from the knees down. There were a few harsh words; it was a one-sided conversation.

After being formally introduced to the industry, it was a short six months from application to acceptance. A friend Dave, also serving on the volunteer fire service, worked briefly for the ambulance service. Dave pointed me in the right direction after hearing about my interest in ambulance work. Everything happens for a reason - there was no crystal ball. Little did I know it would be a career that would span more than four decades.

I bet you thought I was going to quote the exact number of years spent in EMS. I usually do. Looking in the mirror, an aging Traumasaurus is staring back! Many original acquaintances from EMS and the other emergency services have long since moved on, retired, or died. A resounding reminder of the value of an exit plan.

There was no formal pre-requisite to work in EMS, a standard that has evolved for the good of all. Prior experience of a first aid course and a couple of years with a volunteer fire department opened the dialogue with the fellow at the front door. It took several visits to that door to hear the news I longed for.

At twenty years of age, the response to my repetitious question earned the reply, "can you start in two weeks?" The words were paralyzing. There was just one litmus test left: all applicants were required to do an unpaid "ride out" for one shift.

Arriving for the shift, my entrance was met with a snap inspection by Zeke. The German Shepard was the official mascot for the service. He often lay by the door waiting for his favourite crew to return. Other days he would sit in the lounge in anticipation of a treat from a generous medic. I, on the other hand, was a cat person. Thinking the attention was due to the scent of our tabby, I ignored the canine.

It was an eye-opener, riding with an experienced crew, a pair of Mikes. The first Mike possessed the highest medical qualification in the service. Participating in an ongoing study by the government, the improved care level is our standard today, Advanced Life Support. Mike number two, an experienced medic, held the unofficial tenure of best practical joker in the service. We'll come back to this.

We were sent on a couple of transfers where patient contact was routine, with no problems there. I was introduced to the patient as the new guy. It was clear that conversation with a stranger was not going to be an issue. As an observer, the new world of; moving and lifting patients would be different than carrying building materials.

Our calls were completed without any hitches when we stopped at a variety store for a cold drink. With the refreshments barely open (I didn't know we weren't supposed to eat or drink in ambulances), the radio sputtered out a message assigning a "code 4".

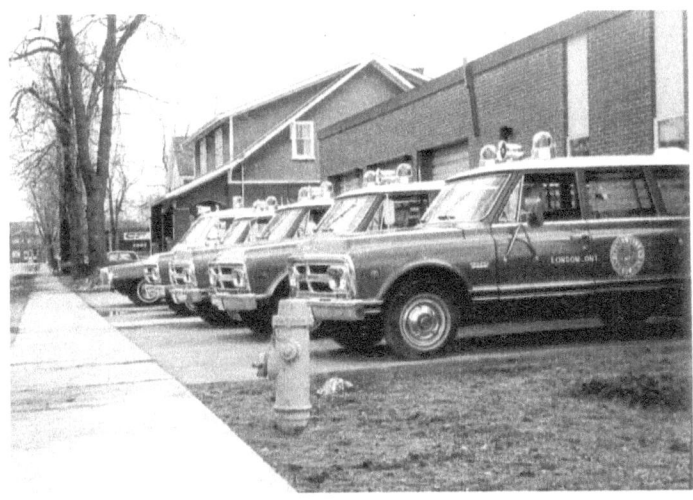

GMC Suburban ambulance

Red and white rotating lights offered their reflection on passing storefront windows. It was a sure sign of the importance of our assignment. The siren? Well, that was another deal. Mike number two, the joker, began narrating his function as the chauffeur. First, he was driving with one hand down Wellington Street, just south of the core. In his other hand was the public-address microphone.

As he drove, Mike imitated the action of shaving his chin, including sound effects. Of course, the microphone was his razor. Depressing the microphone button, Mike sent a buzzing sound out to the public between siren tones. I was thankful he wasn't singing country songs. My confidence was not up to speed yet.

The other Mike was losing it, trying not to laugh. The buzzing sound of the pseudo razor was replaced by the siren when we were in heavy traffic. Ahead was a construction site at the Thames River. A new bridge was being built, the road was divided with orange pylons. In his attempt to thread the needle, Mike made a serpentine-like manoeuvre around every other post.

The evasive moves were in concert with running the multi-function siren to the tune of Yankee Doodle Dandy. It was a skill I would never perfect. The other Mike was screaming in a fabricated horror. In what was better than a slapstick comedy for my initiation to the paramedic's brotherhood, we went on to see my first trauma call.

Arriving at the scene, the crew required some equipment in addition to the stretcher. With the first aid kit and oxygen loaded, we were met by an employee to guide us. The urgency increased as the coworker described a severe injury.

The patient, a warehouse worker, had placed his hand between two pieces of metal shelving as a coworker moved the racks from the other side of the aisle. The shearing action lopped the tips off a couple of fingers. An amputation for my first trauma, neat!

With a small red spot on the first aiders dressing, both Mikes were disappointed. They were unable to show me some gore for the inaugural test. It turns out, today's call for EMS was more for the patient's reaction to seeing his own blood. Our fellow fainted when his first aider friend said there was blood. The microscopic loss was probably a relief to the friend. It was a catalyst for the now-whimpering guy.

It was Friday, said Mike from the front of the ambulance. His advice was to take it easy for the weekend, and it would be back to work as usual on Monday. Considering the humour on-route to the scene, the crew failed to warn our patient not to tap his fingers during the recovery period. I had to laugh at my inside voice - an insight into the dark humour that would follow me throughout my career.

The remainder of the shift was uneventful. Returning to the office, we sat around until it was time to clean the truck and head home. Both Mikes spoke briefly to the supervisor before they said goodbye and left. I found out at the end of the eight-hour shift that the crew was on a mission.

The medic's unwritten assignment was to determine whether I possessed the nerve or stamina to do ambulance work. There were lots of subtle questions and probing statements along the way. As enthused as I was, the emotion was in check. Or was it fear? The action around me looked and sounded more like entertainment. Had I passed muster?

For the first day in a new position, the tension started when I arrived. There were questions from a couple of fellows asking about the volunteer fire department. How had they heard? I had not been indoctrinated into the often strained relationship with firefighters. Looking back at many colleagues, it might have been more frustrated envy than dislike. Several medics moved on to fire careers. Great strides have been made over the years to improve relations with our fire colleagues. In recent times, the two services have become interdependent.

Paramedics today must complete an intense two-year program at a community college. The training out of the gate in 1974 was a mere two weeks. Mentored by Mike's counterpart Ryan, another Advanced Care Paramedic, we worked out of the training room. Basic books offering anatomy and physiology became preferred reading material in the off-hours. The class was informal. The one-on-one approach allowed for lots of questions.

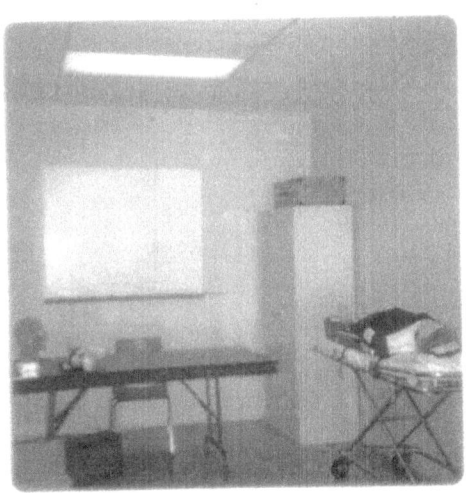

Thames Valley Ambulance training room 1974

The first morning was spent talking about the body's organs, systems and medical terms. This was an extension of first aid training received as a firefighter. I was treating the subject as serious stuff! It was time to break for lunch; I had enjoyed being in the classroom away from the crews.

Mom packed a brown bag lunch, a simple sandwich, and some cookies for the first day on the job. What could go wrong with that menu? Not enjoying coffee yet, I deferred to the hint that there was a pop machine in the garage. A real deal at fifteen cents a can! Leaving my sandwich wrapper opened on the table to go select a drink seemed innocent enough.

Returning to the small lounge, the room was bursting with laughter. After opening the door, I could see a tail wagging from around the corner. It was pointing away from the table and my lunch. Without hesitation, Zeke passed me en route to his post in the garage. A corner of my sandwich hung from his mouth. The overly confident canine tossed his head back in defiance, exiting with the remaining food plundered from the new guy.

A helpful observer informed me that you always left your lunch in the fridge or on a shelf until you were ready to guard it against the four-legged looter. Well, that just made the cookies taste that much better. Following the noon hour initiation, we returned to the pressing matters at hand. Zeke and I went on to be pals, though I am still a cat person.

There were lessons on specific medical emergencies. The instruction and practice on the truck full of equipment seemed endless looking back. In reality, the gear then was so simple. Our modern-day cardiac monitors cost more than ambulances in the early days. Trauma was the most exciting topic. Perhaps this was the result of helping the medics at a few scenes during rescue calls.

The first week covered basic patient assessment; signs and symptoms were a revelation to the untrained. Ryan and I had a few laughs, and he was intrigued during a break when he found out I had been a competitive weight lifter.

Asking for a demonstration, he and another medic broke down when I showed them a pseudo lift. The used uniform trousers issued to me burst in the back. The mishap offered a story for the others once I was out of sight.

Tommy, a supervisor that had the added assignment of issuing uniforms, was on that day, so a quick dash into the supply room netted another used pair of pants, a slightly larger size this time.

Arriving on Monday for the second week, I was introduced to the new guy. Unable to start the same day as I had, Ryan introduced Art to me. Missing the first week would not be as bad as it sounded. Ryan had the gin on Art; there was some medical training in the past. Having attended chiropractic college, anatomy and physiology would be a snap. Oh, I wish I had taken more sciences in high school.

Working as a team, the scenarios went smoothly. The discussion following practice was an education in addition to the hard facts. Art already understood medical terms and anatomy. We were both just leaving ground zero with patient care. The pace picked up as we practiced more new skills to try out for different emergencies. We were growing, improving.

The week ended for me with a handshake and another welcome from Ryan. It would take time. We were both given the warning; pay attention to the senior guy driving. He held the cards until we gained enough experience to try out the instinct that "road time" would instill in both of us. Art would spend another week in class, though it would likely go smoothly with his background.

Following the last day of my orientation, Art and I enjoyed a cold beer at the local watering hole, kicking off a new friendship. He spent some time growing up in the Toronto area. With his dad's career, he also lived for several years in a small town. We had that in common. Older than I and married with a young daughter, we would go on to be lifelong friends.

Following two weeks of orientation with Ryan, it was time to be scheduled into a platoon with other medics. The rotation landed me squarely between two seasoned guys. They would keep me under their wings until I was experienced enough to be tested as a driver. As much fun as it sounded, I had already driven fire vehicles with lights and sirens. Some of the mystique was dashed.

I was in no hurry; the real challenge was caring for the patients. "Attending" to patients was the test in the beginning. Fresh paramedics today are trained and empowered with many times the knowledge and skillsets. Rolling out as a new medic in 1974 should have been a breeze; it wasn't. I was ready to begin the real education on the road.

After finishing the training on a Friday, my first scheduled shift was Sunday afternoon from 4 pm to midnight. New medics were cautiously held back to start their career. You found that the schedule was juggled when you arrived for your shift. Assigned to work with the supervisor, they referred to you as the "Joeboy." There was a reason, the "Joe jobs."

As the Joeboy, you were the last crew out. That was a bummer; I was a keener! Empty the garbage cans, count the dirty laundry twice a week and clean the bathrooms. After catching your breath, there were weekly checks to clean and restock the ambulances. The reward you might get to watch TV and get paid when the work was caught up. Finally, there were calls if the other crews were out.

The Sunday evening shift was a total shut-out, with no calls for my first shift. I worked with the shift supervisor Sam. He was a character that let you think he was indifferent and a challenge to read. Sam held his cards close to his chest - a clean freak and a hard worker, taking on a lot himself. I kept myself busy.

Paramedic crews today rarely see a slow shift. Oh, for the good old days. It was a quiet shift all around. I used my time to pick the brains of the other medics for helpful hints. It was soon evident that my nervousness and enthusiasm needed to be held in check.

Just as the TV news started at eleven, the dispatcher Jerry leaned out of the radio room and shouted at Sam that a medic had called in sick. Turning to me, Sam offered the shift. There was no overtime pay, so working a double shift was a downer for most. That practice ceased with the arrival of a union. In those days, we had an association, which held considerably less influence over our employer. I jumped at the chance to work, and oh, to count dirty linen for the first time. Woo hoo!

And it started again; check the ambulance, count the linen, make a pot of coffee, which I had not learned to enjoy yet. Finally, after the linen was counted, it was time to carry out the trash for Monday morning. Harry was the supervisor now, an old military guy, though the regimented approach had faded.

When the work was done, it was often "feet up" on Harry's watch, no busy work. Again, it was a quiet shift. I was eager to hear about the calls the other two crews were returning from. They were not the least bit interested in sharing. It would take some warming up.

We were down to the last hour. It looked an awful lot like a second shut-out. Was it the new guy curse? Maybe this career was overstated. With just under one hour left, Howard, who routinely slept at the desk, finally picked up the ringing phone. Seconds later, there was a call into the lounge, actually more of a bellow. The snapping payroll clock sound that I had been concentrating on was interrupted by "Frank, why don't you take him on this one?"

The call details sent a chill right up my spine. "Head out to Lucas Street, just outside the city. It's a head-on, car and a pick-up truck". Frank had a couple of years on the job and wasn't too happy to take along a kid for a head-on. Leon, his partner for the shift, was delighted; he would punch out on time. Bonus! Harry agreed that I needed a call. Fifteen hours and I hadn't turned a wheel.

Traffic was light this early on a Monday, before the morning rush. The siren was almost silent. The old "bee-bop" European warning system on the government-issued ambulance was not as "cool" as the yelping, wailing sirens. It worked, sort of. On the way, Frank did not have much advice. I was more reserved with him; he had shown his hypercritical side on the shift during several discussions.

Cruising along, I made an amateurish attempt to form a game plan. What was I thinking? Luckily there were several car accidents to draw from as a volunteer firefighter. It was a start. What to take to the side of the vehicle? Priorities…A – airway, B – breathing, C – circulation. Thinking the worst, I stuck my hand through a cervical collar, riding it up onto my arm, freeing up hands for other jobs. Oh, you simpleton!

Arriving, we were greeted by a provincial police officer. He was doing his best to direct traffic, check the patient and avoid being hit by motorists rushing into the city. Standing in an 80-kilometre zone, then 50-miles per hour, the regulation was ignored by most.

Frank was out of the driver's seat and met me at the rear doors; he was silent. Thanks for the help, I thought. We stacked a backboard, first aid kit, and oxygen bag on the stretcher.

There were two patients by the officers reckoning. A nurse on her way home after a night shift stopped at the collision minutes before we did to render aid. Her presence was reassuring, though she had not done much. She stated the patient in the other car was "not as bad." Frank left me and our equipment. Walking off to the other side of the road, he went to check the second victim. Frank would provide care until the ambulance coming from the adjoining service arrived.

Our patient, the driver of an older pick-up truck, was not belted. The vehicle was built before seat belts were offered or mandated. Thank you, Ralph Nader. I'd just purchased my first new car a year before this crash; it came with shoulder and lap seatbelts. The Highway Traffic Act regulated their use beginning in January 1976. Yours truly was ahead of the curve.

The front grille and left corner of the truck was crushed from the head-on impact. Built more like a military armoured carrier, the force did not transfer into the pillar that held the driver's door hinges. A damaged door would have required a rescue, a process that was in its infancy in the seventies. Any delay would add to an already dire predicament. The nurse opened the door with no resistance.

The patient was slumped over the wheel, a man in his 30's, unconscious from the impact. There was a lot of blood draining from his frothing, slobbering airway. I could not see his face yet. "It's all about the ABCs, but if you don't protect the neck, it's a waste of time." That was a Ryan quote! Luckily, sitting in the back of the ambulance on the way, the new guy's plan paid off.

The nurse stood silently outside the truck, holding the driver's head. I slipped to her right and threaded the collar around the victim's neck and under his chin. The opening at the driver's door of the early sixties vehicle was huge compared to today's pick-ups.

Regular sputtering from the patient's nose and mouth confirmed some success with supporting the neck and airway. Blood covered our hands and forearms. There were no gloves for medics then; if we only knew. The bee bopping sound of a siren in the distance meant Frank would be back at my side shortly.

Now that the victim's neck was immobilized, our next task would be to remove him quickly, without aggravating his injuries. Doing a second assessment, the damage was more apparent. The unrestrained driver was thrust forward into the wheel with the impact.

Steering wheels in the day were large and not padded. They were hard plastic, moulded over steel. The steering wheel's backside was covered in ridges, designed to improve your grip with manual steering. This wheel was well worn, cracked, and the top half bent forward towards the dash.

The source of the victim's bloody sputtering jumped off the page. The driver, in addition to going forward, had his head forced downward towards his chest. The energy from his decelerating head had to be abated somehow.

Our patient's head hurtled into the top section of the steering wheel. The man's mouth briefly enveloped the plastic and steel ring, now covered in blood. The power of the impact broke off most of his teeth, both top and bottom.

As if that was an insufficient insult, the wheel went deeper. Leaving more destruction behind, the stationary landmark split each end of the fellow's mouth to the hinge of his jaw. Swelling and displacement were visible on his left side, evidence of a fractured jaw bone. Time was evaporating. What a compelling case retrospectively for seat belts and airbags.

Frank appeared back at my side, surprised by the progress. Back in the day, with neck pain the only symptom, there would have been ample time to apply the straps and short backboard to immobilize the victim. This was not the time to take the spinal protection to the limit. Even my fresh training left no doubt. Frank blurted a quiet "let's get going" I didn't question him.

Sliding the unresponsive patient onto our spinal board, I felt a hand on my back. The police officer looking over my shoulder could see the urgency; he stepped out of our way. The nurse backed away when Frank returned. She was a sight, blood on her hands and uniform. Our good Samaritan was messier from this experience than her night shift at the hospital.

For being the critic, Frank relented. He began a slow but steady patter of helpful hints as we rolled back to load the stretcher into the ambulance. "Get the suction going" was the first.

Ryan would have been proud; we practiced oral suction in the training room just a week ago. His favourite was vegetable soup. Hearing that, I presented a can to call his bluff. "Hardly anyone pukes water," his introduction.

The patient lay motionless, save his rising chest. With the red-stained shirt removed, I could see a broad crescent-shaped mark. Behind it, there was a definite fault line. Highlighted by some blood puddled in the groove, it crossed his ribs and breast bone at an angle.

With blood streaming from the patient's mouth and nose, the chest was rising more slowly. The frothy blood was settling back, tiny bubbles collapsed on his lips and cheek. Suctioning was a surprise. Expecting just the blood, I was shocked when bits of blood-covered teeth refused to be captured by the suction tip. In another first, my shiny new stainless Kelly clamps (some called them roach clips) worked well to pull out larger pieces and whole teeth?? It was back to suctioning for the moment.

The victim's breathing was shallow now. I announced this observation to Frank and took charge, with timid authority, ventilating the patient with the oxygen valve. A simple "ok" came through the window, then there was some noise.

There hadn't been much interference from the siren until we passed through the city limits. The ride was smooth. Frank's pre-emptive announcements for our turns saved me the surprise resulting in missed steps in the patient compartment. There was not much time to ponder the outcome; I kept busy.

The siren silenced. Frank was talking to Howard now after crossing an intersection. Frank switched the radio to the Provincial channel and waited. Ryan had demonstrated radio patching to the ER during training.

Crews relay a report to the nurses in the emergency room when we travel code 4. In some cases, it would be the attendant doing the talking. For the moment, I had my hands full with suctioning and ventilating our victim, not yet able to multitask. Besides, who wants to take the microphone back through the window covered in blood?

For a greenhorn, I stumbled into a hornet's nest of a call. I was out of my league. I was into the sixteenth hour, during which I would typically be sleeping. The adrenalin was amping me up. I was in high gear narrating the patient's condition to Frank. There were no replies. He was either back in the critic mode or just too busy driving.

The patient report was difficult to hear over the siren pouring in through the driver's window. "Head-on collision, facial smash and flail chest" were the highlights. Flail chest went over my head. The more I looked at the man's chest wall, the darker the marks became as we approached the old Victoria Hospital.

Pulling onto the ramp, it was a quick stop, and the back doors were opening. It was like I was in slow motion. Not wanting to stop ventilating, Frank commanded me out of the patient compartment to unload. Did I have a thousand-mile stare? The stretcher came out of the ambulance, and before I could catch my breath, we were doing the two-step into the hospital.

The radio message obviously got their attention. Nurses and doctors were buzzing around the old "OR 1", a room reserved for the worst of the worst. This was one of them. Questions started flying from the charge nurse and the doctor overseeing this case. It was not in any order, but I spit the highlights out anyway. Giving too many details, we were told to get the stretcher out and received a curt "thanks." Still boiling from the adrenalin rush, I continued to talk in too loud a voice. I'd forgotten that we were in a hospital.

The senior nurse arrived behind me in the hall, her white cap adorned with a black stripe. She towered over me despite being shorter than I. It was her authority and experience that were daunting for my first shift. Did I draw the short straw or what? Thinking there was trouble ahead after turning to greet her, my feet were glued to the freshly cleaned floor. She noticed my lack of composure and announced that I did the right things for the patient. She continued with, "just take a breath, then talk," going forward, of course. Whew, there was a sigh of relief, mine.

After completing a patient report for the first time, Frank gave it a quick once over. His reply; "sure, but don't write so small; you don't need that much stuff." The adrenaline was wearing off now; I thanked him for his advice on the call. An arriving police officer attended the ER to monitor the patient's condition. I walked him into the hall outside OR 1.

Nurses and the doctor were removing their cloth gowns now, blood-smeared and soaked to below the waist. Exiting the room, their absence from the patient's side revealed a sheet draped body on the gurney. The floor was covered with drying blood, layers of footprints the evidence of activity around the patient.

The doctor announced to the cop that the patient died as a result of multiple injuries. In response, the officer explained that both vehicles were likely going over fifty miles per hour. The deceased pick-up driver was the innocent victim; he was still in his lane when found. The other driver heading east was likely blinded by the rising morning sun, crossing over into the oncoming lane, he caused the accident.

With our truck cleaned up, we sped back to the office on overtime. Well, extra time. There was no time and a half for a late call. Frank explained that the other driver was lucky. A construction worker in a heavy coat, he was more protected during the impact. He wound up in a field, slowed down by tall corn. It was harvest time.

Thankfully, there were many shifts ahead that provided the opportunity to transfer lower acuity patients. They needed a ride and reassurance more than patient care. True emergencies are a case of being in the wrong place at the wrong time. There were lots of challenges ahead; thankfully, real disasters came in dribs and drabs.

The call's experience provided the unmistakable feeling of confidence seeping in, bit by bit. It would take over a year to accumulate the worldliness that had you walking in for a shift offering a laugh or smile to coworkers.

2

Are we happy today?

No one can maintain that smile, keep their chin up or be happy all the time. Paramedics are no exception to this notion. Two paramedics sitting in a station or driving around between assignments will find time to be sour about something.

We have a great profession, but there is always something to complain about when left to our own devices. If you look long enough, it's out there.

The title of this chapter is an expression of a long-standing peeve. You know the waitress that starts her order with "What will we have?". I didn't remember inviting her to lunch!

The same frustration re-surfaces when I hear a health care provider start with, "How are we feeling?" I think you should have stayed home if you're sick today.

Humour in our workplace follows a similar path. Faced with unimaginable sights, sounds and smells, you can be overwhelmed in a moment. One release for the stress of repeatedly witnessing sadness and human suffering is humour. Our job is not for the faint of heart, nor is our sense of humour. Older medics refer to it as "dark humour." The term is dated.

The temporary state of mind could be misunderstood as disrespect, a lack of empathy, and verging on crass viewed from the outside. For many medics, including the author, it is the last line of protection from the all-consuming pressures endured when serving the public on their first, worst, or last day.

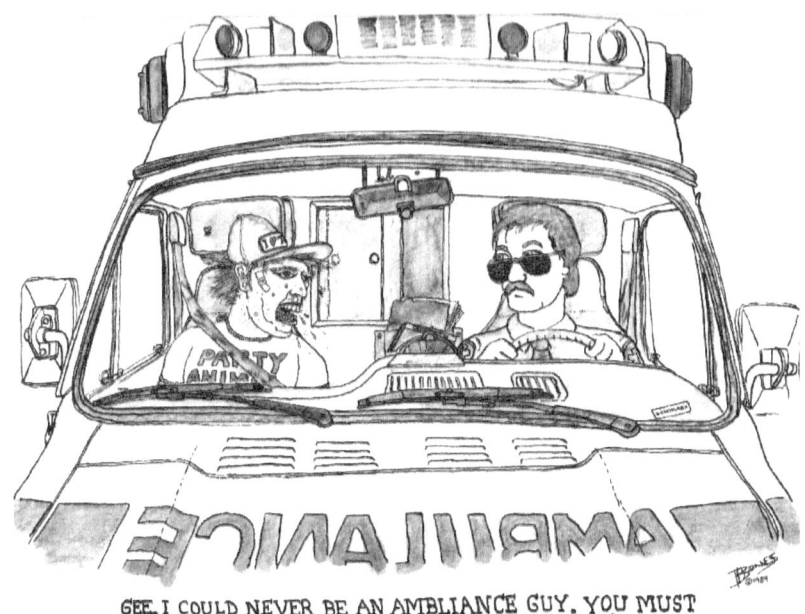

A guest accompanying a patient - credit: Chris "Bones" Skelton

To maintain a balance emotionally, medics must regularly wipe their stress slate clean. Then, paramedics, with their game face on, return to the grind.

There is no way to tell when you are going to have a quiet shift. Responders prepare for the worst and hope for the best. There are times when medics are faced with a stack of terrible calls. You respond, clean up, then return to service.

Following years of trial and error in the attempt to support paramedics, several techniques failed. Today, one early step is to give medics the time to decompress following terrible calls. This technique is one stage within a broader plan to reduce the damage brought on by Post Traumatic Stress Disorder. Many approaches are being studied to treat stress. Rest, diet and therapy, to name a few. And again, though not scientific, humour is another approach medics employ to cope and heal.

Cockaroachathon

Our modern-day EMS stations are improving by leaps and bounds. Purpose-built to contribute to operational ease, they are functional. The often-darkened lounge space is designed to promote a calm setting yet maintain a state of readiness expected of first responders. That wasn't always the case.

Four decades ago, the alliance between the ambulance service and the provincial government was undeniably dictatorial. There was one main base, a brick-and-mortar hub for the operation. Rather than provide the funds for proper stations to serve the remainder of the community, we occupied "satellite stations."

Larger urban ambulance services required peripheral stations to provide a timely service. Rooms were rented or donated to house a crew between calls and keep them out of the public eye. They were a very poorly thought-out fix.

In our city, the provincially funded psychiatric hospital had surplus accommodations. We were the recipients of some good old Ontario generosity. The station was no gift. A small room attached to the old woodworking shop, it was unhealthily warm in the summer. During the winter, the hot water radiators ground out a dry heat that had you coughing, interrupting a quiet evening.

Decorated with recycled furniture from the hospital, it was a dismal hovel, to say the least. Dust from ongoing woodshop activities across the hall stuck to your clothes. The chairs required a pre-wiping before sitting down. Now you have a picture in your head, and we haven't left the station for a call yet.

The wooden, one-storey building was built with a solid but uneven plank floor that rested on short pillars, leaving a meter of crawl space under the entire structure. What a brilliant design to allow for the infrastructure concealed beneath. A floor access hatch in our room answered the long-standing question; our local Storybook Gardens began collecting exotic creatures from the depths below this woodshop, minus Slippery the seal. Well, that's one opinion anyway.

Sitting on gently used lounge chairs that originally served incontinent geriatric patients for years, you could see and hear the "untamed" world every shift. The adjacent kitchen building that prepared food for the institution was adjoined to our castle. Service tunnels carried hot water heat lines from building to building. It was a commuting route for the locals.

Crawling out of nooks and crannies were the cutest little cockroaches in the neighbourhood. The roaches loved the dry heat. We were hosts to an all-inclusive destination for pests.

So, there we sat in the early years of our careers. Art and I were regular partners now, sharing eight-hour shifts serving the east end of our city. The standby location gave you access to Dundas Street and Highbury Avenue. We were buried one-quarter of a mile off each thoroughfare, hidden behind a maze of old government buildings. Ever see a fire station that far off the main route?

Now, add insult to injury with regular creepy episodes as bugs and mice entertained themselves around our room. Cockroaches climbed the walls. It was not unusual in a quiet moment to hear the tap when they fell harmlessly from a wall or the ceiling.

Left to our devices with the off-beat sense of humour many medics possess, our minds wandered, the desire to entertain with a purpose-driven plan. Watching Jerry Lewis one weekend on our 12" black and white TV, his annual fundraising telethon was in full swing. What about a "Cockaroachathon"? I know it's not in the dictionary. I checked.

To identify our displeasure with the pestilent workplace, the thought of a visible competition was spawned. A quick trip next door to the idle wood shop produced some finishing nails. Artie titled the poster, AKA wall, with the term Cockaroachathon. Within minutes we had several entries pinned to the wall. I thought a common steel nail through the body would instantly kill the little pests. Not so.

As we returned to the station for future shifts, the momentum gathered. Other medics could see the rationale and submitted some outstanding entries. Word was spreading, the tote board was growing by the dozens.

The cleaning staff started with a snotty note, choosing not to clean the room. We could find no difference in the cleanliness of the station in their reactive absence. It only took a few weeks to come full circle.

Approached by our boss Donald, the Operations Communications Supervisor. "Ops. Com. Sup." for short, he loved the title; we admitted to the action and gave our rationale. There were some terse exchanges. In the end, we were moved out of the room.

We paid homage to the assistance they lent in correcting our accommodations problem. A close friend took exception to our cruelty. I will always respect his opinion; the behaviour was results-driven. The picture he took of our tote board is digitally memorialized on my computer.

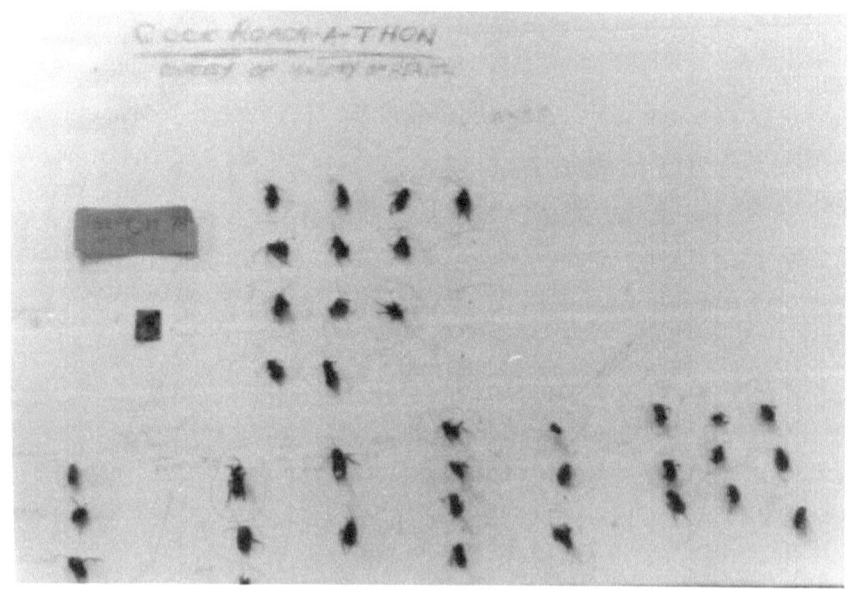

Cockaroachathon 1975 - credit: Chris Skelton

Our host, the Province, moved our operation. We were given a room at the back of the hospital. The change was initially welcomed. It was ten steps or more to navigate the descent to the closet-sized chamber, then back up the stairs to respond. The washroom was clean, even if it was at least one hundred feet away.

We were an emergency service. Maybe that's why we were assigned the subterranean accommodations next to rooms stuffed to the ceiling with outdated provincial disaster supplies. Green crates marked with the Department of National Defence were packed in the fifties. Their best before dates were in the year 1969. It was the winter of 1975.

Just Joking

Two-way radios were "cool" when I was young. I always wanted to talk on one. Then again, I always loved to talk. I joined the local volunteer fire department and realized a bit of a broadcasting fix. Some fire department members had the early citizen's band radios in their personal vehicles. I had to have one, "breaker, breaker," and all that ancient jargon.

Once radios become a regular tool of the trade, their use becomes passe. That is until the unusual presents itself. A faux-pas, a tone of voice, a joke; you get the idea. At times, medics would forget that radios and their use is regulated by the federal government. Oh well.

Steve, one of our dispatchers, had a sense of humour that ranked right up there with comedians of the day. His English accent and wit combined drove the dullest shifts. When the pace was busier, the mood lightened with a well-timed quip.

At a fire stand by early one morning, the blaze brought out the locals. Rubber-neckers added to the entertainment value for medics. There was nothing to do until a patient was brought out to us. Fortunately, that scenario was infrequent. Neither service at the time supplied walkie-talkies for their crews. Before the birth of portable radios in the city, some technical wizard attached the mobile radio speaker to the public-address system in our siren set up.

A great feature, we didn't have to sit in our vehicle or stand next to the door to hear an incoming message. The declaration was broadcast overhead. The downside; everyone within earshot got the message too.

Steve had the worst or the best radio etiquette on record. Note to readers; The Provincial ambulance system requires that you announce every vehicle move. The automatic response from dispatch is usually the iconic "10-4," followed by unit number and time.

A crew clearing from a hospital was acknowledged with "10-4 car 158, London clear at 7:47. Just like the big fucking airplane, Mate." The sound hadn't finished echoing off the surrounding homes before the firefighters were pointing and laughing. The onlookers must have missed it with the fire truck's revving engines propelling water on the waning structure fire.

A television show in the '70s, Kung Fu, brought on nicknames like mine. As the youngest lad on the trucks at the time, the moniker "Grasshopper" stuck for a couple of years. It was reserved for quiet nights.

I was being driven by Kevin and assigned to a "central stand by" late into a night shift. A quiet guy, he was graced with a dry wit like Steve, though more reserved. We were sitting in silence for a while. With only three ambulances on, we were waiting for at least one to clear from a hospital before we could return to the office and stick our feet up.

Relaxing, with our arms hanging out the open windows, the silence was broken with a whisper. "Kevin." We looked at each other when nothing followed and returned to our standby pose. Almost thirty seconds later, "Kevin" was whispered again.

We realized now that Steve was bored, hoping for a response. Kevin slowly retrieved the microphone from its mount on the dash, not wanting to jump at the bait too quickly. He waited, not taking the lure; Steve returned with a third whispered address, "Kevin."

Speaking clearly, Kevin answered, returning with an inquisitive sounding, "What?"

Out of the speaker grille on the radio came the ethereal response, "Your house is on fire." I was taken aback. This was one of the first scripted ha-ha moments early on in my career. Not knowing what to say, I looked at Kevin. He replied in an authoritative tone, "Tell the firemen to save my canary."

I jumped to the conclusion, I might as well take my personal coffee mug home in the morning. Something terrible would come of joking on the radio. The fire chief had warned us years earlier that the feds are always listening. This was bad.

There were a few laughs when we returned to the office a while later. Another medic received the same line weeks ago; he was there to tell the tale now. We were safe.

Years later, Bernie and I were returning to the office one quiet evening shift. The first provincially endorsed Advanced Care air ambulance helicopter had just left town. It was returning to the big smoke of Toronto.

Still a novelty, we hung back at University Hospital to see "799." The old Huey wound up its massive blades beating the local air into submission before leaving the helipad. The thundering departure was announced on the Provincial radio channel. The radio traffic went unnoticed by city crews working on another frequency.

This evening our dispatcher was a part-time employee, Joe. A keen young fellow with no EMS experience, he was totally intrigued by the ambulance service.

He was also a ham radio operator and an auxiliary cop. He couldn't get enough of the action. It was time to throw more excitement his way.

Backing into the third bay, our unannounced arrival was missed by Joe through the window joining the new radio room and the garage. Partially hidden by an idle unit in the middle bay, Bernie and I sat in our truck and reviewed his keen sense of duty. Speedy radio responses to departing and arriving units resembled military precision, crisp and authoritative. This would be a two-person gag.

With a well-timed transmission, the brief rehearsal paid off in spades. Bernie held the microphone in front of me as I started the message. In a Tarzan-like move, I pounded my chest as I spoke. "London, this is 799, over." The background thumping noise sounded like a Huey to us.

There was no hesitation as Joe flung himself forward in the swivelling chair. Turned in our seats, we had a perfect perch to follow the hoax. From his relaxed pose to full attention, he was hooked. Joe failed to notice the signal was coming from the wrong radio channel. He was up for anything. Was the medical helo calling in a Mayday?

"799 go ahead; this is London, over." It was an official response, an air traffic controller would have been proud of. Now that we had his undivided attention, I was lost for a message. The keener was ready to bite the boom microphone as he leaned into the radio console around him.

With the reverberating annunciation at its peak, the helicopter voice lost his nerve. "London 799, disregard, over." Looking sidelong through the window, Joe could see us through the cab windows of the unit separating us. Lost for an intelligent helicopter come back, I just waved. The chest pounding was over. The single-finger response from the radio room was un-military and luckily did not come over the air.

Our return to the lounge was silent. That lasted for less than a minute. Belly laughs all around. The four of us seated acknowledged that the keener got the message, loud and clear: chill out.

Shot in the dark

There was never a boring shift with Mike. He was the leading practical joker on our team. Coming to London from an adjacent ambulance service in St. Thomas, his humour led the way. Quiet at first, when you met the tall, lanky medic, looks were deceiving.

Seated next to him, you always took a good look around if you were the only person, not laughing. The joke was likely on you. A hand gesture behind your head, a roll of the eyes as you finished a story, he made us all laugh.

Of course, if he could attract an accomplice for his gags, the blame could be shared. His efforts were always successful. One spoof that never grew old was to write across the top of the lenses of someone's glasses with a wax crayon. As the spectacles sat idle on the table next to their snoozing owner on a night shift, a message would be crafted.

The notice to the opposing person, a patient or hospital staffer, drew laughs until the wearer realized there was a reason for the snicker. Just out of the host's visual range would be a "Help me," "I'm a loser," or the owner's name.

Returning to base in the middle of a night shift, Mike coasted backwards into the garage with the ignition off. The near-silent approach earned the element of surprise for the scheming prankster. Asking for my assistance on the way back to the office, I had never heard of this one. Involving a sudden noise, the shock would surely bring on an incident of incontinence. None of the sleeping medics in the lounge was known to wear adult diapers.

In the storage room outside the lounge, medical supplies stood ready to restock returning ambulances. Next to the storeroom door sat our oxygen supply. In a rack were small, white steel cylinders, the type we carried in the resuscitation bags.

Picking up a six-foot plywood spinal board from the supply room was the easy part. Managing the task silently was a new skill. The steel supply room door squeaked when opened too quickly. Mike removed the small tank from the storage rack. He found a spare wheel needed to open the valve at the top. The element of surprise was still in his, our favour. I, too, would be to blame.

Opening the lounge door by a returning crew was commonplace. It was dark; no one stirred. Standing shoulder to shoulder in the centre of the room, I slowly set the end of the plywood slab on the floor, starting with the board almost vertical in a state of readiness.

At my side, Mike suspended the cylinder close to the floor, prepared for our surprise. Lying sprawled around the room on couches and chairs were four resting medics. A dispatcher reclined in an almost dark radio room off the lounge.

Realizing Mike sprung this gag before, I asked for advice on the assistant's role during the drive back to base. The timing was everything. The spinal board hitting the floor flat simultaneously as the rolling oxygen cylinder released its blasting hiss was essential for the gag to be successful.

As instructed, I released the board from its vertical standby position. As the plywood reached the midpoint on its way to the floor, I placed my foot partway up the board, pushing to sharpen the impact.

Mike, at the ready, held the cylinder inches above the floor to introduce the escaping gas. With split-second timing, he opened the valve, dropping the tank, rolling it towards the wall. The hiss that followed the steel tank hitting the concrete floor was in concert with the wooden backboard smacking the smooth surface.

Startled medics came to life. Two fellows lying on the couches were longer than the furniture. Their feet stuck out the ends around the steel armrests. One faltered. Catching his foot on the steel support, he wound up with two hands on the lounge floor, still engaged in the furniture. The other escaped, landing in an awkward stance. He ran out a couple of steps to avoid a fall.

The two medics slouched in the chairs bolted to an upright stance. A coffee mug that once rested on a lap skittered along the floor. The broken handle not travelling as far as the remaining shattered parts. The surprised dispatcher's feet fell off his desk. Hitting the floor, the socked feet tilted him to attention. Expletives were bursting like fireworks.

There was no doubt who the leader was. Mike retrieved the still whistling cylinder. It stopped by the wall next to the door into the radio room and idle front office. The sound was silenced.

I stood the backboard up and dragged it to the garage. Though I was in on the joke, I was laughing the least. Tommy, the shift supervisor, wound up on the floor in a pushup stance. He was not the fitness type. After a couple of nasties, Tom settled down and poured a cup of over-brewed black coffee to soothe his nerves. He was forgiving. Funny, he went on to be an ordained minister.

Definitely ham, not turkey

Early on, our tiny fleet was split between small vans and the original versions of an SUV. The vans did not have the extended roof that later units did to permit standing in the patient area. The SUVs were similar, only smaller inside. The stretcher had to load with the patient's head lying flat. A position that often panicked short of breath victims. With no headroom, doing CPR on pulseless patients was like working in mom's freezer.

Medics loved the utility-style vehicles. They were equipped with the yelping wailing sirens and cornered on a dime. A move that was near impossible in a van. The other feature was that both driver and attendant could ride in the cab. The front to rear divider was a split window that slid open.

The vans had the front passenger seat pulled. In its place, some of the less used equipment was stored. The attendant always rode in the patient area. To be a part of the team, you talked to the driver through the small window divider.

Early on a warm morning, Dwayne and I were returning to the office. Our patient safely back in the township nursing home, we were headed back for a coffee. Some ground fog was hanging around in the low-lying gulleys. Cruising along Riverside Drive in our Suburban, we chatted.

As I drove, we talked about the service he left after a brief period to come to London. Dwayne worked in the same hospital-based setup that Mike came from. Their employment at the hospital had not overlapped.

Something distracted me. A set of high beams flashed in the rear-view mirror. There was good visibility out the back through the sliding glass divider and rear windows. Trailing close behind were Hugh and Stewart in another Suburban. They were assigned to the Byron station, a dismal room. For some reason, we were both headed downtown. They caught up unnoticed. There was nothing on the radio.

Dwayne, a real joker, sported a great sense of humour. Maybe it was the water supply in the Elgin General Hospital. There were always funny quips and sayings. Describing childbirth as something akin to pushing a watermelon through a buttonhole, he was in awe of the miracle. He had already delivered a baby early in his career. I would have to wait. The description gave me something to look forward to.

We hadn't travelled a quarter-mile, and Dwayne's mind was in overdrive. "Can you hold this thing steady?" he asked. "Sure," but I hesitated, thinking; if he climbs out of the moving vehicle, we would be in trouble sooner than later if blood loss was involved.

Getting up on the bench seat, he balanced himself with one hand on the dash. You couldn't do this in a van. Where was he going with this move? He offered no explanation or warning. Without introduction, he pulled his uniform pants down and pressed his butt cheeks against the sliding rear divider.

I kept my eyes on the road. The thought of a partially clad coworker next to me in a moving vehicle was startling. "What the hell are you doing," I asked? "Giving them a pressed ham" was the reply. I was in tears now at the thought of what the sight was from the rear of our vehicle.

Hugh driving, and Stewart, the unsuspecting passenger, knew of the new guy's sense of humour. Neither could have seen this coming. You couldn't un-see this. I was praying for the intermittent foggy patches as we passed the golf course on our right to block the approaching motorist's view.

The road surface changed as we bounced over a poorly repaired pothole. With a one-word curse, Dwayne sat down, pants still lowered. He laughed like a hyena. The radio microphone clicked from the witnesses behind us. The moment passed, the pants were quickly returned to their uniform position. Huston, there was a problem.

Looking back over my right shoulder, there was a change. The pothole that suddenly returned my passenger to his seat had thrown him briefly against the partially closed divider. The glass was now cracked. Spreading out from a small finger hole used to open and close the portal was a spidery mark extending to the middle of the glass, something we would have to report.

I was at a loss for an explanation. Along with an expert sense of humour, Dwayne had a good memory. Returning to the office, my coworker took the bull by the horns.

Standing near the workbench in the garage was Monty, the fleet supervisor. Walking right up to him, he explained the damage.

Our first call of the morning was right around the corner from the hospital, a patient with a bad attitude. The police had offered him a simple choice. Go to jail for intoxication in a public place, or go to the hospital for his obvious behavioural issues. He climbed into our unit with no physical ailments to avoid adding to a long history with the law.

I had spoken to our patient during the brief taxi ride to the emergency room. During the conversation, I turned quickly to check to see if he was swinging at Dwayne. Busted. Not me, the window. Dwayne later told me that he had received a small cut to his nether end from the incident. Being the conscientious medic, I asked if he needed a ride to the hospital. There was no offer extended to provide first aid.

Pie

One lasting mantra describing a good medic; look after yourself. You're not much of a paramedic if you get wet, cold, dirty or go hungry on a shift.

Life is not perfect. Complaining about things you can change is a waste of time. Nothing makes a medic happier on a shift than their food. That is almost all the time.

The shift with Ethan at our Byron station one evening would be a bore. The conversation was good, but the calls were scarce. The tiny black and white television was balanced on the corner of the table near the window. A small chrome antenna tilted towards the window attracted a snowy picture from CFPL, the only channel available. Neither of us brought food. Both single, we lived at home and were over the brown bag lunch experience.

We each considered ourselves connoisseurs of fine fast food, though I was not familiar with choices around the city. Ethan stepped up to the plate and suggested pizza from Byron. This presented a challenge. No calls were going on at the moment. We could escape detection if we picked up something on the way back to a base. Asking to go on air and drive to pick something up was an absolute no-no, my, how things have changed.

Ordering was an issue too. Before the cell phone era, the only phone available was the now obsolete rotary dial phone in our room. There were no direct lines to dispatch in the beginning. Our station phones could make outgoing calls. The dilemma, if you were calling out, dispatch could not call you. The answer; brief calls, and don't give anyone the number.

Calling for a pizza tonight was easy. The "pizza" yellow pages were lying on the table, just the pizza yellow pages. Evidence of a medics missed opportunity and no pen. Ethan dialled up the shop and ordered. The person on the line knew where our room was on the old Children's Psychiatric Research Institute's property, CPRI.

Ethan issued simple directions; if we were out on a call, the money would be on the sill of the slightly open window. Take the dough, slide the pizza onto the table inside and; "keep the change, you filthy animal." Sorry, the quote was a line I always wanted to use. It was nearly fifteen years before the young actor sent those words from the pseudo vintage movie through the mail slot in the film "Home Alone."

The shift continued to be a wash. The phone was silent. We counted the minutes down until the hot meal arrived, along with a couple of cans of cold pop. With the window set to receive the pizza, the unspeakable happened. Two rings broke the silence. The old green plastic dial phone jingled with an assignment.

Business was bustling downtown. We were needed at our standby location to cover. Assigned to sit at the old Westown Plaza Mall, the name later changed to; Cherryhill Mall on Oxford Street. From there, we could balance our availability between the core and the west end. It was pouring rain as we got into our Suburban. Approaching headlights turned into the driveway to our station.

Luck was with us; the pizza had landed. We grabbed the pie. The driver, knowing the drill, retrieved the cash from the station's window behind us. There was no spare room on the front seat.

The meal got the position of honour, our stretcher. Fastened to the Hudson's Bay red wool blanket with a Velcro strap, we headed off through the rain. Both of us prayed to be passed over for an accident call. It was a sure thing; you were getting soaking wet when you stepped onto the road in bad weather.

Pulling into the lot, the rain eased up. There was no room to open the box between us in the front cab. We were destined to dine in the rear of the ambulance with no headroom. The pizza held its heat for the short ride. The corrugated top hit the ceiling protecting the pieces in the box. There were no paper napkins, so it was towels from the cabinet beside the stretcher. Sitting in the truck, the light rain continued.

Between the hot pizza and the closed windows, the back of the ambulance steamed up quickly. Sitting in a small seat for the attendant and Ethan sitting on the bench, we dined in cramped quarters. The radio microphone was dangling through the divider in anticipation of an interrupted meal.

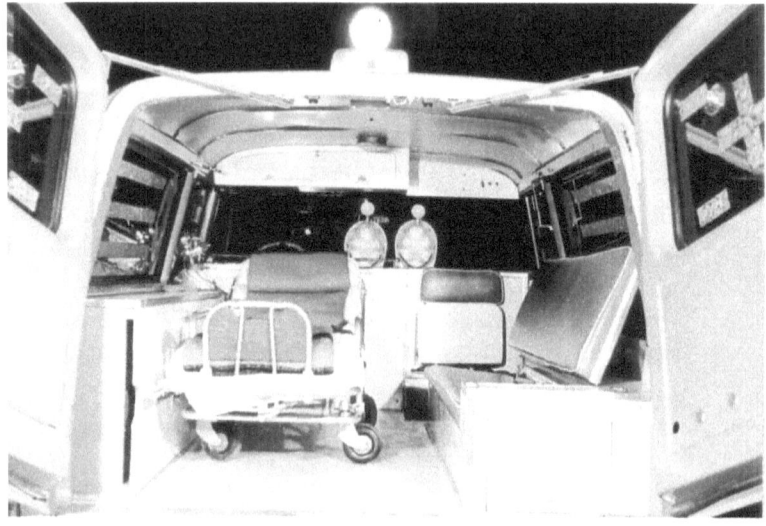

GMC Suburban patient compartment - aka dining room

Hot cheese ran off the pizza, necessitating its rescue with bare hands. Runny grease from our delicacy ran down our chins. What a treat! The small white towels were soon stained a dull red from the liquid sauce.

Eating our fill, the remaining pizza in the box was stored under the stretcher between the wheels in the event we got a call. We sat in the cab later, laughing about the feast and our dinner setting. It was almost an hour before we were directed to a call.

The ailing patient had only been in the ambulance on the way to the hospital for a few minutes when she asked. "Do you smell food?". I chalked it up to passing a restaurant; the patient was satisfied with the answer. The box was long gone; our stained dinner napkins were hidden safely under the bench seat.

Bullseye

Who says supper time is a totally safe experience? Part of the successful meal process for a first responder is quick access to food. The corresponding component to a perfect snack is getting it down before being interrupted. The combination is not always within reach. Attention to detail can fall through the cracks. The result can be painful.

Before a series of unfortunate circumstances resulting in crinkled ambulance roofs, medics often used the drive-through approach to expedite their mealtime practice. Henry and I were on the way back to our broom closet-sized station in the ER at St. Joseph's Hospital. It was time to make a pick-up. It looked efficient; we didn't have walkie-talkies, so we were on top of the radio in the event of an emergency.

Stopping at the illuminated board, Henry was up for the chilli meal, and it was to be a burger for me. The old guy and his pigtailed kid would be our hosts tonight. Drive through in its day was all about convenience. Safety was not on the radar. The life expectancy of the containers for fast food ranged from milliseconds to hours for medics. The packaging was not military-grade.

Making our purchase, two orders meant that we did not have to even up the change later. Our window-bound server was pleased to help us. During the transfer, the bag with the chilli struck the outside of the ambulance door. The opening was higher than the counter she had lifted it from.

With both orders safely on the floor between our seats, we returned to our station at St. Joesphs Hospital. Pulling up on the steep ramp, it was less than two minutes since we received the food. A quick "10-7" on the radio begged for an uninterrupted break. Before I could hang the microphone back into its clip, there was a groan from the passenger's seat.

In a split second, Henry exited the cab. Was the groan in anticipation of a steaming hot bowl of chilli? The expression was followed with an expletive that was not from a famished medic; was it from pain? You know the difference between when your kid is pissed and hurt. This was a liberal dose of both, though not sounding terminal.

My partner disappeared around the back of the van, leaving the cab door ajar. Henry hopped into the rear of the ambulance in a split second. Meeting him with my drink and burger in hand, the sight affirmed we would be on a delay before dinner. The thin paper bag carrying the steaming chilli failed. The lid sprung off the paper bowl when it hit the cab door at the drive-through, spilling the hot contents. The rest is history.

Wiping the grub from the front of his uniform pants, his expression said it all. His ordinarily calm exterior was broken; luckily, he wasn't hurt. He was pissed at losing the food. The paper bag sat on the ground by the open side door. With a quick cleanup, we launched from the hospital ramp.

Fortunately, the line disappeared in the nearby drive-thru. We skipped the order part; the window opened at our official presence. A soggy, stained bag went back through the window with a sour look. The current lapse in activity propelled the crew into a race car pit stop resolution to our dilemma.

Emergency averted; we returned to the ramp and chowed down without further delay. The EMS gods were kind. With the snack finished, Henry vanished to give his crotch a second round of cleanup. It took a while before the ordeal was remembered as funny. At the time, being able to finish our meal settled the mishap.

I used to think medics were a unique subculture until I was invited to a couple of police social gatherings. We have a lot of the same values and need the same things to maintain an even keel. Regular breaks, including food. Time to decompress following the demands of our profession. Finally, a good sense of humour. Life is not perfect, far from it. Humour helps!

3

Poor Fido

The downtown base was affectionately referred to as "the office." Working there was a pleasure for some medics; for others, it was a pain. Senior management staff also worked there. The station's location provided regular excitement derived from a variety of unusual but recurring calls. The city's core was home to the usual vices and disorders: substance abuse, mental health and the irreverent theme of; violence.

The experience was almost magnetic. Adrenaline junkies enjoyed racing for a few blocks to the scene and then off to the old Victoria ER. Always a quick turnaround in the day. No delays handing off your patient; you were right back on the road for the next run. The strain of a wearisome call load was compounded by the predictable weekday scrutiny from "white shirts." The environment acted like a caustic substance, repelling medics that some might consider less hearty.

I always enjoyed the theme, the hustle and bustle of the calls we responded to from the office. Was I a keener? There have been medics that worked the core off and on for years. Leaving, then returning as if refreshed by a less burdensome workload at a satellite station out in the "burbs." Like moths to a flame, replace "moths and flame" with medics to the action.

Imagine the dedication of medics that found it gratifying to swap out the downtown "crazy" calls for that ever-present groundswell of garden variety medical calls, chest pains, shortness of breath, abdominal pain and generally unwell runs. Medical hails are the real challenge for emergency care skill sets, a paramedic's patience, and at the heart of every EMS system.

Most medics enjoy a break from the routine and jump at the chance to respond to unusual requests for assistance. Where do they find such men and women? (note the trace of sarcasm!)

On a warm night, standing in front of the three garage doors, you could occasionally hear our next call happening in real-time. The foreboding commotion pre-empted that all too familiar telephone ringing in our radio room, the dispatcher's voice spilling from an open door, validating the request for assistance.

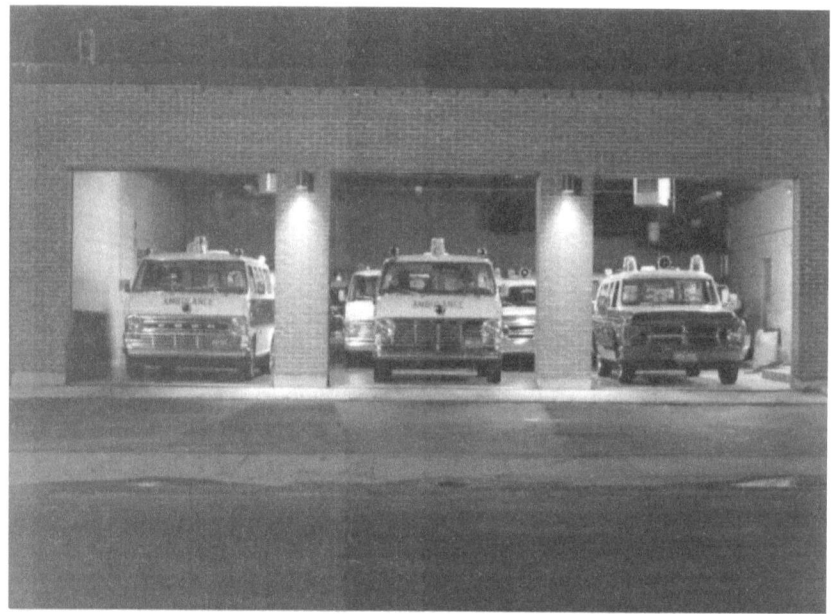

"The office"

There was the soulful screech of tires followed by metal impacting metal. It didn't need to be a weekend to hear a loud party or fight break out from a nearby house or backyard ruckus. On one occasion, the premonition for the call for help, detecting the unmistakable smell of smoke from a nearby structure fire. We transported a few victims from that misadventure. What an image to conjure up a macabre quantification of job security, "just another day at the office."

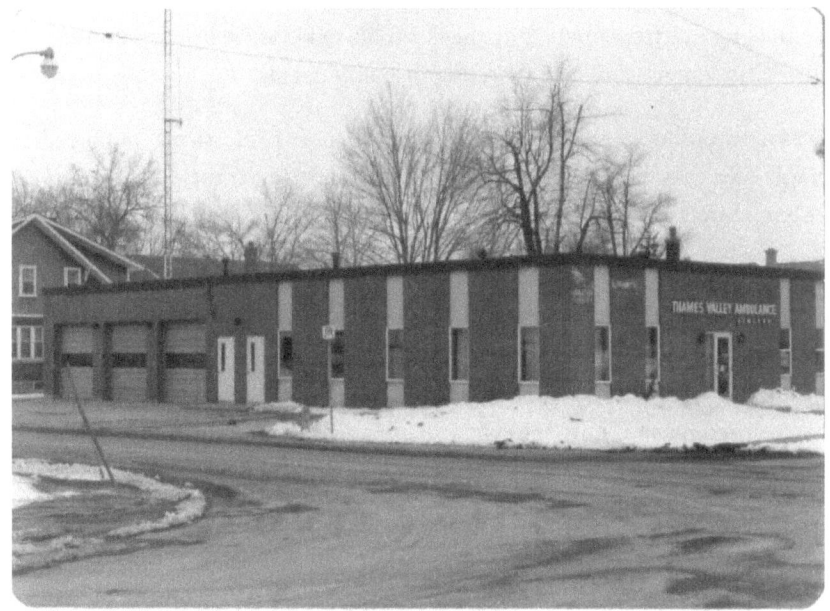

Standing outside, with your back to the bay doors, if you turned to your right, you were facing south. Your view was blocked, but south Street and its ancient Victoria Hospital were out there in the distance. A few blocks south of the office, a small wartime house sat quietly; who knew.

A voice bellowed out of the dispatch room into our meagre lounge. No one needed bells, whistles or horns to alert us to an impending request for service.

We were eight feet away. Less if the communicator propelled himself out of the narrow room broadcasting from an ailing wheeled chair.

The dispatcher today was an old fart. Howard working in the business since the fifties was an old east coaster. Leaving the roadside of our service with bad knees and a failing back, he chose the comfort of a chair. I witnessed an earlier ambulance response of his before joining EMS.

Anyone that has ever stopped at a gas station for directions would appreciate his simple edict: "Youze fellas go up the street here code four. See the guy out front there and check on his neighbour. I'm sendin the cops". Now here were some riveting dispatch details.

The communique reminded me of his profoundly professional radio call a couple of weeks earlier. "153, this is Lundah, check out the guy that just fell on King Street in front of the Market Parkin buildin. The caller thinks he has a busted leg or somethink". I understood him; we all got used to it. I mean, what could you dare say to the guy to improve those broadcasting skills?

Setting down an unfinished cold drink, I made my way out to the truck. Dave closed his homemade keyboard, an attaché case version. He constructed it to practice his piano keyboard drills between calls, thankfully minus the sound.

Dave had more time on the road than I. He was streetwise beyond his time, having lived on his own since he was sixteen. I could hear his little voice, "what a waste of time."

I turned the emergency lights on but hesitated to use the siren for the single stop sign and cross street on route to the "check the welfare of the resident" call. There were no other cars on the road around us. EMS dispatch protocol dictates lights and sirens when answering the call taker's question "Is the patient conscious?" deviates from" YES." "I don't know" gets the same rapid response.

EMS regularly receives these calls from concerned neighbours. Sometimes inquiries come via the police from relatives living in a distant city. Today, children of ageing parents pay alarm companies to act as surrogate caregivers. Technology offers a necklace or wrist fob that users activate when they believe they are in distress. The word "believe" is in the previous sentence with good reason.

Remember the commercial "I've fallen, and I can't get up." Most paramedics could easily substitute that line for: "can you send the boys over? I can't reach my water." The emergency medical services get calls just like this daily; it's a wonder we don't resort to jumping out a window.

Oh right, it's the seventies. I am currently sitting less than three feet off the ground in the cab of a van.

The city police officer arrived in his black cruiser without the assistance of lights or sirens. In fact, at the time, the London police cruisers did not have sirens. They had been removed by order of a senior officer. Someone complained of the noise late at night.

Emergency warning systems are a necessary evil. They are an overused feature on ambulances and not by any design of the paramedics. The architects of the system assign the lights and siren priority to more calls than not. Working for the emergency service is a little like working at a candy factory. Everyone is envious.

You like the "treats" (substitute lights and siren). Soon after, the novelty wears off, and it's time to get down to business. A respected friend and medic, Ryan, once ranted about driving: "you can teach a bean bag to drive with lights and siren. The real work starts when you climb out of the truck". In a nutshell, an experienced responder will tell you; driving an emergency vehicle can best be described as hours of boredom occasionally interrupted by seconds of terror.

In an unremarkable situation thus far, we engaged in a conversation with our caller, the neighbour at the curb, showing no urgency in his introduction. Our four-way discussion revealed the obvious. Several weeks of advertising flyers and newspapers appeared to be trapped between the front storm door and the residence entrance. The garbage visible on the porch, evidence of the absence of activity in and around the house.

Spilling out onto the concrete stoop was a library of windblown, wet and faded material. If you were really curious, you could have conducted an autopsy on all the paper from the bottom up and discovered the London Free Press's oldest edition to establish a timeline. I love a challenge but not my job!

Our host lived beside our call address. He offered up that the resident was an elderly widower. The resident had not been seen in weeks, two at least. He was last seen walking to the variety store a block and a half away.

Questioned by the police officer, the caller denied having seen or heard anything that lead him to believe anything nefarious had taken place. I ventured up the sidewalk taking in the scene; the front windows displayed curtains yellowed from smoking. All were closed, filthy both inside and out. Again, the grime on the inside of the glass suggested a cloudy film from cooking or smoking.

As I climbed up onto the porch, I sensed the end was near. Turning to Dave and the police officer, out popped, "yup, he's in there." I asked the cop if it was ok to try the door? He stepped up at this point and assumed control. It is much better if the police open the door, less court time for the medics if something comes of this call.

I had not shared the latest news with either of my comrades: my sensitive nose picked up on "that" smell. Kind of like raw meat, combined with a festering open wound with some feces thrown in for good measure. That could have been what you found in a garbage can after missing the last pick-up on a warm garbage day. It was faint but an unmistakable stench.

Pulling the storm door out of the way, some of the papers sheltered inside spilled out onto the cop's feet. It just shows that there is a modicum of skill in residential flyer delivery. The inside door, its wood finish faded from the sun, did not yield, even with a vigorous push. It would be all too simple if the door swung wide open, revealing a crotchety old geezer in his comfy chair yelling: "get the fuck out of my house." Like we haven't heard that one before.

I took one last shot at an easy-in. Peeling up the corner of the wet broadloom carpet, acting like a doormat, nope, there was no hidden key. The cop was surprised by my detective-like curiosity. The brief comment revealed some envy.

We were disappointed with the result. Inches of soggy newsprint giving way to; a few of last year's bugs very wet, dead or still in a state of hibernation.

I made a quick retreat here, walking back to the ambulance. Dave yelled: "where are you going? Getting ready," I grunted. What I really meant was, I was preparing to take a hit for the team. My outside voice buried well behind the conspicuously embroidered *Chris* above my right breast pocket.

Getting to the truck, I removed the fuel cap and inserted an index finger into the filler neck. Picking up some gasoline residue, I quickly applied the moist petroleum to my moustache in the hopes of avoiding the brunt of the odour, patiently awaiting my return. The others were oblivious to the significance of the preparation.

Time for the "360", a walk-around assessment of the exterior of our scene. In this instance, if we were lucky, the stroll might reveal a simple way in. The east side offered up a big fat zero. The windows were behind unkempt cedar bushes and secure, wood frames painted over like they hadn't been opened in decades.

There was a back door entering a mudroom of sorts. Visible through the windows, the collection of junk against the door, lending ease to the decision to carry on.

Reaching the west side of the house, the neighbour stopped. He pointed to the remaining window that we stood in front of. He had been inside to visit before and knew that behind the curtain was a hallway.

This was going to be easy. An old-fashioned double-hung sash window, already partially open. Blocking our path, a storm window affording little comfort to either security or heat loss. The single sheet of glass was held in place by screws through an aluminum frame.

I suggested to the officer that I could enter through this last option avoiding damage to the home. The neighbour spoke up, recognizing the fastener type, quickly disappearing to retrieve a screwdriver to assist. Turning to Dave and the officer, I said, "he's dead in there and starting to rot!"

Dave, disputing my proclamation, replied, "how the heck can you tell?" For a second time now, I leaned over to the side margin of the poorly affixed aluminum framed storm window and sniffed. I suggested to both that they take a whiff. Neither took me up on the offer; *what, is there a problem here?*

Returning with the missing link, the neighbour offered to remove the window fasteners. Turning his proposal down and taking his screwdriver, I directed my lucky assistants to be ready. It was up to them to support and remove the window when the screws were gone.

It was a stretch to get the top fasteners out. I wasn't worried when the shaking tool left a few scratches. The screws holding the side frames came out with less effort being within reach. Finally, the bottom piece proved to be the lynchpin.

Two of the screws were beyond their best before date. The previous handyman's efforts had stripped the heads. Getting frustrated, the police officer endorsed the removal of the window by force. With a vigorous yank on the frame, the lower aluminum strip stayed behind. A move that would prove to be my undoing. What a difference authority makes.

In a split second, my earlier assessment of the situation came to fruition. The partially open window released the strong but undeniable odour of a decomposing body from within. This wasn't garbage!

From beyond the now moving curtain came a sound that always gets my undivided attention, a pissed-off dog. I would come to find out that it wasn't as pissed as it was traumatized by the experience. Trapped in this once sealed residence.

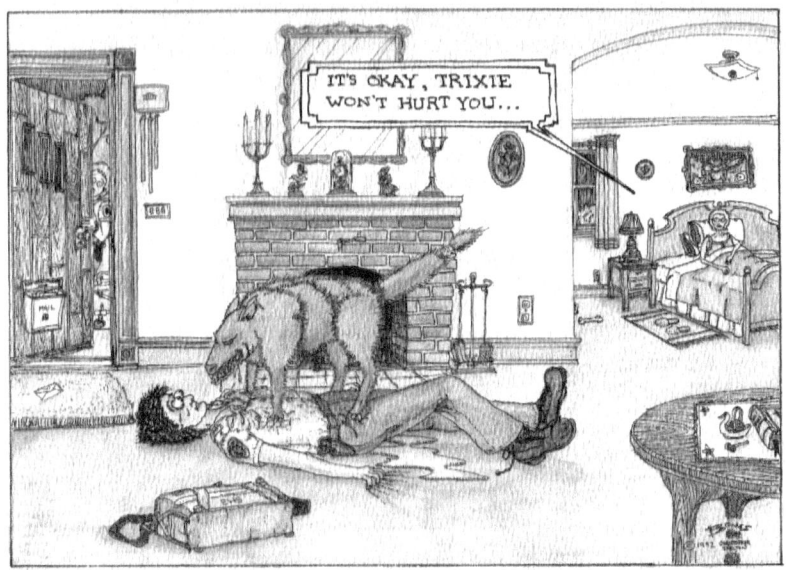

A pissed off dog at the scene - Credit: Chris "Bones" Skelton

The neighbour was nowhere to be seen. He was likely the victim of his own nose working just fine! The police officer stood back, taking our lead; he remained silent. Dave looked at me, pointing his piano playing finger at his chest. His quiet announcement, "not me."

I had already decided I would do the deed. Besides, I just had to go to the front door and open it to admit the madding crowds, all waiting to gawk at the seemingly obvious.

It took quite a push to get the top half of the old window up and out of the way. But wait, there's more. There was still the agitated dog to deal with. It was running up and down the hallway previously described by the now absent neighbour.

A quick sideward swish of the curtains revealed my opponent. Fido was barking like I was a burglar. Lacking both the criminality and agility to be a thief, I needed a distraction to avoid clashing with my brown adversary. By my feet were a few rocks left behind by the gardener.

The first attempt was a test; I was no Blue Jay's pitcher. The toss barely pushed the projectile through the now-waving curtains. The rock landed a few feet to the right. Chasing the stone, the dog remained curious for a few seconds. He quickly returned to his post, barking, proclaiming his disdain for our presence.

A larger stone might go further for the second pitch, buying me time to avoid the dog and get through the window. At a svelte 220 pounds in those days, it would be a challenge tantamount to entering a biathlon. Simultaneous throwing and jumping were not my skills.

I dispatched the rock with a substantial heave in through the window towards the rear of the house. Bouncing noisily in the distance, there was a dull metal clunk. Fido was off to the races as I grabbed the sill of the window.

It was a poor attempt at a jump, the best this overweight paramedic could muster. Beyond my comprehension, the event now evolved into a triathlon. Adding a western roll from public school track and field days to clear the sill. Shit, that hurt.

My left thigh caught the pointed aluminum strip left behind from the forced window removal. Look at me, ripped pants and a gouged leg. As if that didn't add enough insult to injury. I was under the gun to pick myself up and run like the wind towards the dog.

Skipping down the hall in a few steps to a long-abandoned summer kitchen, an open door offered to isolate my opponent on the other side. Luckily the projectile skittered behind something.

The last thing I could see from the door was Fido's bum up in the air, tail wagging. He was looking under an old fridge concealing his prize. Mission accomplished, though he voiced his disapproval.

Checking my thigh, it was a relief to find that other than a slightly wounded ego and a badly ripped pair of pants, the damage was minimal. Later that day, it would take a brief whisper in the ear of a great ER nurse and a sign-off from a doctor to receive a long-overdue tetanus booster. Avoiding an accident report, it was on to business. I hated paperwork.

In the opposing direction to the dog, the front door lay straight ahead. Off to my right were three doors, a bedroom, next to a bathroom, last and the closest hall door to the front of the house, a sitting room. The smell was hedging on overpowering; thankfully, the leaded gas did its thing.

As I crossed the third door, a sidelong glance caught the long-passed resident. He was seated peacefully in a lounge chair. It was well worn and now soiled with the by-products of his death.

Reaching the front door, it was secured with the only option left to its elderly owner. A kitchen chair pushed up against the door under the doorknob. The original lock in the handle missing. The chain back up to the door lock hung freely, screws pulled from the frame.

The floor in front of the entrance was surrounded by deposits of now dry dog poop. Fecal land mines lay everywhere. I didn't use to think of the neighbourhood as being that dangerous.

Dave and the police officer silently welcomed me at the front door. They stepped aside as if to say, why aren't you running out to the fresh air. In turn, I brought them up to speed with a brief report. "He's in the small sitting room down the hall in the first room on your left." Both offered a deadpan response.

"No," I said with incredulous inflection, "he's dead in the sitting room." I was waiting. The young peace officer finally entered, following me. He made it halfway to the sitting room, lungs pleading to be refilled. With a quick about-face, he disappeared past Dave. I turned to see him at the doorway, leaning over the newsprint-littered garden.

Dave was less inhibited in his pursuit of the truth, following me to the patient. He peered into the door of the one-time bedroom, now sitting room. Our patient sat slouched in an old green brocade cloth chair. A partially shredded newspaper draped over his lap. Strips of newsprint lay on the floor around him.

The home seemed deserted now, the mystery solved. The lonely barking companion's mission shifted to being a bodyguard. The low noise was eerily distracting in the background, offering no risk to intruders.

Across from the man sat a small, 12" black and white television balanced on a chair. It silently displayed a poor-quality picture. The set had been on a long time.

Our other responder returned a little green from the obvious. I was ruminating, then recanted the urge to blurt out, have a look at this; you haven't seen anything yet!

The realization of what we were looking at when directly facing the fellow was just setting in. It could have been simply misinterpreted as a decomposing face. The ambient temperature in the house was warmer than you, and I would take comfort in.

Our patient was beginning to swell. The victim's body was producing the gas associated with decomposition, giving him a rather portly appearance. In keeping with physics, the resulting gas found or created pockets to conceal itself in. That was until the surrounding tissue could no longer contain it.

Bubbling up to a higher position, the gas took the path of least resistance. Finally, exposing itself, the vapour found body orifices or points where the skin broke down. Further sanctioning its foul-smelling escape.

This patient proved to be one of the most grotesque presentations of a deceased person in my career. It is sad to say, Fido played an unwitting role in facilitating this ghastly sight. The loving pet sensed the emergent nature of his one and only pal. Coming to his assistance, could he predict death?

In a futile attempt to rouse his pal to play or be let out to run and relieve itself, the canine licked its owner's face. The move was intended to offer care and affection to his unresponsive master. He innocently disfigured the pensioner.

In the early days, the dog's rough tongue surface likely just scratched the face of his owner. The skin began to break down, aided by the dog's saliva. The tissue soon gave way and was consumed by the sympathizing caregiver.

Repeated jumps up onto the man's lap were evidenced by the shredded paper on the victim's clothing and the floor.

The dog returned to check on the now silent resident. In addition to working away at the face, Fido licked the back of the man's hands. The patient was approaching a state of moderate decomposition. He was now missing his nose and most of both cheeks.

The backs of each hand were also stripped of skin from the affectionate lapping. Exposed were the once concealed tendons and other connective tissue. All the attention was a naive attempt on the canine's part to comfort its master and elicit a response.

Adding to the vision was the greenish-brown discoloration of the flesh, mingled with the oozing body fluid. The purulent liquid was exiting our patient's face through the now deformed but patent airway. The secretions were being propelled by gas entrapped below.

Admittedly this was one of the most empathic turnarounds in my experience. I no longer had concerns for the gentlemen, now relieved of his meagre lifestyle as a retiree. His career had long since passed. Our patient's loneliness was compounded by the loss of his wife, leaving one companion behind. What an end.

What happens to Fido now? For the record, I am a cat person. Able to cuddle the little feline in my life and talk baby talk to eight pounds of fur and fish breath. There's a revelation my comrades will pounce on like a cat to a ball of yarn. Read it and weep, my friends.

It was now time to ponder the future of a loyal guardian, who shouldered the protection of its master up until minutes ago. I found myself more emotional than in past cases of facing sights of suffering. It wasn't the gas fumes that made me sit back and reflect.

The police officer stationed at the front door summoned his Sergeant for assistance. It was not his first call for a "natural causes" death by his own admission. He looked relieved to be on the outside of the front door.

From the entrance, we could hear the now muffled and waning sound of Fido. There was no reward here. He was confused over his confinement, following such an admirable performance of protecting his best friend.

Dave returned to our ambulance. Sitting with the cab door open, he called in our results from the "check the welfare of" assignment.

The radio update likely included a delay at the scene, pending an officer taking our statements. I couldn't hear his radio message. This was long before EMS was equipped with walkie-talkies. Sometime in the future, it would be a welcomed and sometimes despised asset.

Arriving without fanfare, the seasoned police supervisor approached. His forage cap confidently tilted high on his forehead. He was sporting an accompanying swagger. He listened closely to the report from his officer.

The constable very recently regained his composure. There was no sign that his initial overview of the scene of death resulted in such a retching response. A reaction he needed to resolve before his supervisor showed up. His calmness now, a show of assurance to the Sergeant that he had the situation in hand. The secret was safe with us.

Offering few details as if this were an ordinary situation. I was disappointed when the constable belittled the reek of the home's interior, stating, "it smells in there, Sarg." It wasn't up to us to reveal his reaction. I did giggle under my breath.

I turned to see Dave returning to our scrum, hoping for a quick resolution. He had seen and smelled enough, wanting to return to the office for more piano practice.

With nothing to be done for the patient, my advocacy turned to the now-imprisoned dog.

The Sargent announced he would call animal control to have the dog destroyed. Wait a minute. Fido wasn't accused of repeatedly biting the local kids. The neighbour that disappeared had not labelled Fido public nuisance number one. The dog successfully maintained a protective barrier around his charge, no matter how disturbing it looked to us today.

The supervisor was unwavering in his intent to have the dog removed and destroyed. In his mind, any issues at the scene would be resolved. My animal-loving sentiment dragged me to the left side of the argument. He was making the case without a trial, finding the dog guilty of consuming human flesh.

Our Sergeant assumed that the risk of spreading infection outweighed any benefit of its rehabilitation at the pound. We found out later, the dog's fate rested in the hands of a veterinarian. There was some small consolation that a qualified practitioner would make the correct decision.

Heading out to the first patrol car to give our statement, a curious neighbour approached. She cautiously inquired about the resident that we appeared to have left in the house. Surely the public must have some intuition here. The police officer hesitated in responding to the curious lady. Dave and I walked away from the discussion, leaving the details to the cop.

Besides, if asked, I would likely be a little too graphic, one of many self disclaimed faults. The officer quickly followed, laughing under his breath at handing the neighbour off to the Sergeant. "Maybe she likes dogs."

In succession, Dave and I gave statements of our observations made at the scene. Dave's declaration was sharply shorter than mine. I stopped and recanted part of my technical description of the facial decomposition. Working with a paper report, the constable was noticeably but silently pissed.

The term "nose" worked just as well as the medical expression nasal pharynx when the first attempt to spell it stalled. Proboscis was out of reach as well. It was added trouble with the report being handwritten on a carbon copy form, circa the late '70s.

We cleared the scene, glad for the fresh air, as we returned to the office to pick up where we left off.

There were still bubbles in my can of warm pop. Dave clicked away on his faux keyboard in the lounge as I sat in the radio room. Perched in the only spare chair with squeaking, failing wheels, I shared the call details with Howard. It was a miserable and failed attempt to bring a fresh new story to an ambulance veteran.

He was the same fellow that laughed last month while sitting in identical positions. Howard took great pleasure, launching into the tale of a recent clean-up. The gruesome task followed the discovery of a suicide victim in an unplugged chest freezer in a basement.

It was an overdose, compounded by a "last call" drink with the empty 26-ounce bottle found beside him in the closed freezer. A nearby note under the pill bottle told a brief but despondent story. You know, a failed marriage, a shitty job, there was probably more, but it got lost in the translation. The now liquid contents of the old thirty-two cubic freezer sat idle for weeks.

Howard was a storyteller, describing how he and Sam, one of my supervisors, stood chuckling as they smoked fat cigars in a putrescent basement.

Never having been a smoker, the solution; a trace of gasoline under my nose. It was another one of the great tricks the pair shared to cope with a foul environment. This was one of those rare times and a profession where I wished I had been a smoker. NOT!

The senior medics compared notes, scheming how to get the freezer onto its end to pour its contents into an aluminum sealer.

A "sealer" is a container used in the funeral industry to package a body in just such a state of decomposition. Only medics or funeral home staff faced with such sights could truly appreciate trying to cloak the sound of laughter. All the while diligently maintaining their coarse sanity far from misunderstanding eyes and ears. Oh, why did I take a run at the master of clean-ups?

4

You Know… Stuff Just Happens

We have all experienced "that" moment. You make an innocent mistake or oversight. You forget the procedure, maybe a brain fart: nothing serious. No one is injured; nothing gets broken. Sometimes you get away with it, no witnesses. Then, there are the times it catches up with you.

Long ago, practical jokes and stunts were a source of entertainment in our industry. No one got hurt; we were lucky. In some cases, there was a little too much time on our hands. Idle minds wandered.

Today, with occupational health and safety legislation and in-house policy and procedure manuals thick enough to double as a phone book, those Ha Ha moments have all but disappeared.

Younger medics missed that by a decade or three. A moment now is "Lol" or "WTF" on a phone screen. I get it or got it with my daughter's assistance.

The resulting embarrassment from a mistake is magnified when it happens in front of a friend or co-worker. "Tell the truth, and it shall set you free." Someone omnipotently famous said it; I can't take credit for that line.

With so many years in the same industry, there were times where I was the cause, other times the witness to someone else that could take the credit or be assigned blame.

There are only so many tools in your vehicle, medical kit or carried on your belt. At one point or another, you must improvise to solve a problem. Making it up as you go can also set you up for "stuff" happening. Sometimes the consequences are humorous; other times, not so much.

A Couple of Keystone Cops

Remember when you were a keener? Always the first to stand up and volunteer for a job. It wears off, doesn't it? It took some time for me and was not without its costs.

Art and I were paired up early on when I was checked out for driving, and the summer holidays arrived. Drivers have a couple of extra jobs. Making the stretcher with fresh linen and returning it to the ambulance are two that come to mind. Junior drivers should have a checklist.

Art came "two-stepping" out of the ER doors. "Got a VSA." It took a couple of giant steps to catch up to him and throw myself into the truck. The address was close to the hospital, easy to find. We had not worked a cardiac arrest together yet, so we quickly worked out a game plan.

Plan your work and work the plan. Someone with the bigger picture thought that one up. Our scheme was already doomed. We just didn't know it yet.

Arriving at the old wartime home, we went to the rear to get the stretcher and oxygen bag. Opening the first door, my first thought was to sit on the bumper and cry or slap myself.

The stretcher was not there. It was still sitting right where I left it in Victoria Hospital; "shit." Exchanging expressions, you can only imagine.

Plan "B" take the oxygen bag and check the patient out. Running into the home past an anxious wife, we found an elderly fellow sitting on a couch. He was obviously not in cardiac arrest but short of breath. Art started oxygen and did the basics, including taking a history.

Our victim was weak and had laid his head down, exhausted from his difficulty breathing. The dispatcher's question, "is he speaking?" drew the answer no. With the wife's first answer and patient history, the dispatcher decided the victim was pulseless. This fellow weighed a hundred and thirty pounds with his pockets full of nickels.

Telling Art I was going for the stretcher, he looked back at me like I intended to return to the hospital. I had a plan. We could improvise; we had a portable stretcher stored in the front cab. The suspense marking his face was worth keeping the secret for the moment. I disappeared without an explanation.

One of the demands of our profession includes being masters of improvisation. Like the marines, we adapt and overcome. Reappearing behind Art in record time, he quickly realized I hadn't gone back to Victoria. Unfolding the "number 9" stretcher, he caught on without a word.

Placing the cot on the small living room floor, we moved our patient down onto it without losing a beat. The concerned wife looked on, but there were no questions.

We lifted the aluminum frame like an army cot from the ends with the oxygen bag placed between his feet. On the way back to the patient, I left the front screen door propped open with the pneumatic arm.

It was a short trip to the ambulance's rear doors, where we set the cot down from the ends, and each grabbed a side rail.

The open rear doors accepted the stretcher onto the floor. The only change, we had to step up into the ambulance and lift the cot a second time onto the bench where the attendant usually sat to care for the patient.

We secured the cot, preventing a second disaster. In a New York minute, we were down the road with Artie sitting behind the patient's head, awkward, but it worked.

Arriving back at Victoria a couple of blocks away, I ran into the front entrance and grabbed our original stretcher. The wheeled bed was designed to carry our portable cot without a hitch.

The move drew a couple of concerned looks from the charge nurse. She surely thought being the Samaritans we were, the stretcher was used to assist a patient arriving by car at the entrance. We were called upon to help occasionally.

Opening the rear doors, Art just laughed over the patient's shoulders. The plan worked, and the secret was ours until now. We reversed the move and pushed our patient into the department. We lost no time.

Sometimes you can make a great save. Other times there is a price to be paid. We lucked out!

LOOK OUT BELOW!

Honestly, we do have a lot of tools in our kit. Sometimes we choose not to use them and improvise. The adaptation can save time, then there are times you can get caught short. Using our stair chair is a great example.

The original, light, folding aluminum chair had wheels. You could wheel a patient out of a confined room instead of carrying or use it going downstairs.

Ethan worked for a couple of years in the ambulance business before I started. He had a good sense of humour.

It rained most of the night, so there was mud around. Ethan was wearing his old-style galoshes, the overshoe type with the zipped front. With the zipper down, they had a tongue that flopped open. I chose a laced combat boot, a style the cops wore, practical.

Assigned to pick up an elderly woman to transport to a nursing home for admission, these could be difficult calls. Ethan and I talked on the way. For some patients transitioning from their homes to assisted living was like going to prison.

If a patient's faculties were intact and mobility was the issue, they fretted. If their memory and thought processing was failing, it was not a shock, just confusing.

This was a full-on fretting case. Our patient was upstairs in a beautiful century home. Well kept, her husband received some help. Holding his cane, he was sitting with their daughter when we arrived at the front door.

The daughter briefly explained that we might get some resistance, taking mom from her room on the second floor. Mom knew we were coming but thought her daughter could continue to stay with them to look after her.

The live-in help started a few weeks ago after a fall. With a husband and children at home, the daughter's plan was, at best, temporary.

We set up our stretcher in the living room at the landing by the stair's bottom. Following the daughter, we found our patient on the second floor in a chair next to her bed.

Setting a book down, I got the feeling she hadn't been reading it. A distraction at best, our patient sounded annoyed that her daughter couldn't continue the live-in arrangement. Explaining that "Dad" would be joining her as soon as a double room was available, our patient's anxiety level faded.

Our host explained that "the boys" were here to give her a ride to the nursing home. The patient's latest conundrum after our introduction was, "how will you get me down?" I explained we would be carrying her.

Ethan and I looked at the lady, sizing her up. When I threw the term stair chair out, he shook his head. We checked out the chair she was sitting in; it was too heavy. Sometimes a light but sturdy chair was all we needed.

Choosing the stair chair would mean another trip out to the ambulance. This lady was a "lightweight," tipping the scales at around one hundred pounds. We would lift her without the chair, simple.

A patient's anxiety during an ambulance call can often be reduced with comforting statements and a simple explanation of what's to come. The unknown is often frightening for people in crisis or changing times.

The sign of a good and experienced medic is their ability to comfort patients and tell them just enough.

Our stretcher was set up on the main floor. Ethan had a clean bed sheet over his arm, looking more like a waiter than a medic. He was closest to the patient's back. For this lift, we switched roles. It would be my saving grace.

I asked the lady to hold her arms down at her side as Ethan reached under them to hold her wrists. It was a simple two-line request. I appealed to her to relax for the lift.

The attendant usually lifts the patient from behind. The driver would cradle the patient from behind the knees, leaving a free hand to steady the trip down the stairs in this case. We call it a "fore and aft" lift.

With the lift explained and sheet placed over her lap to ensure the lady's modesty, it was up and away. Reaching the top of the stairs, we hesitated until we lined ourselves up, each taking our bearings for the descent.

The patient's back was against Ethan's chest as he leaned away from the stairs to steady his descent. A step at a time, we started down. So, did something else.

Changing our patient's position during the lift promoted some trapped gas to begin its exit. The noise of the escaping vapour was undeniable. Professional faces on, we kept our composure. It was like a good comedian trying not to laugh at his own punch line.

It was all good until the punch line changed consistency.

They say, "where there is smoke, there is fire." The same principle can be applied to the presence of gas.

I was cradling the patient's legs and could hear the change in tone. The signal was interrupted by longer pauses between the "putt-putting" sounds.

The military would describe the situation during an artillery barrage as; "Danger Close." There was no place to go; we were halfway to the landing.

Taking a brief look up at Ethan, we acknowledged the inevitable. Looking down to avoid eye contact, I caught the movement from below.

I could hear the daughter's alarmed reaction to the noise, apologizing for her mother's lack of control. That was the least of our worries now.

Incoming!

Freefalling past Ethan's knees was a brown blur. For the rest of the world, vomit, urine, and feces are just an accepted part of health care. Caregivers take it in their stride, though no one looks forward to the experience.

One upside of a bad situation is when the opportunity presents itself to revisit the predicament later. In private, recalling the lighter side often relieves the nasty part of our job. We refer to it as dark humour.

If you can't laugh at yourself in our industry, the pressure will get to you. That can be a career-ender.

As if it wasn't bad enough that the lady lost control. In this instance, the brown blur lodged itself in the flopping tongue on Ethan's boot. I looked anxiously to see if more poop ended up on the carpeted runner on the stairs. The poop Gods were not kind.

Crediting my composure to the proximity of the woman and her daughter, we reached the main floor. It was a quick transfer with our patient to the waiting stretcher. I kept up a conversation about how friendly the destination would be for our patient and her husband.

There was a brief moment our eyes made contact, though I was expressionless. There was also the matter of the ordnance on the stairs behind us. The daughter and our patient were unaware of the presence of the bomb or its target. My partner would be informed when we had reached the truck.

The daughter was left to deal with her father and lock their house. Our plan was to meet in the admitting area of the nursing home. Reaching the back of the ambulance, the patient was lowered and then lifted into the rear. The unexpected change for Ethan, I closed the doors before climbing in.

Bending at the waist, I let loose with a belly laugh out of sight of the patient. This punch line had run its course. Straightening up, I looked at Ethan and motioned to him to look south. There, running down the inside of the fanned tongue of his boot, was a lump. Even he laughed.

Climbing into the ambulance, I handed him a small towel so he could stop the poop from reaching his shoe. There would still need to be some cleaning. He removed the boots and left them inside the rear doors. Was it punishment or convenience?

Ethan went on to be a dispatcher, a great one. A large part of his success in the communications centre is owed to his experience from time spent on the road. We have remained acquaintances to this day.

The story would remain idle until the evening of his retirement. Someone foolishly asked if anyone had a funny story to tell friends and family at the gathering. A lawyer once said; Never ask a question that you don't already know the answer to.

Veteran Paramedic – Not Veterinarian

Being the cat lover that I am, has come to bite me a few times. The soft spot has netted me a couple of scratches from a pet at a call scene. No one likes to see an animal in distress. When confronted with an injured animal, paramedics face a decision. There are unwritten rules that our services are reserved for human patients. Thankfully it was dark outside.

We are routinely sent to the scenes of working fires. You would think the priority is for residents. Instead, the dual purpose for the response is; to treat patients rescued from burning buildings. Secondly, in the event, a firefighter is injured. The latter happens more than you would think.

Late one evening, we were sent to standby at a house fire in the core. There were no patients tonight; it was a precaution to be there. For the most part, we would stand around, waiting for the worst. It is common to leave the scene empty-handed, thankfully, not having to deal with fire victims. We were getting ready to clear on this occasion.

Jogging toward us, a firefighter cradled a small object in his arms. Your mind immediately runs to the dark side. A dead baby, the result of smoke inhalation, was found when the air was cleared. Stay away from me; I am a catastrophist.

Sometimes victims hide in unusual places; that's why they can be missed on the primary search. Kids are known to choose underneath beds and in closets as safe havens. Paramedics are in the business of treating sick and injured people. The hiding information comes from training as a volunteer firefighter years ago.

Imagine our relief when the firefighter unfolded his arms to reveal a gasping tabby cat. Hiding under the bed, the distressed kitten found refuge during the initial stages of the fire. Doing the right thing, the lone resident left immediately, leaving the cat, escaping without incident.

When the pumper crew exited the house, the anxious homeowner asked if anyone found his cat. Two men went back inside to give it the old college try. There under a bed in a spare room, the cat made some noise in response to the search team.

Our patient did not look burned. Kitty was hiding or trapped in the smoke-filled room, too frightened to escape during the firefighting efforts.

Nearby residents retreated to the comfort of their homes. Relieved their neighbour was not injured, they were heading back to bed. There were no more sirens and loud noises.

It was good for us; inquiring eyes were gone. Ben, my partner for the shift, was not a pet owner. I was on my own.

We were in the shadows beside a pumper. Our only witnesses were other responders. Time for some oxygen, the straight hose blowing in the small cat's face just scared it. A child's clear oxygen mask worked, though.

Laying the cat on one of our blankets on the ground, the oxygen looked like it was working. Kitty was lying still. Our patient's chest looking more relaxed now, not heaving in distress. I never thought about assessing an animal before tonight.

Patient assessment for a medic involves asking questions, listening to and observing responses. One finding to judge breathing distress is to count the number of words in the victim's response. Describing your observations to the hospital staff; "Our patient has three or four-word dyspnea." Nurses get that.

"Our cat mews once and a while" not so descriptive. There would be no report to a vet.

Getting back to basics, I spoke to the cat and petted the side of its head and lay my hand lightly on its stomach, then chest. Humans in respiratory distress will have heaving chests, and the stomach will draw in when their chest is too tired to assist in the respiratory effort. The cat was recovering.

From behind the fire truck, the homeowner appeared. His concern shifted from the damage to his pet. We had done about as much as we could; our advice was not a professional diagnosis. Find a vet as soon as possible to follow up.

Receiving a handshake, I was relieved. It turns out the man lost his wife this year, and the pet was his remaining pal. The effort cost us some oxygen, a mask and a blanket. A small price to pay; he already lost the use of his home for a while.

This service might provide some comfort on a terrible night. I was just relieved; neighbours and the press missed the save. It was no time to be mistaken for a hero.

There is a limit to my generosity. Several years later, would find me at another fire scene. More serious, this time, one resident was taken to the hospital. We responded as a second crew to stand by for the responders until the fire was out. Working the shift with Art, we were both animal lovers; he owned a dog, I was between cats.

Running from the side door to the house, a frenzied firefighter called his friends for some help. In his arms was a patient; for a moment, I thought we were looking at a burned kid. Sprawled over his arm as he turned was a small dog. It looked lifeless. Here we go again with the oxygen.

For some reason, I hesitated. The lifesaver stopped at the curb adjacent to the pumper, still supplying the water to the working fire. What I missed from my position down the street was the camera. The Platoon Chief standing nearby could see his firefighter with the patient in his arms but made no move to summon us. We stood next to our stretcher at the ready in the event there was a human patient.

Coming from the sidewalk to the curb, a newspaper photographer approached the firefighter. Another firefighter joined the group, looking on like he was on a mission. Taking the dog from his co-worker, he listened at the dog's mouth. Without hesitation, the smokie did something that made me gag, the unthinkable, he started mouth to mouth. There was a flash.

I considered approaching the action. When the resuscitation started, that was a game-changer. It was daytime with lots of witnesses. We decided as a crew that we were not up for direct contact with an animal. Animal CPR was out of my scope, a choice shared by Art.

The story got some laughs at the office. Most agreed they were not up for doggy CPR. The act of kindness did not go unnoticed. The next morning's paper's issue had a great big picture of the rescuer doing mouth to mouth on the dog. Bravo to the firefighters! It was a move that preserved our innocence. Besides, what nurse would kiss a paramedic that kissed a dog for a photograph? I mean, really, Lol.

Foot in Mouth Disease

Over the years, I have stuck my foot in my mouth; just ask family or friends. Equipped with a loud voice and an opinion, the result was sometimes embarrassing. So, when someone else commits a boo-boo, it just earns a laugh under my breath. I am not cruel or without conscience; if the opportunity presents itself, I will save the person.

Art and I responded to an abdominal pain call. The discomfort was several days old. It was a good thing the hail was not assigned emergency status. We were driving slowly. The radio crackled a couple of times; neither of us recognized the barely audible voice.

The interference cropped up again, now clear as a bell. Ryan and Randy were sitting at "central stand by." The last available unit in the city, they were positioned to go in any direction. It was London's last hope, with only one ambulance available. Sitting at the corner for a while, they were showing their boredom. Randy's right knee resting against the radio microphone button went unnoticed.

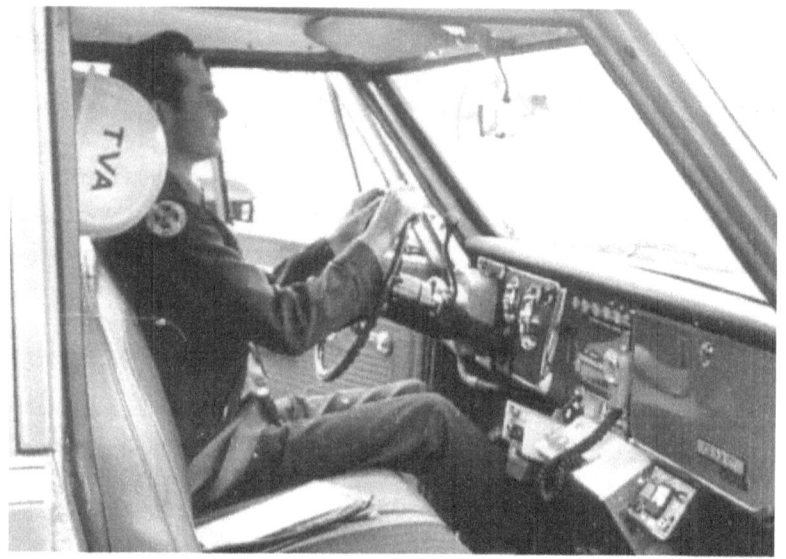

Ambulance cab interior/radio & siren next to driver's knee

Our service recently changed hands. The owner, when I started, sold to the lead supervisor and an entrepreneurial medic. For their first days, everything was okay. It didn't take too long before things went sideways. Labour management relations plummeted; some saw this as a double-cross.

Sitting with too much time on their hands, the newly acclaimed union president and a slightly sour but immensely humorous medic arrived at an inevitable topic. In a slapstick fashion, both threw out barbs about our boss Fred. Maybe we were all envious of his newfound status. It was a conversation that resurfaced for years.

Fred passed through the lounge a few days back, sporting a new suede jacket. Pointing the purchase out to staff, he was looking for a compliment. Instead, crews were left to chew on the subject after he disappeared into the front office. No one really cared. But in the face of failed contract negotiations, you didn't need much more to sour the environment.

Back and forth for the duration of the transmission, Ryan goaded Randy over the jacket. Randy jumped at the chance, exclaiming it was cheap and not really a refined garment. His crowning comment; "I told him I bought the same one at K-Mart." Both medics laughed at the observation. The radio briefly went silent, then crackled regularly enough that the dispatcher could not get a warning out.

Art and I arrived at the residence for our abdominal pain during the longest transmission. We were riveted to the conversation, belly laughs all around. I thought I would pee my pants at some of the comments. Coming to our senses, the dispatcher was beyond rescuing the pair. Knowing Steve, he was likely doubled up on the floor, hoping the tape recorder didn't fail for the Spanish inquisition ahead.

There was one possibility. We all knew where the crew was sitting. At a street corner outside our favourite variety store, a husband and wife team were the owners. Unable to announce our arrival, we entered the patient's residence and split up.

Art went for the patient; I asked the husband to see the patient's medications. Adding that I needed to use the telephone, the request grew stranger wanting to use the phone book.

Looking up the number for the variety store was simple. Getting the owner to understand our strange request through their thick Greek accents would be a chore. Since we did not have walkie-talkies, I was unsure of the state of damage we were at.

Helen and Nick were great folks; newer to Canada, there were times when it was a chore to explain something. We lucked out today. Helen answered the phone, laughing when I explained who and why I was calling. The introduction drew a chuckle. Helen always thought I had Greek blood and addressed me as "Creese." She recognized my voice. Her news, Steve just called, Nick was already out at the ambulance talking.

I thanked Helen and went back to business. The topic would occasionally surface if someone arrived for a shift in a new coat. There would be future radio faux-pas; that is the business. I still chuckle at the topic of suede coats.

Chubby or Cute

Languages are still a bit of a mystery to me. High school French took a turn for the worst. I resigned myself to the reality I would not be bi-lingual after a dismal conclusion to the grade nine subject. Most people from Europe have me beat by a mile in that they speak at least two languages; some, many more. Envy, not jealousy, makes this tale more valuable in illustrating my point. Thank you, Aaron.

Before some medical specialties were readily accessible, London was host to an eminent neurosurgeon with a unique skill. People came from around the world to benefit from his surgical specialty. Pickups at the airport were a daily, sometimes hourly occurrence. He researched and perfected the resection of a basilar aneurysm.

"Who Cares?" I heard that; read on.

The surgeon was the most down-to-earth fellow in the hospital. He would greet medics addressing them as equals in the hallway. Patients arriving at his floor in our care would get a warm greeting. He knew the patient's names without introduction; the comfort he spread was legendary. The good doctor would go on to receive national awards and recognition.

Aaron and I worked this day at the station in the east end, closest to the aerodrome. It was a routine call to go to the "Shell shack," where visiting aircraft were greeted and refuelled. The twin-engine turboprop plane rolled up and stopped, cooling the engines down.

There was no rush; the procedure took a couple of minutes. We had lots of time while they did their pilot stuff and lowered the stairs. We returned to our ambulance and waited to be summoned out onto the apron.

The pilot waved us out after the chocks were set against the wheels to stop the idle plane from rolling. The second aviator assisted a female passenger climbing down the few steps to the concrete parking area. The look over her shoulder towards the open door in the aircraft told me she was a relative or friend of the patient.

We rolled our stretcher to the bottom of the steps as the pilot still in the aircraft gave us a brief report. Aaron was attending, so he took the medical chart from the flyer. The stable female patient was accompanied by a friend acting as an escort.

I guess that was the aviator's version of a medical report. She was coming to see our neurosurgeon. How stable can you be if you need an operation that involves opening your skull and cutting your brain? I think I oversimplified the procedure.

The escort spoke to her friend in French. I was out. The conversation went back and forth for a minute, including a few smiles and hand gestures. Luckily for me, Aaron, a long-time friend and co-worker, was born in France and is fluently bilingual.

Understanding the opening but foreign conversation, Aaron was silent. Something made him hold his cards close to his chest, a real poker player. If I was him, I would have blurted out some greeting in French.

Both ladies switched to English as quickly as they had exchanged French when the pilots said goodbye. I knew they would at least understand if I had an important message for them. The French returned, loading the patient into our ambulance. For the twenty-minute ride to the hospital, the escort rode upfront with me.

I spoke to my passenger, receiving a nod instead of a verbal acknowledgement. Overhearing Aaron getting information from the patient, he had the necessary stuff in the patient's chart. He was just making conversation.

Our passengers began a conversation in French. An exchange that went back and forth from the cab to the patient compartment for minutes. Speaking rapidly, the ladies laughed at times in response to the other's statement; I was at a loss.

I never once heard the French word for pen, ruler or thanks. The singular words were the sum of my bilingual retention. Still silent, Aaron's absence of French spoke volumes.

Arriving at the hospital, we met at the rear doors to unload the patient. During the lift out of the ambulance, two words uttered from our patient evoked another laugh from her friend. We hadn't faltered, lowering the cot out of the ambulance; there could be no criticism?

Aaron's timing was better than a comedic punch line, almost nonchalant. No one ever likes a joke at their expense. We were between the ambulance and the hospital doors when my partner stopped the stretcher and addressed me in English. "Darbs', I am having trouble; which one of us is the cute one? And which one of us does she think is chubby? We both have beards."

There were audible gasps as Aaron began a sentence in Parisian French, a purer version of the language than I had been witness to, on and off for the last half an hour. Both women were aghast when they became aware of my partner's roots. Their expressions were worth a million dollars.

His address included his understanding of their exchange and his European upbringing. His statement was in a quiet, respectful tone. Unfortunately, though, I did not comprehend a single word in French. His explanation later over a coffee was amusing.

There were no apologies in the elevator after leaving admitting. A brief exchange at the nursing desk and the patient's bedside was purely obligatory on our part. Aarons parting farewell in his mother tongue was French to me, though his articulation was terrific. He niced them out in French.

If memory serves me correctly, there was a brief snicker as we entered the elevator to depart. The best surprise is a well-timed one.

No Traction

Death is always seen as so sad. It really is a gloomy topic. Paramedics do their very best to take every step within their scope to prevent it. In the early days, and you will hear several versions of a person's end in this writing, we transported nearly every pulseless patient, regardless of the situation's hopelessness.

Education and experience today in the medical community have established that after approximately eight minutes of being in a pulseless state, the chances of survival reduce on a sliding scale. Even in that circumstance, the patient would have to otherwise be in a low-risk group to make it. There are exceptions.

With a poor medical history or risk factors like smoking or obesity, the odds are stacked against the patient. Add a series of unfortunate events in this scenario, and it probably didn't help the outcome; the optics were terrible. This is one such story.

Working in poor weather, the public always asks, "Were there lots of accidents last night?" "Nope, but we were delayed getting to calls, slipped several times, and every call was a test." That reply does not sell papers; it is just the truth.

We responded to the cities edge in heavy snow; that sucks. For the VSA patient, it stinks to the power of ten. A fifteen-minute response time from downtown is never a good thing for a patient that is not breathing. Like I said, add risk factors, and the die is most assuredly cast.

Pulling up to the scene, the snow was coming down so heavily, the home was almost whited out. We were delayed looking for house numbers; some had numbers, some were hidden behind shrubs. There was no one at the door to greet us. Finally, an opening door in the middle of the night was our best guess.

An older woman greeted us. Our stretcher in tow, the steps were too slippery to take the chance of climbing the hazard until we had a look at the situation. We left the cot on the sidewalk, quickly being covered in large fresh flakes. Oxygen bag in hand, Art and I entered the home in search of our patient.

This would have been the perfect call to have some help from our friends at Fire. Unfortunately, we did not have a dual response to these calls yet. We could have used the extra trained hands. Our patient was in the washroom.

Sitting on the toilet, the unresponsive patient was as deep in the room as you could get. The room was tiny when you deducted the unusable maneuvering space occupied by the bathtub and vanity. This was going to be a challenge.

To begin any care, we had to get the patient to the floor in a larger area. We needed room to properly start the resuscitation. Some time had elapsed since the lady's breathing stopped. The event was unwitnessed; the patient's skin darkened from the lack of life-giving oxygen. Since the victim was still warm, we were obliged to transport her.

We slid the patient off the toilet in an awkward move, then worked our way to the door. One of my feet started in the bathtub until there was room. It took a couple of minutes. Imagine three people in a small bathroom standing. Try laying one person down and not receiving any cooperation with the move.

Where were the police? Officers usually responded to these calls? They were trained in the new CPR standards. Art and I recently qualified as instructors in cardiopulmonary resuscitation.

As great as the skill is, it was taught in a large room, in good lighting. Paramedics are professionals that bring real expertise to the field. Addressing the roadblocks such as extrication, obese patients and reducing scene time, the desired result is improved patient outcomes (in some cases, the patient cooperates). And that was before Advanced Care and defibrillators. That's in another chapter.

Our patient was not responding to CPR on the hallway floor. The only option left now, rapid transport to the closest hospital. Even if the odds were not stacked against us, and they were, this was going to be a real challenge.

Our assignment tonight: transport the patient to the hospital and let the physician pronounce death.

I returned to the front of the house to get ready for transport. A nearby snow shovel on the steps improved our chances of getting away with the call and not slipping or falling. There were only three steps and a small concrete porch to clean off.

Art stayed behind to keep up single-rescuer CPR. The patient's daughter paced nearby, asking when we would get the patient on the way. There was no one else to help us; the core task was to safely transport the patient, including our safety.

With the walk and steps cleaned down to the concrete, I called out to Artie. He appeared at the door and rolled his eyes. The job was obvious, the projected outcome a given. We manoeuvred the stretcher into the home, leaving a trail of snow falling from the wheels. I brushed the snow off the linen and blanket outside, but nearly an inch of fluffy wet snow had fallen since we arrived.

The lift from the floor was the least of our worries. As heavy as the patient was, there were no obstructions; we were loaded in seconds. There was more CPR, keeping up the effort. We made it out to the porch, and I was down the stairs at the foot of the stretcher with ease. The stretcher was still on the higher surface.

Here was the tricky part; I was two and a half feet lower than Art now; we would both be on slippery ground. We had to inch our way off the porch in order not to pull each other over. Sliding to a halt behind us was the first police officer. Seeing us struggle with the stretcher, he left his forage cap in the cruiser. A no-no if his supervisor attended the scene under any circumstances.

We had done this before; the slow but sure pace kept us out of trouble arriving on the lower level quickly. A brief stop for a few chest compressions, and we would head down the walk to our waiting ambulance. The patient's daughter was leaning out the front door, watching as if to see or hope for a change in her relative's condition. There would be no change, at least one for the good of all.

The police officer met us on the walk. We weren't about to stop to give a statement. There was not a word spoken. That was a mistake. The concrete path was alongside a hedge covered in over a foot of fresh snow.

The walk also had over a foot of snow on it; its shelter created a taller, peaked drift right down the centre. We were not struggling with the extrication, so my reasoning later went with the cop wanting to look helpful in front of the onlooking daughter. Without asking if he could help, the constable grabbed the side hand railing and lifted the stretcher. The results were catastrophic.

The obese woman on the now imbalanced stretcher caused the top-heavy load to start an unstoppable roll towards the hedge. I am a big guy, so I used arm power and weight to fight the rolling motion from the foot end. Art was a flyweight at the time, and he grabbed and hung on as the spin progressed. He was fighting the force caused by the twirling stretcher and the patient's upper body weight.

The last I saw of Artie was the bottoms of his shoes as he cleared the hedge. The cop was pulled over the side of the now upside-down stretcher tight against the snowy bushes. Four black wheels pointed straight up at the local snow squalls; we lost control.

From the open doorway, our patient's daughter wailed, "Oh, Mother." I was speechless. Artie picked himself up out of the snow and hopped over the hedge; he was a mess. The cop now hung over the undercarriage of the stretcher when he did not let go. I helped him back up, he waited for our direction. This would take a little finesse.

The hastily made plan was to collapse the inverted stretcher's undercarriage, the last couple of stops. The cop was like a fish out of water. You could see from the look on his face, he knew he caused the rollover. With the undercarriage lowered, we had to power the stretcher back on its wheels.

Assuming his original position before the rollover, Artie held the stretcher frame at the head end. An angle that I hoped would block our monitor's view from the door. How bad was it going to be? Fortunately for us, we always took the patient's security seriously. The straps were fastened tightly across the chest and waist, pulling the patient down into the mattress. The darkened, snowy sidewalk worked in our favour.

Artie told the cop to reach across the stretcher and wait for our order to pull the cot back over. After getting positioned, we rotated the stretcher back onto its wheels. The whole fiasco took about a minute. It was a minute longer than we wanted to be under the riveting eyes of the daughter. This call was full of challenges; sometimes, stuff just happens.

The moment of truth would have been humorous if this was a scene from a modern-day staged Youtube video. The patient, now righted, had accumulated a rather round compacted disc of snow covering her face. If you were around in the fifties, or if you search "Soupy Sales," you will get it. The slapstick comedian was famous for smacking his victim in the face with a crème pie. Totally harmless but bound to get laughs. This incident did not get laughs.

After the initial comment from the door, there was no gasp, so I begged the EMS gods to spare the daughter from seeing the insult. A simple flip and the packed snow released from the victim's face. The short journey to the rear of the waiting ambulance was uneventful. The cop asked before grabbing again if we needed help; we accepted the assistance.

The ER trip was slow going in the snow squalls. Nothing changed; the inevitable took place. The ER doc took one look at the patient after reading the strip from the freshly connected heart monitor and listened to our history. The resuscitation was discontinued.

We were locked into directives and legislation that dictated we transport every lifeless patient with few exceptions, even at the expense of their dignity. Thankfully things changed, progress intervened, and the medical community relented. It was a relief for patients, their families and paramedics.

Cuffed

This is probably not the time to ask. Have you ever been arrested? When you are suspected or accused of committing a crime, the arrest process is sobering, to say the least, having witnessed a few arrests. I have never been arrested, but I have been handcuffed once and pepper-sprayed, more than once.

Paramedics often respond to calls where crimes were reported to have taken place. In tandem with crimes, victims, the accused and sometimes responders get injured. Old school medics were more likely to dive in to help the police in their time of need than the younger responders today. It is not a criticism, just an observation.

Working with a younger medic one warm Saturday evening, we were called to an outdoor patio bar for a disturbance. There was a report of a person under the influence of drugs and alcohol that injured another patron. Two ambulances were sent.

Arriving at the establishment, the patio was an oversized outdoor sunken living room. Directed down several steps into a pit-like setting, we were the first unit in.

Off to the side, sitting by himself, was a fellow with a nasty cut above his eye. His "T" shirt was blood-soaked. My partner walked up to assess the injuries and dress his wound.

In addition to being part of a crew, I was supervising the shift. There were several police officers at the scene. Most were gathered around a fellow sitting boldly at a table across from a young lady. I took the position; she was his date. That was before the disturbance. I decided to check to see if the fellow with the police was injured. Or was I in "nosy supervisor mode?"

When alcohol is involved, men, especially the younger ones, often exhibit token chivalry. You either are chivalrous, or you are not. I have long believed that; some behavioural traits remain in a recessive mode with sobriety. Alcohol rarely brings out the best in people. Not professionally trained in psychology, these are my observations.

Police always have the lead at a crime scene. We are there to treat and transport patients and support the officers if they require it. A story was floating around that the fellow seated at the table was not so demure before the first responders' appearance. The word was that the sweating patron went face to face with the victim and hit him with something.

Police posed the story to the seated patron regarding the confrontation. That was all this fellow needed. He decided to leave. Standing, he was reminded that he was the subject of a police investigation and to remain still. An officer standing in front of him asked for his name and to produce his identification. Swaying now, after a quick move to stand, he motioned to walk away, the wrong move.

Having a hand gripped tightly around your wrist by a police officer would make most of us stop in our tracks. This fellow began to struggle. Forgetting that he was on a crowded patio, it also slipped past him that several police officers were present. Finally, two flights of stairs to climb and affect his escape; the reaction was poorly thought out.

Raising his voice, the surrounding crowd lost their collective, festive ambience for the moment. Onlookers had the advantage now, having seen the outburst earlier. This action was closing the loop.

The young lady sensing that her date was long over, picked up her belongings and retreated to an open area by the bar. The struggle escalated, a chair in our fellow's departure path turned over with a pull intended to launch himself past the furniture. More official hands reached out for the suspect, who had clearly been told to stand still.

Looking over towards my partner, Gord, the patient's head wound was dressed. The victim was riveted to the action, a missed opportunity perhaps. Retribution was currently being dispensed legally. The struggle now escalated to a dog pile.

Our struggling assailant was in a full sweat. The police were losing their grip on his wrists. Their attempts to wrestle him to the ground only slowed his progress towards the stairs. Surrounding table and chair legs screeched on the concrete patio as patrons dashed to avoid becoming the next victim.

My sometimes co-worker Artie was forever reminding me when I was on the cusp of a decision to act that; God hates a coward. I was in. Stumbling on the way to the scrum, my hip struck a table corner. The approach was only delayed for a second. Police forced the fellow down on one knee now, looking more like the submission pose from a losing wrestler.

When someone is struggling, you can sometimes anticipate their moves. An intoxicated patient is decidedly more predictable. Someone on drugs or alcohol can be many times stronger. The fight was on. I was sweating; my athletic ability now exceeded its capacity in the scramble.

There were two hands on the suspect's left wrist; one was mine. On his back from his persistence in evading his captors, the fellow was trying to roll over to stand and escape custody. There was a knee on one thigh, the red stripe on the side of the pant leg announcing its ownership. I was on his left side; the other wrist belonged to a cop now on the wrong side to attempt a rollover to handcuff the perpetrator.

The twisting and rolling played into our hands. Letting the suspect roll to his right, I could hold onto his left hand with my left. Rolling the wrist over, it went onto his back at his waist. Another hand quickly assumed a position next to mine above the wrist. A sergeant getting into the fray now brought the right hand behind the prisoner's back at his waist.

Slightly under control, the dogpile gathered momentum. We were up against a table. Other hands appeared, one bearing an open handcuff. Arms covered arms, we were all sweating, a forage cap with a chrome badge rolled sideways, evidence of the conundrum in progress.

The first cuff clicked shut and was ratcheted up to a tight fit on his left hand. This was no time to let go. A cop once demonstrated to a couple of us the potential for disaster during an arrest. If a cuff gets applied to one of the suspect's wrists and the cuffed hand gets loose before the other cuff is secured, "danger present"! An open cuff swung in a violent motion could cause real damage.

Using my other hand, I grabbed the fellow's loose hand as the officer holding it moved to allow for the cuff. Sensing the freedom, the suspect pulled his free hand towards his right hip. If he got it under his belly, the move could assist him in righting himself. Two other officers grabbed for the feet to prevent the attempt to stand.

In an awkward move, my right hand grabbed for his right hand. With the twisting, there were now two hands gripping the same wrist. The click happened so fast, I didn't feel the stainless bracelet encompass my wrist. Snapped shut and squeezed, I was caught. A simple "shit" announced my annoyance.

Pressing down harder on the still loose wrist, I was the only remaining restraint. Attached to the only bad guy in the room, it was time to explain where we were as far as I was concerned. "Wrong guy," I blurted out. But, unfortunately, the Sargent realizing the missed opportunity, was too close to do anything more than help restrain the fellow from bucking like a small bronco bull.

The police were recently trained and equipped with a new tool on their belts, oleoresin capsicum-OC, "pepper spray" for the uninitiated. Most medics had seen the canister holstered in the small leather pouch.

The accused, at his peak now, attempted to spit on any target within range. I heard the letters "OC" proclaimed. The call was intended to warn you to turn your head if you were close and weren't part of the offensive on the escapee. I never got that training bulletin.

It didn't make the squirting sound you would expect. Out came the spray in a narrow stream, a yellow aerosol. Sticking like mustard on our skin, it quickly ran with the beads of sweat. The suspect, Sargent and I were hit with the yellow agent. Glad that I was amped up with the excitement, the grip I had around his right hand did not loosen. The Sargent held on too. I could hear change jingle over my shoulder.

From a police officer's pocket standing next to us came his handcuff key. I couldn't see out of my left eye now. The seconds it took to uncuff the author and cuff the suspect up seemed like another whole minute. I heard an "ok" and let go.

Before me was a snake's den of hands. Forgetting the help I had been, it was time for some self-aid; that's selfish first aid. The coughing was not as bad as I thought it would be. Not the only collateral damage, several eyes, throats and lots of skin were the unwitting recipients of the noxious weapon.

Wimpishly walking to the bar, I knew exactly what I was looking for. Have you ever seen the wet cloth a waiter uses to clean a tabletop at a restaurant or bar? As dirty as it probably was, I grabbed the one from behind the counter and wiped my closed eye.

Providing no relief, I headed around the end and behind the bar. Oh, for a cold beer now. I settled for cold water. The tap next to the bartender ran continually while he mixed drinks throughout the melee.

The mess was secondary now. Rinsing my hands under the water to get the pepper spray off, I cupped a hand and, leaning over the sink, threw water in my eyes. Both were stinging. It was getting better; somewhere along the way, tears took over.

Returning to the patio floor, I was glad to see the fellow being led away and our patient standing, ready to exit with Gord and me. The date was nowhere to be seen. Cancelling the second unit that had been coming slow time, we would handle this minor injury. The drive to the hospital was silent as I continued to tear up.

The Sargent stopped by the office later. We had a good laugh when he realized medics were never trained on the defensive side of the spray procedure. Police are sprayed in a controlled training exercise to give them the experience. The command "OC" probably saves many officers once they know the drill. Turning away or holding their breath until the aerosol has settled would save the grief most of the time.

The suspect under arrest had to wait until he arrived at the police station cells before seeing relief from the irritant. Unable to remove the sticky mess, the ride in the patrol car would stick in his mind. The frustration of the constant stinging would not hurt like the punishment for hitting the victim with the beer bottle.

Accepting a career as a paramedic is not as simple as providing first aid, CPR and driving. Anything can happen. The longer you serve as a medic, the more likely you will take in the unusual. With training, hearing war stories and keeping your eyes and ears open, your situational awareness will sharpen. That helps keep you out of trouble. There are few guarantees, except to say again: stuff happens.

5

ABC

Airway, breathing, circulation. The rudiments that paramedics aspire to. It seemed so simple the first time it passed by my eager ears. The first cardiopulmonary resuscitation training (CPR) was offered before there were provincial standards.

Most individuals pursuing a career as a paramedic begin their training with first aid and CPR. It doesn't get any more basic than that for your first two steps. Some approach the career after achieving status as a lifeguard or volunteer firefighter, also a great base to work from.

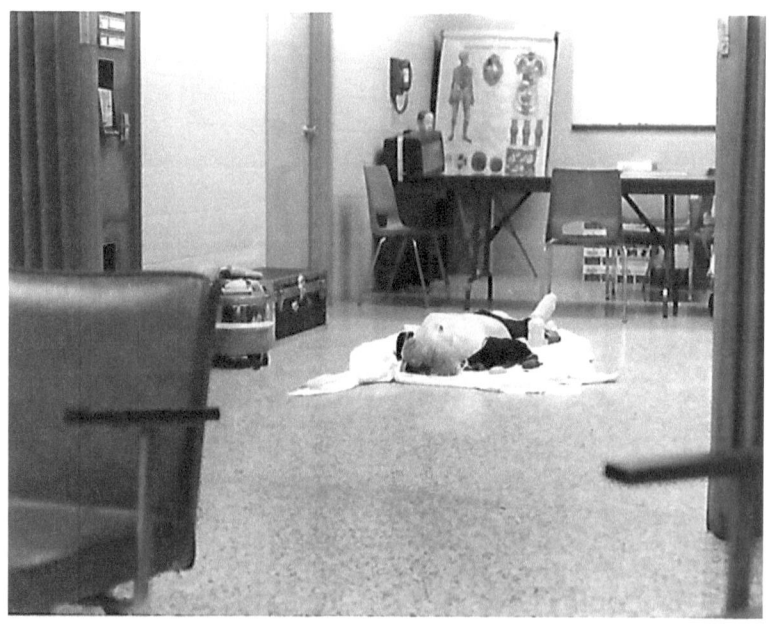

CPR training 1974

In the seventies, the skill of CPR came with the proviso; don't break any ribs. There was a myth that all first aiders were covered under the blanket of a "Good Samaritan" law. Ha!

The fear factor was reinforced with; you might not be backed if things don't go right. In the beginning, things didn't "go right" that often. We didn't know any better on the street; no one was sued.

Resuscitation was included in the basic ambulance training conducted at the Canadian Forces Base Borden. It came with a similar contingency. Researchers knew then that rhythmic chest compressions, along with artificial respirations, would help.

A patient's window of survival could be extended. Ambulances could get these patients to a qualified person who could provide more substantial intervention. What, doctors reign supreme? Are ambulance attendants chopped liver or what?

The internet aptly points out that CPR standards began in the '60s. It would be 1973 or 1974 before the basics were recognized in Canada. In 1975 a local anesthesiologist mounted the attack against cardiac arrest.

The generous doctor slipped over to Michigan to take the then three levels of training. His patience and dedication led to sharing the skill with local paramedics, police and firefighters. Thanks, Doctor Anthony Webster.

Three volunteers from each emergency service were sent to the first two levels of training. Along with two EMS colleagues, we emerged with an instructor's ticket. It was the second official step in the battle that paramedics waged against cardiac arrest.

The first was to send two of our medics to an advanced care course designed to be a pilot program in pre-hospital care. The designation "Kingston pilot program" left the provincial pundits in the position of being able to cease funding or curtail the "pilot" project. Step one did not go the distance initially.

Although there are no accurate stats locally, it seems a safe bet to say that the rate of cardiac arrest has increased per capita over the decades. That sounds terrible, so with an explanation in layman's terms, this is how it looks. Reporting for pre-hospital cardiac arrest locally was not a priority in the early days.

The guidelines for the Province's ambulance services for treating cardiac arrest were all-encompassing. For years, if your head was still attached, you were not split into two pieces or bloated and floating in a pond; Casualty Care Attendants were compelled through legislation to transport you doing CPR. Taken almost literally, the Ambulance Act saw to that.

Only a physician could pronounce death. In a legal sense, that is still true. In practical terms today, graduates of a paramedic course, accredited by the Province to practice in our Ontario, can presume death if they follow revised regulatory guidelines. What a relief. It's an exception to bring dead people to the ER anymore. If that sounds gross or negligent at first glance, there is a method in the healthcare system's madness.

Before full-time college courses were widely offered, two weeks of training seemed enough time to give a newbie the basics. Working with an experienced medic, you could take their lead, right. Four months later, after passing the "smoke test," I was sent to Canadian Forces Base Borden for the month-long Provincial Casualty Care Attendants course.

I realized then; there was a mountain of detail to patient care that escaped me beyond the professional education under my belt to date. Jumping at the chance, coworker Artie and I enrolled in the brand-new part-time Ambulance and Emergency Care course at our local Fanshawe College.

A couple of years later, after challenging the Provincial exam, successful candidates were formally registered as Emergency Medical Care Attendants (EMCA). It seemed that attaining the title of paramedic would take decades. Alas, I digress…

During the first two weeks of employment, training included basic instruction delivered by several seasoned medics. Each trainer had a specialty and its application to our craft to pass on. One such fellow was Tim. He came from a hospital job that specialized in the patient's airway and breathing. They called him an inhalation therapist in his day. Today the profession is referred to as a Registered Respiratory Therapist, or RRT.

Tim sported that "ambulance" sense of humour, a trait we all learned from. His craft's finite technical details were not much use to us on the street in the day. We did not have ventilators or advanced devices in the field. His ability to transfer his specialty to a grassroots level was remarkable.

Tim led us through oxygen therapy, clearing difficult airways and resuscitation techniques, such as they were in the day. His understandings of the basics were the best.

Who thinks of oxygen as dangerous? Tim's demo of the properties of the clear, odourless gas was convincing. You have heard of the patient falling asleep with an oxygen mask lying on linen and a cigarette igniting the bedding. One exhalation of a lung full of pure oxygen through a lit cigarette did it for me. The cigarette disappeared in a couple of seconds. Lesson over.

During the second day with Tim, our training was interrupted. Tim and his partner for the day, Mike, were also required as a crew with our limited resources. During training, they were assigned to be the last ambulance out of the base.

Used only in a dire emergency, one presented itself. The dispatcher for the shift, Kelly, came to greet us at the door. He assigned the call but was also snooping to see what the current lesson was.

Initiation day

We left the base for a quick ride to one of the senior's apartment buildings downtown. Mike and I met on my "ride-along" a week ago. Paired with Tim, this would be a real learning opportunity. The break from a classroom was a welcome gift on this sunny fall day. We were responding to the report of an unconscious, pulseless elderly male.

I was shaking at the prospect of assisting with some CPR. I rode in the back of the van with Tim and was given the task of carrying the small gym bag with the oxygen cylinder, masks and suction required for resuscitation. Was I ready for what lay ahead?

Some residents sat on the bench at the circular drive out front. We received what I came to realize later was the standard greeting; "what apartment are you going to?". Having to plead ignorance on behalf of the impending patient, we passed through the lobby and into the elevator. Barely large enough for our stretcher with the head sitting up all the way, our quarters were cramped.

The stainless-steel-lined cage was representative of the building standards of the day. Who knew that effective CPR was not possible with the patient sitting bolt upright? The building code would be a standard that would evolve over the decades. Today, residential elevators are large enough for two medics and firefighters to do CPR during their descent.

Arriving at the apartment door, our greeter was the next-door neighbour. She was accompanied by the patient's wife. There, in the hall of the small apartment, were a couple of glum expressions. Tim, attending the call, asked immediately where the patient was and what had happened.

In a strong English accent, the neighbour explained that she had been summoned. She responded when the wife of the patient came home from a visit with her daughter. The spouse came next door to tell her friend she found her husband unresponsive. Hearing the wife speak up now, I realized there was an added bond between the women. Both spoke with the same accent.

The patient's wife returned from an overnight visit and found her husband sitting in a chair. We passed both residents to start a patient assessment. Tim stepping to the side to let me in on the process, narrated his actions.

It was a gift; this was only the third time being within an arm's reach of a body. Seeing my grandfather in a casket was the first. Helping the fire department recover a drowning victim the second.

With some trepidation, I reached out to check for a carotid pulse. The man's cold neck told a story; there was no pulse, bristling whiskers, a red herring to my overly sensitive pulse-taking fingertips. I felt the back of the patient's cold neck, then moved the back of my hand over his nostrils, searching for exhaled breath. Breathless.

It was almost twenty-four hours since the couple exchanged words. It was too late.

Turning to the ladies, Mike offered some direction, instructing the neighbour to take the wife to her apartment next door and make her a cup of tea. Something a Brit might appreciate in the worst of circumstances.

Tim explained to the victim's wife that her husband "passed." The term has since been replaced with "died" so that there is no doubt. The plan was to send the police to meet the wife when they arrived.

Paramedics today have been trained in death notification. The guiding principle is to be kind and empathetic but be direct. Leave no doubt that there is no coming back. Using the expression passed was an innocent oversight in our early attempts as the conduit for the worst of news.

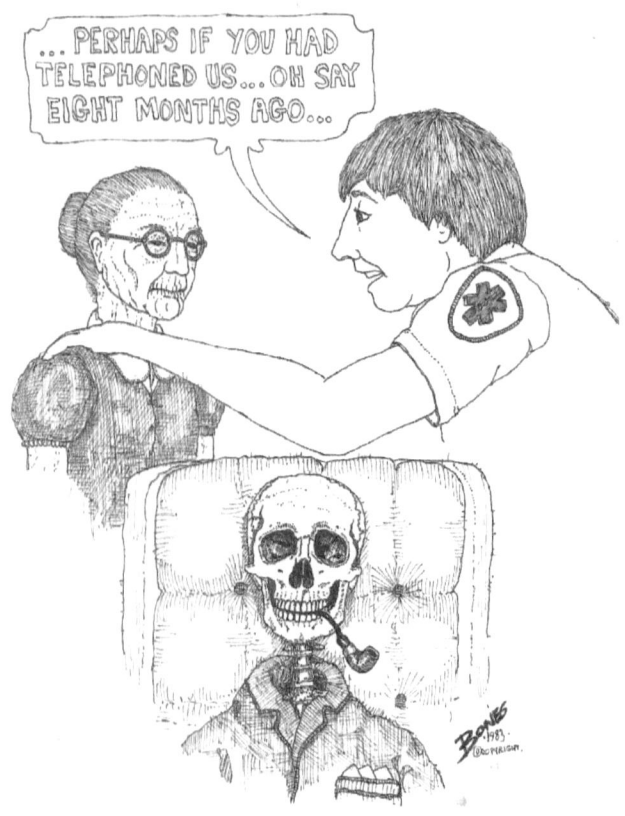

An early version of a death notification

As the door closed behind the ladies. I was silent, waiting for some follow-up learning points. Instead, the lesson was pushed off.

The next move was to notify the dispatcher of the call status. Kelly took a brief message from Mike to inform the police. The call was over before I realized it.

Quicker than you can say, abracadaver Mike went for the rotary channel knob on the idle television. Alive now, the snowy black and white image was the local afternoon show. With a couple of channel clicks, the baseball game came up. Mike blurted out, "oh, look, the game."

Tim explained it was a waiting game now. Our obligation; to hold the scene of death for the police. With no estimate of the police response delay, my mentors demonstrated how to pass the time. I was as nervous as a cat and paced.

Mike, in his usual laid-back fashion, sat down on the couch to the patient's right. If he wasn't a baseball fan, and this was his attempt to goad my nerves, mission accomplished. Tim quickly took Mike's lead and sat to the patient's left. A new newspaper lay on the coffee table; it looked undisturbed. Tim began reviewing the sports section.

As I paced around the small living room, I took the opportunity to look out the window down several stories to the circular drive. No police yet; I was growing anxious. It turns out the delay we were experiencing was par for the course. The report of a natural death drew no elevation of anyone's blood pressure at the police station.

Minutes later, a young constable arrived with a soft knock at the door. Television off and the three of us standing, he entered the quiet scene. Tim gave a brief report of what we encountered; it sounded so routine. I would learn later; there are times and places for lots of details and intense descriptions. This was not the occasion.

We all walked next door and introduced the officer to the patient's wife. It was my first Code 5 call, an "obvious death."

Taking Ho Ho to oh oh

Just over two months later, I was assigned to work the day shift. It was Christmas day. I was not offended to hear it was my turn to work on the holiday as the new guy on the block, single and not a care in the world. The family agreed to hold off on the festivities until the tour ended at 4 pm.

Another single medic, Matt, took me under his wing for the day. We were assigned to work out of the small room donated to us by University Hospital. I was over the jitters that most medics started with.

Nearly eleven weeks under my belt, there were a couple of serious collisions; chest pain calls were plentiful. I was beginning to get the gist of diabetic emergencies, and there were a few seizures too.

Matt picked up the phone; with a couple of umm hums, he hung up. He was a cool character. All I got was a "let's go, young man." On the way out to the van parked under the ER ambulance entrance, he announced we had a VSA. The acronym for vital signs absent, it is synonymous with cardiac arrest. The ambulance service is rife with shortened terms and phonetic substitutions.

The ride was a blast; Matt was a driver. He was trained as a driving instructor and loved nothing more than a "zoom," as he called them. I learned a lot from his lead. The drive took us to the edge of the city. Backing into the driveway, our afternoon arrival disrupted the caller's early Christmas dinner.

The woman who met us at the sidewalk let us know it was her mother-in-law in distress. Pulling the stretcher to the door, a male from within yelled out that our cot would fit into the living room. The introduction led me to believe our colleagues had been here before. The voice instructed us to the dining room.

Lying on the floor was an elderly woman. Family encircled the room, the festivities sadly interrupted. The man at her side briefly let up on the pace of his CPR, explaining he had been providing care since the woman collapsed. His report included that she was a resident at a nursing home, signed out for Christmas day.

The call went so smoothly; I thought it was too good to be true. Taking over the ventilations with our oxygen and pressure-driven ventilator, we continued with two-rescuer CPR. After another couple of minutes with no change in our patient, it was time to leave. I attempted compressions on the way out; furniture blocked the sides of the stretcher leaving the room.

The helpful man's assistance did not go unnoticed. Before we cleared the door, the Samaritan offered to continue compressions for the trip to the hospital. Looking at Matt, he spoke up, glad for the assist. Matt put him in through the rear doors after I jumped in.

With my hands busy, Matt did the quick radio patch to the ER. The resuscitation was uninterrupted, an experience that was almost impossible when you were on your own doing single-rescuer CPR. I was hoping for the best, it was my first VSA, and it was Christmas. The family needed a save.

Arriving at the ER waiting room, a nurse held the heavy door open. Our efforts were continuous, right to the resuscitation room. The nurse spoke up to our civilian assistant, advising him he could not enter and thanked him. To our surprise, he announced he was the patient's son. I was shocked. He was as cool as a cucumber for the call.

Thinking that the woman's relatives were still back at the residence, I assumed our helper was a family friend with some hospital training. When he spoke up, he advised he received the training through work. Both Matt and I were floored. In a conversation later, we both agreed we would never have taken him if his identity was known at the scene.

As it turns out, the woman's fate was pre-destined with a long history of heart issues. The escort did not share that with us earlier. We never did see him again. He was placed in a quiet room to wait for the doctor to share his Mom's outcome privately. In some respects, seeing his Mom through to the end provided closure. Way more than the average son would ever be witness to.

Trust me, I'm a paramedic

The government had a way about them. They endorsed and licensed the private operation of ambulance services around the Province. The word was, it cost less per operational hour than a "Provincial" service run directly by them.

In contradiction to their mandate, the folks from the head office in Toronto still wanted to micromanage the privateers. Overbearing regulations were abounding. Some were good, others disruptive.

The original VSA call here was not mine. It vividly illustrates the conundrum that the city hospitals faced following my coworker's experience. The subsequent cardiac arrest calls threw the cities ERs into a tailspin sending shock waves directly to Toronto. A feat not easily repeated. The patient I responded to added to the enigmatic regulations in the Ambulance Act.

On another Christmas day, a crew with lots of experience responded to a VSA call for a young male. Finding a fellow in his twenties living on his own, his absence went unnoticed. That was until he failed to show for Christmas dinner with relatives. He was deceased for some time. The crew was confident of their findings following a physical exam. The coroner attended, pronounced the patient dead, and that was the end of it.

The attending medic Dwayne was very qualified, participating in the process of certifying freshly graduated kids. The exam team was a position that I held in high regard. So, did his coworkers from the head office that selected the team with Dwayne as a leader. All was well until someone stirred a pot.

Some six months later, a family member spoke to their physician, and the death topic arose. A call to the regional coroner did not net any information, so the doctor wrote the government. He inquired through the ambulance regulators about why the patient did not survive the medical distress.

No one ever related the details to the inquiring doctor of what was told to the attending coroner or anyone. You would think that the attending coroner would have raised a flag at the time if there were issues. The ball was rolling.

Officials landed in the city and immediately suspended Dwayne from his position on the certifying team. It was so far after the fact that someone was on a witch hunt. Although Casualty Care Attendants were not permitted to pronounce death, there was an "or otherwise" clause. Early on, the article in the "Act" gave medics latitude to leave patients that were hopelessly beyond survival, a common-sense practice.

An after-the-fact judgment by investigators placed the blame for this death firmly on the medics. The move called our powers of discretion squarely into question. No one of good conscience would do any less than their level best for every patient in distress. It is only after consensus between responding medics that a patient is presumed deceased. Any ambiguity results in transporting; "let the doctor decide."

The spin-off was horrible. Medics, unable to exercise the powers of discretion, jumped on the proverbial "bandwagon." In response to the interim findings, paramedics agreed amongst themselves to follow the legislation to the letter. Every pulseless, breathless patient was transported to London's ER's. Doctors looked on in horror, thinking we could not see the bleeding obvious.

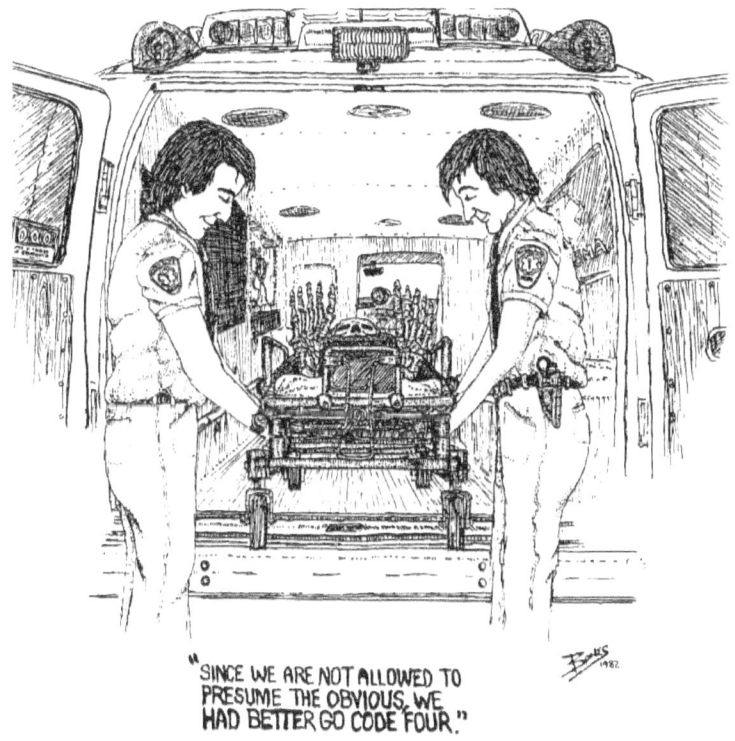

Credit: Chris "Bones" Skelton

An emergency doctor we all received training from and respected came forward after several mildly decomposing patients were deposited in his resuscitation Room. It took about a minute to explain the challenge in our operational criteria. It turns out he then checked with the other ER docs around the city. All were reporting the same recent phenomenon.

Patients were arriving with contracted, discoloured limbs. Other victims were starting to smell from days of decomposition. Police were questioning why their scenes of death were being disturbed. The simple explanation to all, "government regulations."

Working with a summer student the same week, we arrived in the emergency room with a fellow who was hours and hours beyond a successful revival. He was frozen in a pose, fit for a "special effect" in a horror movie. Our patient would not lay flat on his back. His hand stuck straight out behind him. A position he wound up in when he collapsed unnoticed between a bathtub and toilet.

Finally, great minds met. The investigator was directed to close the investigation. Dwayne's embargo lifted; things went back to a normal that gave medics credit for their professional judgement. To this day, if the same issue re-surfaced, medics could resolve it by taking the same course of action.

I Smell Dead People

Warm spring day shifts are not always full of sunshine and lollipops. The suckers would leave you with a pleasant aftertaste. We just finished a couple of low-priority transfers to outpatient clinics. With any luck, we would make it back to base for a hot coffee and a break.

A fascinating aspect of the job is the absence of predictability. Just when you get your heart set on an albeit short reprieve from the routine, things go south. This day would be no different.

Working the shift today with Jo-Ann, she was past her infancy in the business. At least that's the picture of confidence and the tone that the chatter painted, that conviction to step up and make a connection with patients. For the less experienced, one of the most challenging parts of the learning curve demands you take the lead when addressing patients.

You need to be willing to and know when to ask a question on the fly or take a hint or direction when faced with something new…or face the music. As the radio started to squawk, reason fluttered out the window, replaced with a brief whine from me about lost breaks.

"Car 159, this is London. Five-nine go ahead. One five-nine, you're 10-8 code four to 779 Bast Street. A next-door neighbour checking on a vacationing neighbour's house found their son on the garage floor. Possible code five".

Code 5, take your pick; deceased, expired, cardiac arrest, any or all. A brief ride to the residence ended with the surprise that the police arrived before us. Most spontaneous calls find us at the scene first. Something that only works when no hazards are lurking behind a door.

The neighbour and officer met us at the driveway's end rather quietly, given the call's nature. I think the young cop was a little hesitant to race in, considering the story. No one was scrambling to give us the scoop. What did they know that we needed to know before we went strutting in?

Walking up the lane, pulling our stretcher and equipment, the neighbour described having the owner's key to let him in the side door to the garage. He stated that the owner and his wife were down south for a few weeks. They left the inside door unlocked from the garage to the kitchen to have the friend check the house.

The neighbour's only task: was to check the furnace and look around the basement for water, conceivable during a spring melt causing a flooded basement. Something not uncommon in our "Forest City." Our guide spoke up and was surprised to discover the neighbour's son at the door leading into the kitchen. The fellow was startled to find him at home. The patient was a student supposed to be in residence facing spring midterm exams.

I could smell traces of exhaust at the side entrance to the two-car garage; an engine had been running but not recently. Only one car was parked inside, taking up the bay closest to the exterior entrance door. A biting presence that often burns the eyes as much as your nose and throat, the dregs of carbon monoxide became obvious. The exhaust was all but dissipated for the uninitiated.

A familiar odour met my senses on the tail end of the exhaust. Turning to my partner, I offered up my impression, "CODE FIVE." It went right over the cop's head. The best bet would have been to announce "10-45," a police radio code for a deceased person.

An older sedan blocked our preview of the lower part of the slightly open interior door to the house. As I looked through the rear window into the car, I could see the driver's door ajar and a key hanging in the ignition. Question answered.

Before reaching the patient, I turned to the officer, motioned into the car and whispered, "carbon monoxide – suicide." I guess you need the gold shield with the title detective across the top. It must have sounded like I was an amateur sleuth. Maybe the suggestion seemed premature and out of context. Did I block his view?

Walking around the sedan, the patient came into view as we cleared the car's rear corner: my partner, me and the officer in a single file. Two small steps bridged the difference in floor heights between the garage and kitchen.

The patient collapsed, now positioned awkwardly on the wooden steps. His fingers were stuck through the narrowly open door, a forearms length above the threshold. He lay almost on his stomach, his head on a precarious tilt back, caught on the edge of the door sill.

He was a heavy-set fellow in a "T" shirt, jeans and running shoes. From the side of his face, he looked to be in his early 20's. Jo-Ann standing in front of me, set the oxygen case down and stood silently, looking at the patient.

How long is this going to take, I wondered? She turned to the officer, impassively declaring his condition beyond treatment. Adding, "he's starting to decompose." The officer looked at me like, "what's with you two?" I shrugged, my inside voice offering, "it's an ambulance thing."

Halleluiah, here's a teaching moment. This had to be one of the first decomposing bodies my partner and the cop had seen from their reactions. The neighbour standing at the outside door spoke up and said he would be next door. Thinking about it later, the situation caught up to him when he realized what he had seen. And smelled.

The police officer gaining confidence, closed in behind both of us. The patient had a large neck, with a couple of rolls and wrinkle lines traversing above the collar of his "T" shirt. Now step back a minute.

Thankfully most of you have not been eyewitnesses to a decomposing body, a couple of tidbits here for the uninitiated. When something dies, human or animal, putrefaction occurs. The protein and bacteria go to work with a couple of by-products. First, a rather malodorous smell and second, there is some gas.

In this case, there was lots of gas. It is often trapped below the skin or in a temporarily sealed body cavity. Not for long, though. Some advice: don't poke the bear.

Paramedics or other responders who have had the experience will agree, the smell is unique, something your brain or personal olfactometer permanently records. Imagine opening a garbage can full of rotting leftover meat products in warm weather. This is decidedly worse.

The experience can work in one of two ways. First, to prepare you for future exposures. Morgue attendants and pathologists must enjoy this ability. Second and less desirably so, to make you want to run like the wind. Unlike rotting food, the effect of gas from a decomposing body goes well beyond turning up your nose.

The odour is so unique. That must be why cadaver dogs can be so accurate in their professional pursuit. It is a sour smell that can be so intense in a closed space I have seen medics wretch without warning.

Sitting around on a night shift, one of the old farts (a medic from my EMS childhood in the '70s) shared a temporary remedy. After encountering something that does not agree with your nose, you have a couple of choices.

You can retreat to your ambulance and open the fuel cap. Insert your finger into the opening, getting a small amount of gasoline or diesel residue on your finger and rub it on your top lip. If you carry a lunch pail, then following your first experience, keep some Vicks or A5-35 handy and use it instead of the gas. The foul smell disappears into the medicinal one. But alas, I digress.

Ahhh, the gas. A decomposing body creates liberal quantities of it, filling up the body's hidden cavities in a relatively innocuous manner. It creeps around, looking for a secret place, hoping to remain unnoticed until it has nowhere to hide. This process may take days, depending on the circumstances of death and the local temperature.

Then rather like a metamorphosis, the affected areas slowly begin to swell. You will remember that gas will rise in an enclosed liquid environment to its highest available space from your first science or physics class. When it comes to the human body, nothing is off the table. We are chock full of nooks and crannies.

Depending on the position of the deceased, the enlargement can almost look uniform. This is common when you find people who have died lying on their backs in their sleep. For this poor fellow lying on the steps, gas seeped up from the abdomen and chest into his back and neck.

It has been my experience that when the skin is wrinkled and under some tension, it tends to break down first. In this case, it chose to break down in the deepest part of the wrinkles on our victim's neck, the final twist. When the trapped gas, odour and pressure combine forces, it is the perfect trifecta for a mess. I could see it from several feet back, looking at our patient from the side. He was slightly silhouetted by light pouring in the open side door to the garage behind the now silent car.

A fine spray of body fluid erupted from the wrinkles on the young man's neck. Pinholes in the decomposing skin propelled the liquid and odour we were alerted to at the side door moments earlier. Now to bring it home. Remember the sound produced when escaping air from the neck of a balloon is restricted? The vaporizing body fluid was making a similar, almost inaudible sizzling sound.

Jo-Ann was aware of the odour now, but it was time for this teaching moment to pop. I asked her if she could hear it? With a negative response, I motioned for her to close ranks. Now I am not mean at heart. When she leaned closer to the patient, I kept her off to the side.

At this point, not being sure she heard the sizzle and could see the escaping body fluid, I placed the palm of my hand between her shoulder blades to get her within range of the inconspicuous sizzle. Withdrawing quickly, the effect was achieved, the lesson over.

You might view this as a nasty trick. Future patient assessments will include looking from all angles and remaining at a safe distance to avoid getting sprayed. This is not the time to follow the most basic patient care standards; who needed to take a pulse here? But when the lawyer asks you to describe your observations, after you state the patient was in an advanced state of decomposition, there will not be a settled or doubting stomach in the courtroom. Guaranteed!

An educated guess, sad but likely accurate. The stress of spring exams and some pre-existing issues overwhelmed our patient, the preverbal straw, and camels back analogy. To abort the suicide endeavour, the recanting fellow exited the idling vehicle.

Already severely affected by the toxic environment, our victim attempted the short but unsuccessful journey to the kitchen door. He collapsed on the steps in a failed effort to open the door and escape the deadly atmosphere. He was close. The fingers trapped in the narrow opening between the door and its frame told a story. The door wasn't open enough to make a difference.

The victim lay next to the only source of unpoisoned air, on the other side of the door. There might have been some slim chance for salvation if the car had not continued to churn out more noxious gas. The sedan's ignition was still on when we entered the scene. There was no way of knowing how long it continued to run before finally exhausting the fuel supply.

Completing the government's green patient form from our ambulance's cab, there were a couple of dozen tic boxes to choose from. Three lines to narrate, describing the patient and scene. Only a medic on the same call could draw the inference of the brief, disjointed words, abbreviations and canned responses to satisfy computerized fields. Oh, the eighties.

It was off to the base for a break and unwind before the next run. Safely back at the office sitting in the lounge, the all-important details paled when compared to the sitcom crews were watching. Rehashing the response was chicken feed considering the experience of the EMS veterans in my presence. Besides, why ruin a laugh with something most had likely already experienced in one form or another.

This had been a career-building opportunity with a learning experience thrown in for good measure. Calls like this were challenging when going home to loved ones after the shift. I dare say the reiteration would ruin their night sharing the details. It can be very stressful for a medic when you inevitably ponder the human side in the aftermath. You can only polish the callus you call experience, hoping to maintain that awkward balance between professionalism and empathy.

The "doc" in a box

With time comes progress. Well, most of the time. It was the eighties, CPR was now a household term, the public was on board for citizen CPR. Mass classes for instruction were given in schools, malls and at special events. Suddenly there was money for research studies to no end.

One of the first findings that encouraged citizen's enlistment was an education on the risk factors causing cardiac arrest. With a positive public response, a study on early CPR drove the next step. These were keys to the future but viewed by medics as baby steps.

Following the American model, early defibrillation became the subsequent study then hurdle. Get medics to the scene to get that first shock in following citizen CPR, and you had a real plan. With the data in hand, pundits found the money to train and equip Emergency Medical Care Attendants around the Province.

Our initial training sessions in the mid-eighties landed us an early model of a defibrillator. The first machine took all the guesswork out of the equation. It was referred to as a Semi-Automatic External Defibrillator or SAED, measuring a foot square and half a foot high. Known as the "1000," our "doc in a box" made the job a no-brainer. Medics did not want to hear that.

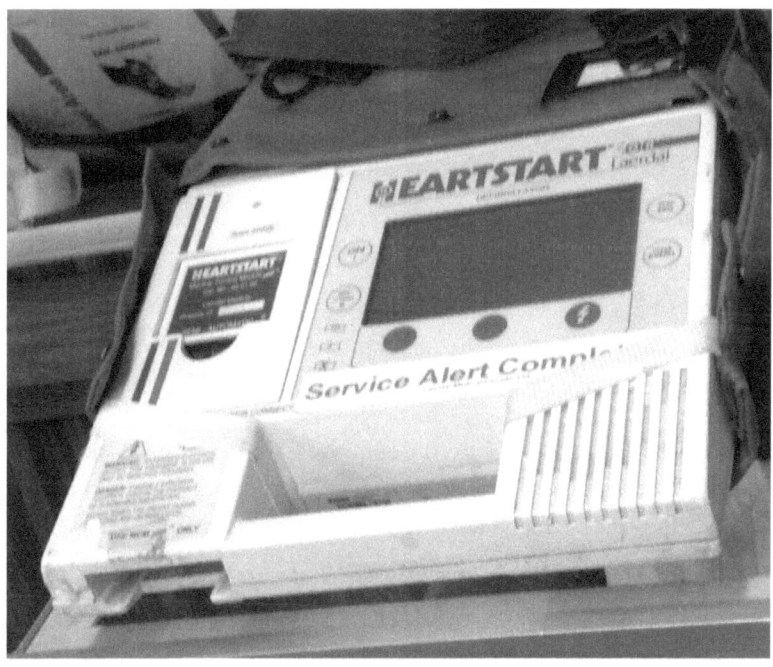

Doc in a box - defibrillator

The old salts in the industry wanted, no, were pleading for some user satisfaction. They dreamt of holding the paddles with the coiled cords against the patient's chest, yelling, "CLEAR." Too many of us watched with untold envy the American show "Emergency" in the seventies.

The iconic Los Angeles fire medics used an original manual monitor defibrillator. Calling out the patient's heart rhythm in a dramatic tone, they saved everyone. Indeed, we must sport the same tools of the trade.

With another piece of equipment to check at the start of each shift, our patient care arsenal was growing. It only took a minute and a few tic boxes on the daily check sheet. We felt empowered.

Stories of the medic's first field experiences were shared with great interest at the station and hospitals. Some of the nurses in the ER had their noses out of joint. We could defibrillate, and they couldn't. Go figure.

It took a couple of months to encounter my first vital signs absent patient after the training. Working with a part-time medic, Gord received the training as well. He carried the added responsibility of working at a second service.

Responding to an older subdivision, it took a few minutes to roll up on the scene of the two-story home. I went ahead of Gord with the oxygen kit and the shock box. He trailed behind with the stretcher.

A distraught wife met me at the door; her husband in his fifties lay in the bedroom upstairs. Our victim was sitting on the foot end of the bed when he collapsed. Falling back on the bed, his legs hung over the side with his feet flat on the floor.

Appearing in the doorway, Gord brought the CPR board in. We were graced with yet another toy. A small, orange plastic oval-shaped board with hand holes to place under the patient's back. A cupped area at one end allowed the head to tilt back, opening the victim's airway.

Doing CPR on a patient lying on a mattress is futile. The force of compressions on the chest pushed the victim into the bed with no actual chest squeezing. As a result, no blood was forced through the patient. In later years we scrapped the board and placed all victims on the floor.

Ken and I secreted a CPR board out of the office one evening. Using the orange board at a tobogganing outing with nurses provided a great solo ride. Everything should have two purposes.

With a few breaths and some compressions in, the patient was hooked up to the box. There was no time to explain to the patient's wife; she was probably surprised to hear the unit announce, "stand clear" as it charged. Surprise, a police officer appeared at the door over my shoulder. With an audience, the defibrillator issued its first shock at 200 joules.

As if the electronic voice wasn't enough, the result of the shock finished our relative off. The woman let out a yelp as the patient started to sit up and kick his legs out. It is a typical response to a jolt of power passing through the body, tensing the muscles. Usually, relatives are not present during resuscitation. Times were a-changing. A quick pulse check, no luck. Back on the chest for more CPR.

We continued with another couple of minutes of CPR. The police officer could only stand back and watch the latest advance in patient care firsthand. The analyze button was pushed again, followed by the warning to stand clear. As the machine dispensed its shock, the command followed to "check pulse." You could hear his wife sobbing in the hall. No pulse.

I took over CPR while Gord and the cop brought the stretcher to the bottom of the four-step route to the living room. When Gord returned, I analyzed again, likely a futile attempt since the first two were unsuccessful. The third shock was a little more dramatic; our fella got 360 joules this time. No pulse.

Loading the patient, we enlisted the officer to carry some equipment out to the ambulance. Since he was there, Gord asked him to transport the victim's wife to the ER. With the wife unable to hear us, our observer asked if everyone did the "arm and leg thing" with the shock.

I had to be honest since I had dispensed very few shocks; "I don't know, this was my first time shocking someone in a laid-back position." Something made me think he wasn't expecting that answer. Gord spoke up, saying that he had seen limbs pull up using the competitor's machine at his home service. His patients received shocks while lying supine or flat. Sounded like the devices were similar.

Transporting the patient, there was no change on route to the hospital. ER staff were unimpressed with our efforts. The experts took over the patient's care. Employing several advanced techniques to salvage our victim, the care had run its course. He was pronounced.

Sing-along

With so many calls to draw on, you only want to hear about a few notable runs; some departures are more memorable than others. To say it is just another day at the office would be trite, approaching insensitive.

Medics must move on. Learning from most calls, wanting to forget others. Some runs are remembered for the light that they bring into a sometimes-dark career. Trust a medic to make lemonade with a lemon.

Did you ever find yourself driving along, radio turned up, singing to the music? It can be somewhat cathartic. It was years before there were enough ambulance stations to cover the far reaches from the downtown. We had to get in our ambulances and drive, and drive, and sometimes drive some more.

This was one of those calls, travelling about fifteen minutes to get to the scene. Add to that the processing time for the call details. Then there was the delay when the caller didn't do the 911 thing right away. He wasn't even at the patient's side yet. It was a hot summer night.

Dispatch received the call for a male, unresponsive. The patient's family received the original call from his wife, then drove to the patient's location and had a look. That's when someone dialled 911. If no one ever shared this with you, after about eight minutes of cardiac arrest without resuscitation – irreversible brain damage starts. Give or take.

It was a lovely night for a drive, stars out, windows open, arms hanging out kind of night. Besides, the rig we were working in had no air conditioning. In the heat of the summer, you attempted to cool the ambulance interior by unlocking the bottom latch of the hinged windows in the back of the ambulance. They tilted out.

Arriving at the mobile home, Brandon and I knew we were in for a workout. Family milled around outside smoking. A relative, with a distressed look on her face, met us at the door. Her husband echoed the sentiment as we passed, entering the older mobile home. The man identified himself as the son of the patient.

Led to the bedroom, we realized our second curse on the call. A waterbed. Who puts a king-sized waterbed in a room barely able to contain it? You know the place is too small when you remove the only entrance door and the closet doors to get the pseudo wave pool in. Was the portable dwelling even built to support the weight?

Lying in the center of the bed was our victim. Curses, you could see that he vomited. You couldn't get to him without climbing onto the mattress. To get into bed to sleep, you had to crawl over the foot rail and take your place. The doorless room afforded no privacy. What was the upside to this setup?

We couldn't treat the patient in bed. It would be like doing CPR on a raft in the ocean. Time was wasting. Leaving the gear behind, Brandon and I climbed onto the mattress, boots and all. I hoped we wouldn't puncture the vinyl bladder; the mini tsunami would surely result in a lawsuit.

The wave action created by two men stepping on the waterbed mattress must have been a sight from the door. Good thing it was an emergency. The silent patient rocked back and forth regularly as we stepped alongside. Yup, he vomited. Looking Brandon in the eye, I could hardly keep a straight face. Could our luck get worse?

Too far out of town to call for help, the family was our only source of manpower. Using the bottom sheet as a hammock, our assistants could pull the patient to the foot end. I spoke up now and asked the son at the door if he could find another person to help. His wife volunteered from outside the room.

There was no time to apologize for our water walking act. I described how we would get the man out of the bedroom and onto the living room floor. From there, we would begin resuscitation. All hands-on deck, it was a real job.

As we pulled the four corners of the sheet towards the foot of the bed, water rushed around our unresponsive patient. Oh, and did I mention he was a three hundred pounder?

It was about two am now. Why was that important, you ask? When you eat a late-night supper, that is about the time digestive acids begin to work. Breaking down the food in your stomach, the result is a sour, acidic odour. Air, belching out around the escaping food and liquid, can be nauseating. This was a classic example.

Our victim's bum hit the floor first with a thump going over the end of the bed rail. Using the sheet, the couple outside the room pulled the man out of the doorway. As we made a less than graceful exit from the water feature, we kept his head from striking the floor.

The sheet was soaked in vomit. The small mobile home hosting a pungent flavour now went well beyond the smell to your taste buds. Kneeling on either side of our victim, we rolled him over onto his side between two recliner chairs and a television.

Brandon retched quietly. Gravity worked much better for clearing the volume of regurgitated food than our puny suction unit in the orange case beside the patient. It was back to the basics. This was a minor nightmare.

Some CPR and the attempt to get some oxygen into our victim revealed he had aspirated some supper. For the untrained, aspiration is the term for getting foreign material into the airway and lungs. Yes, it is terrible. The rattling from within his chest and upper airway as we ventilated illustrated that the damage was already done.

Brandon was retching again. I thought he was going to lose it. Our patient needed deep suction at the hospital. Chest compressions caused the foul odour coming from our victim to waft upwards. The cloud struck every sense we trained ourselves to ignore. We desperately needed fresh air.

Connecting our SAED was another near futile assignment. The peel and stick defibrillator pads required a dry surface to attach to the chest. Some vomit and sweat and the skin needed to be wiped for the adhesive pads to stick. Supper on a hairy chest, yuk. Calling out for a towel, the daughter-in-law reappeared with a cloth. The pads attached; would they last?

"Analyzing" ……." no shock indicated." In a brief repeat, we did more CPR for a couple of minutes. The second attempt to shock the heart yielded the same results. Working at the head ventilating, Brandon was almost at his limit. He was a grey that only nauseated patients get. Just before they barf.

Time to move. Our standing orders were complete for now. The next job was to get the guy to our stretcher. From there, it was a routine call. We used the bed linen as a drag sheet to get the fellow to the door and out to the stretcher enlisting some help.

Mobile homes were not designed to get uncooperative patients out of horizontally. Tight corners and personalized modifications that did not meet the building code blocked our way. Finally, dragging our unresponsive patient to the two steps outside the door to the trailer, we could get him onto our waiting stretcher.

With the head of the stretcher pulled up to the steps, it bridged the gap. The rotting hand railing wavered with my weight against it trying to maneuver the victim onto the stretcher.

It was only a few feet to the ground if it broke. The small wooden landing groaned under the combination of the patient and rescuer's weight.

We just wanted to get out of there now. It took several minutes longer than it would on a routine call to get this far. The game clock was in overtime. Loading our patient into the ambulance, I instructed the family not to try to keep up behind us.

We explained that we would be using our lights and siren to pull through traffic. I hoped that this would paint the positive picture that we were doing everything possible. It was all about getting their loved one to the hospital. We had, and we would.

One of the rear tip-out windows closed on the way to the call. With a slight pull, the worn latch popped back into the locked open position. Closing the door behind Brandon, my heart went out to him; the air was thick. The extra opening wouldn't save the day. There was never enough fresh air for these calls. The sound of more retching slipped out through the small space.

Dispatch was quick answering the hospital patch request when I passed on the information for Brandon. He was busy; besides, his hands were a mess from the obvious.

A history of high blood pressure, chest pain, and distress were expressed by the patient to his wife before becoming unresponsive. When I said the patient vomited and aspirated, it was an understatement.

The retching was regular now. I could hear Brandon through the small pass-through window dividing the cab from the patient compartment. He was struggling. As the patch ended, I hoped that the ER nurse would not ask if someone was barfing in the back. I could hear it clearly.

Shit. I turned my head to look in the rear-view mirror, a feature not left in the cab, to see who was in traffic behind me. The reflected image was for monitoring the attendant and to improve communication in the event there was trouble.

Brandon was breathing in my ear and retching some more. Head through the small opening, he was a mile away from the chest for CPR, regardless of the futility.

"I can't do it, man," he was puffing from the dry heaves. To get him back on track, I sent him back through the window with a promise; "We just need to get your mind off it." The AM/FM radio, a recent addition to EMS, was turned off earlier. It was never supposed to be on during an emergency call, right? Time for some music.

It was the middle of the night. The local station must have been on a nostalgia kick. As the news ended, an old tune from my first year in high school started. Turning up the volume loud enough to distract Brandon, Otis Redding began to whistle then sing, "Sittin' on the Dock of the Bay."

Singing without accompaniment, a sharp bark at Brandon through the window drew a weak response to start. As his singing came to pitch, the retching subsided. I remember both of us laughing; it was working. With the ambulance up to speed, the air quality was probably a lot better. The air was rancid in the mobile home and the back of the ambulance to start.

The song ended before we reached the ER. With his mind off the offensive odour, Brandon's mood became calm for the most part. We arrived at the hospital only a little worse for the wear. The staff made no mention of the background sounds during the radio patch. As predicted, our patient was pronounced deceased when doctors viewed his flat heart tracing and had the timeline described.

There was a real mess in the back of the ambulance. The paperwork for this call would take a few minutes, but it had to go in right away. The crud and puke in the back was mine to straighten up. Brandon regained his stride and did the best he could with our victim's airway.

Brandon needed to finish his form and throw it into the envelope for the base hospital folks. Little did we know that we set our own trap. The devil is always in the details.

He looked better, now sitting at the desk. The air was fresh in the small room we used for report writing. That's not saying much; it's a hospital.

The shift finished rather uneventfully. The topic of our VSA came up with the day crew, discussing the access in the mobile home, not the retching part. Brandon's experience was safe with me.

During my days off, the phone rang in the kitchen as I was sipping the first coffee of the day. Without call display, there was no time to prepare or ramp up a guilty feeling. Something that might happen today if you had an inkling of who you were about to talk to. My conscience was clear.

Laughing their greeting at the other end of the phone were two familiar voices. I just had to untangle them to figure it out. Calling today were the Base Hospital program's head, Doctor Smith and his program manager, Martin.

Oh, the details. Wondering what had gotten into them both, I asked why the call? Technology, mostly old technology, caught us. Well, it was new at the time.

Defibrillating patients is a delegated medical act. Doctors are the only health care providers with the unrestricted right to shock a patient's heart. Meeting the goal of getting that all-important "early shock" in; doctors "delegate." Empowered, subservient levels of caregivers perform the procedure following training and certification.

Delegates like paramedics and nurses. Paramedics shoulder the responsibility of this empowerment to perform more of these restricted technical skills than any other healthcare provider, short of a physician.

The original defibrillators did not have a screen to witness or interpret the heart rhythm in the field. The assessment, decision and permission were all made electronically. Our "Doc in the Box (sorry, Dr. Smith) announced audible prompts when the time was right *to shock or not to shock*. That kind of sounded a little Shakespearian for a moment.

"Document, document, and document. The standard in health care is "not documented, not done." Keeping paramedics on the straight and narrow with the low-tech/high-tech shock box, the inventors included a small cassette tape recorder. It logged two details.

The device stored the patient's heart rhythm, and then there was an audio track. Medics were to narrate their findings and actions during a resuscitation. Receiving the paperwork and cassette, the medical control folks could see and hear secondhand what unfolded on the call. Busted. "Nice singing" was all I heard from Martin as Dr. Smith chuckled in the background.

Discovering the entertaining audio rendition begged an explanation. The description of the timeline for our response and extrication of the patient from his watery grave only made the story worse. This was one of those calls that could not have been improved, given the delays and challenges we encountered.

Quickly getting over the trepidations, we agreed that the call went as well as it could have in the circumstance. Brandon would laugh and be relieved with the news. The recording of the call escaped me when Brandon submitted the tape and transporting documents to Base Hospital. It was probably better to be received without an introduction.

Hugs help

Receiving a message from a crew the other day, their text summoned me to the ER. Without any idea of why the guys wanted me there, it was a little concerning. Supervisors hardly ever get the call when something goes well. It's usually quite the opposite.

Sandy and Jordan are always calling about something. Mostly good news, but they were faced with some strange calls to resolve. Expect the unusual with their requests. This would be the exception; maybe the tide is changing.

Passing through the ambulance entrance doors, Sandy was cleaning his stretcher. Jordan was in the report room, clacking away on his laptop. "There's someone in the back bubble that wants to meet you," Sandy announced. "Like who?" was my first question. Followed with, "what's it about, a complaint?" Always the doubting Thomas, the master of "doom and gloom."

"No, she says she remembers you from a call twenty years ago." "It's not an old girlfriend?" "Nope, I don't think so."

Entering one of the primary patient areas, I walked past several cubicles. The curtained bays were left open for passing doctors and nurses.

They could monitor their patients from workstations in the center of the room. The cloth dividers were generally closed when an exam was underway, or the patient wished privacy.

Warned about passing this spot, a patient called out, "Are you, Chris Darby?". Turning around, I could see my summons was under the scrutiny of several doctors and nurses within earshot. Addressing the lady on the stretcher, I offered my apology for not recognizing her. Was I supposed to know her?

I met her friendly outstretched hand, waiting for my return greeting. The lady acknowledged I should not remember her. "We met over twenty years ago; I have never forgotten your name." Now I was scared. At least there would be witnesses.

"You took my baby to the hospital; she died that night." On the "what do you say to that?" scale of one to ten, it barely topped out at a one? That revelation is the last thing a paramedic wants to hear with or without an audience.

It was impossible to conjure up a natural response other than offering my condolences; it was so many years ago. Saying I was sorry for the mother's loss was the best I could muster at the moment. I felt disingenuous.

Probably looking a little shaken at this point, the lady sat up on the stretcher and asked to hug me. It was a different request. Still off-balance, I obliged. Puzzled, I felt compelled to ask a couple of questions. With the address and date, the story jumped off the page in a couple of sentences.

For all these years, this lady remembered a name. One that by all accounts should have brought up emotions and terrible memories better left buried. Literally. It happened early one morning.

Working with Callie, we were steady all night. Even if the calls were coming in slowly, supervisory duties filled the gaps. The tour couldn't end soon enough; I was dragging my butt.

We just returned from a south-end nursing home. Calls like this came in threes. There was a brief dry spell, thankfully.

A mother awoke, her instinct telling her something was wrong. The missing sound; a baby crying for an early morning feeding. Running to check the crib, Mom faced the worst tragedy of her life. Lying lifeless, her baby, just a few months old, stopped breathing during the night.

There were no signals, no long medical history. Not a single reason to make you stay up keeping watch, no time to prepare. Without warning, the worst day of her life.

Calling 911 is always a nightmare. A police dispatcher answers the initial call; they hear your request. You want to blurt out the details. They tell you to stay on the line, announcing they are transferring your call to the ambulance dispatcher. Delays, this is not the time. Just send the ambulance.

An EMS call taker answers, asking for the address. Their next question: what is the nature of the emergency? You want to reach through the phone and drag the paramedic by the ear to your door. What is taking so long? They make you go through the details in a methodical, step by step fashion.

The dispatcher needs to get it right the first time. Anything less will cause a preventable delay. Hearing the nature of the problem, emergency medical communicators are trained to offer first aid advice or instruction for starting CPR over the phone. Sometimes it helps. Then, there are times when it understandably goes right over the caller's head.

Behind the scenes, the call taker passes the early details of the call electronically to the ambulance dispatcher in the same room. In seconds, the closest ambulance to respond is chosen, the crew is notified. In many cases, the ambulance crew is in the process of responding before the final information is received by the call taker.

At the 911 center at the London Police headquarters, their communicator checks for officer locations and status. If there is an officer close by, one is sent to assist. They know CPR and first aid. There are more steps to dispatching; check out the other stories.

The ride to the far corner of the city was simple but in the opposite direction from Children's Hospital. The distance was a complication in this case. Contrary to outdated beliefs, paramedics must drive within the limits of the Highway Traffic Act. Locally, we can exceed the speed by 30 kilometres an hour. Having to stop for red lights is a "must-do."

Arriving at the scene, the modest home was quiet for a baby in distress call. A police officer was seconds ahead of us; he was already at the baby's side. Nothing was being done when we walked into the nursery. A distraught mom stood holding the baby beside the empty crib. There were knowing tears on her cheeks.

Callie scooped the baby out of mom's arms. CPR was started on the walk to the driveway. We were outside, standing next to the running ambulance in seconds. That low rumble, a thumping in the distance, was getting more noticeable to me. Callie and the cop missed it. Now here was an opportunity.

Using the portable radio microphone on my shoulder, "London, this is 173". From the morning air above, NHX, our local medivac helicopter, was bearing down on us. It was sitting on the helipad at Victoria Hospital on Commissioners road when we passed earlier on the way back to base.

"173, go ahead; this is London". London is that NXH that I hear overhead?" "10-4 173, they are on route to the airport".

"Tell them to set down at the mall just around the corner; we will be there in a minute with a VSA infant." With another quick "10-4," the dispatcher was off to the Provincial radio channel to relay our request to the approaching helo crew.

Helping Callie into the ambulance, she had a puzzled look in her eye as I closed the door. Turning to the police officer, I told him to take Mom to the Children's Hospital and shared the plan. We were off. Two blocks away was a large parking lot. Empty this time of the morning; it would be a quick drop, stop and away. A fraction of the time that it would take us driving to Children's ER.

Arriving at the mall, our warning lights gave Scott the low down. Doing a last-minute tail turn, the helicopter pilot headed to the corner of the striped lot, not another car to be seen. Coming in for a rolling stop, the thundering forty-eight-foot blade span kicked up the requisite dust.

You always waited for the cloud billowing out from the whirling blades to pass before approaching the running machine. I have seen eager cops eat a pound of grit, being too keen to greet an arriving helicopter.

Walking, guiding Callie to the machine, she kept up the CPR as we crossed the parking lot. The chopper was noisy; they kept the jet turbine engines up to speed. There would be no time for a meet and greet here.

Now under the moving blades and whining engines, the door opened to a familiar face.

Jessica looked out from the cabin, headset on; she motioned for Callie to hop in. We all knew each other; Jessica worked with us on the land ambulance. Some of my days off were spent as a medic on the machine. Today I was earthbound. I wasn't jealous of this run.

Both medics, busy now. I strapped Callie into a seat and closed the door behind her. Not expecting to end her shift at five hundred feet doing one hundred twenty knots over the city at dawn, I would catch hell when I picked her up for the ride back to base.

As I stood less than arm's length from the pilot's seat, the flight crew looked back into the rear cabin. The action from both pilots was continuous. Scott, one hand on each control, I tapped the plexiglass bubble window with my palm and gave a thumb up. His glance my way acknowledged the buzz from the unique in-city scene call.

Without hesitation, the thrill-seeking Australian aviator eased up on the already engaged collective pitch control giving the blades lifting action. The machine hopped into the air, still right next to me. Only a few feet off the ground, the aircraft transitioned quickly to forward flight. Passing a silent hamburger joint just below, it was good that this brand was not yet serving breakfast. A startled customer would likely have dropped their hash browns.

The chopper arrived at the hospital before I could get halfway there to pick up my startled coworker. The machine sat silently out on the helipad in darkness. The emergency was over until a fresh day crew took over back at the airport. Orange approach lights were still on around the pad; the sunrise was about to drown them out.

In the department, pediatric nurses were charting their recent attempts to revive the patient. A doctor sat, explaining some of the details from the resuscitative process. The teaching hospital never stopped, using every opportunity as a learning moment.

Back in the report room, Callie and Jessica sat writing rough notes in silence. It had been too long since the child was breathing on her own. Doctors worked for a while, their exhaustive efforts in vain. Everyone gave their best. The outcome was disappointing but a relief knowing the attempt had been made. It did not go unnoticed.

With a slightly caustic, hello, I got the stink eye from Callie. Jessica let out a sarcastic snicker for sending her on the unscheduled ride. I could sense Callie liked the experience, though. Despite the terrible outcome, there was no criticism for the choice. During the few minutes drive over to pick Callie up, I began to wonder if someone from the hallowed halls would question the "city" pick up for the baby?

The local private medivac helicopter has since been replaced with a shiny orange hot rod. Did I spell that right? Looks like it; there is no wiggly red line under Ornge.

Today, policies and procedures are abounding. Requests for the Critical Care Flight Paramedics from Ornge within an invisible boundary for miles around the city would be denied.

Rightly so, most land paramedics did not have advanced skill sets back in the day that this call took place. Most medics, including the author, still thought speed replaced skill. Our Provincial air medics are world-class. The Advanced Care land paramedics in our Province are also ahead of other programs.

It was still a "cool" call remembering back. Mom would not let go of my hand as we spoke. She reinforced that I should not feel bad about the outcome for her child. She went on to say that the police officer and she spoke during her ride to Children's Hospital. He explained the exceptional lengths everyone was going to and the quick ride her daughter was getting. She said it helped her grieve later.

It had been more than a couple of decades since this Mom's catastrophe; the hug was a reward to be cherished.

On scene

You can't imagine a more hopeless feeling in the world than seeing a person take their last breath to the power of ten when it is a child. Your adrenaline is pumping like a fountain, and you do your best. With "basic life support," your only skill set, the options are limited.

Working one day at the airport with a crew on the medivac helicopter, it was a slow start. Andy, our engineer or mechanic for our aircraft, kept us out of service for the morning to complete some routine maintenance. You get used to it with helicopters. Who wants the blades to stop whirling around when the cars and people below are the sizes of ants?

Scott and Nate were the flight crew today. Scott, an Australian with lots of flying experience, a seat of the pants pilot. Nate was the conservative type relying on the numbers. He had been flying in the military for years. There was always a colourful conversation when they worked together; it got interesting.

Noon rolled around; we were still grounded. Finally, the decision we had been waiting for, a test run-up. Engineers often wanted an engine start after maintenance to confirm that all the temperatures, pressures and gages showed the aircraft was operating correctly. On some occasions, there was a test flight, really. Not a time to ask Andy what those extra nuts and bolts were for that were still sitting on the tool bench.

Nate dispelled my technical questions long ago; I was a hangar rat. "You're just here for the free ride, so don't ask questions about anything mechanical." My job was as a door manager in the back and primary care. Nurses or doctors would be on for the ride if anything serious was to break out.

For the most part, Nate was right. Our machine was assigned hospital-to-hospital trips. The aeromedical attendant looked after more stable patients. For the critical victims, the trauma or neonatal unit sent out a team. That was until you got a scene call. We also covered the region when an incident required rapid transport from a highway or remote location.

The sun was overhead now. The sky was dotted with a few of those puffy little clouds hanging around. With the aircraft pulled out of the hangar, the start was typical. Heads sticking in the flight deck door for a few minutes had me wondering.

As the machine sat doing a run-up outside, one of us had to stay back in the office near the phone to listen for a call. With a couple of rings, I asked the caller to speak up. The noise coming in through the open hangar door was not helping. The dispatcher was happy with the noise, telling me we had a call if we were off the "out of service" status. I gave up, telling the dispatcher the pilots would call back in a minute.

Running out to the helicopter was not the norm. You always walked out and stopped at the edge of the rotor blade arc. They wanted us for a call that I couldn't accept. I was in a hurry. I appeared at the pilot's door like I was selling Avon, tapping on the plexiglass window.

Unable to turn the engines off and get rid of the loud noise, I was reduced to yelling in Scott's ear as he held his headset away to hear my request. With a "hold on" wave, he spoke to Nate, who disconnected his headgear and exited the aircraft.

The test run-up was still underway as we walked clear of the blades. Nate's palms up "what gives" signal drew a blank. I couldn't answer his question. He called dispatch to get the call details.

Nate came out of the office, waving me over, "Got your stuff," he asked? "Yup," was my response. Sometimes during maintenance, we removed the pedestal bed and patient care equipment from the cabin floor to allow access for repairs or test gear. Today, we were ready to fly.

Opening the side door to the helicopter, the headset was the first order of the day. The noise was terrible. Sitting with the door open, I had one foot on the ground and one on the cabin floor. Just keeping my options open in case Andy came running out with a handful of spare parts again.

I could see the map over Scott's shoulder. Our main Provincial highway is a regular source of business for the ambulance services along its path. A lot of folks think that the bad weather brings out the accidents on the four-lane route.

There are terrible accidents in good weather; people drive faster then. Their slanted logic that clear roads are safer is a myth. Going more quickly gets you to the scene of the crash sooner.

The intercom came to life, and Nate relayed the story. "We are going to a crash with a van. There are kids involved". I left the door open and one foot on terra firma while the machine was run up to speed. An indicator light on Nate's instrument panel gave away my casual start to the call.

As I closed and latched the door, the machine started to taxi out to the apron in front of the flight line. I was the radio operator for ambulance dispatch. The crew was not supposed to know more details once we were underway. This was a scene call.

The crew contacted the tower, so we just kept rolling, doing a running takeoff. Medivacs have priority at the airport when the nature of the call is declared. Besides, we could fly low and in any direction under other traffic. We would clear the control zone with the controller's blessing with all eyes peering out of the aircraft's windows.

Announcing to the ambulance dispatch centre that we were on route, the communicator's update was immediate. One ambulance was on the scene, another was on the way. The first report was that one seriously injured patient was still in the vehicle. We were airborne for five minutes; the crew estimated ten minutes to landing. I passed the ETA to dispatch. It was a sunny day, a real myth buster to the "bad weather" believers.

Approaching the scene, Scott was sizing up his landing choices. Sometimes the Provincial Police held the traffic for air ambulances. Their selection for a landing zone wasn't always the same as the pilot's view from above. This was one of those cases. Our two twenty-four-foot blades required twice as much clearance around them to avoid an accident.

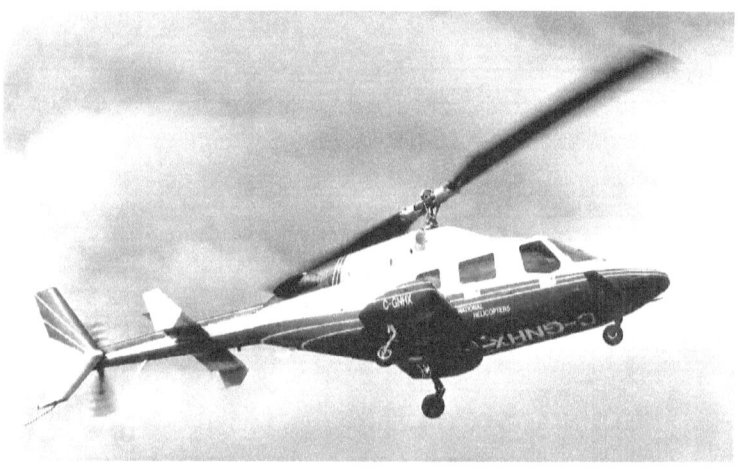

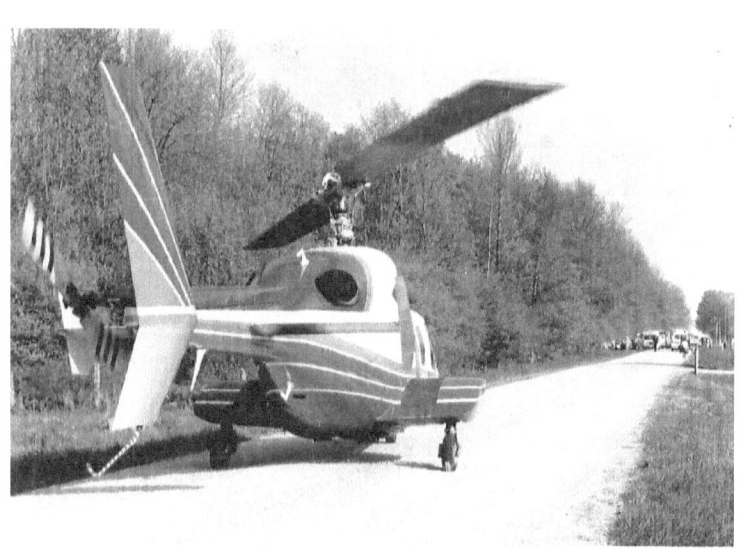

C-GNHX – credit: Ian MacLeod

When you are standing on the ground at the airport, the blades are at least ten feet off the ground. You get used to the clearance. You still bend over at the waist when you get out near the blade tips. They have been known to swoop down at slow speeds. Landing on a hill or uneven ground, blades can be closer to the ground on one side than the other.

Landing today in a shallow ditch, well, that was a new one for me. We came in low, Nate calling out the clearance expecting Scott to land on the road. Scott didn't like the blade tips near the median between the east and westbound lanes. Who was I to question? I'm the door manager, remember!

Setting down in the grass, a farm fence lined the opposite side of the aircraft to my seat. With a shallow rise next to my door, I knew this would be a different setup. Opening the single door, dust from the virgin ditch was blowing around. I put my sunglasses back on. I usually ditched them; I am no Tom Cruise in a flight suit.

Getting my feet back on the dirt, I quickly realized we would be loading from the opposite side. It was several feet up to the edge of the grass where the shoulder of the road started. Arms full of gear, I walked forward to get away from the blades.

Local paramedics and a couple of police officers looked at me as I walked away from the running aircraft. Looking back, I could see why. Scott had the engines up to one hundred percent. With engines at reduced power, rotor blades can droop. We were sitting so low in the ditch he kept the "paddles" up to speed, holding them flat. There wasn't much air between the blades and the ground.

The rolled-over van spewed its contents around the ditch way out ahead of us. Papers, maps and clothes blew around, partly the result of our recent landing. Several first aid dressing wrappers blew away as medics and cops milled around the scene.

The second land ambulance arrived. The crew stayed in their vehicle for the moment, avoiding the debris and dust rolling downwind.

A medic I recognized motioned me over to a van-style ambulance's rear doors, opening one door. Inside was a child on a folding stretcher. He had a collar on and was immobilized to a backboard with straps and medical tape. An oxygen mask covered his face; under it, a plastic airway coming from his mouth. The kid wasn't moving.

The crew just finished their extrication and placed him in their unit to avoid the dust storm from our landing. The report was that he was not belted in the back of the van. Tumbling around in the rollover, I was figuring a head and neck injury for a start. There were a couple of minor lacerations. It was inside our victim that was likely the real issue.

Sitting next to the female land medic, she reported the child was not conscious. I looked at his eyes and quickly checked his breathing. He was very pale, arms and hands cold to my touch. He would be going with us.

The land crew agreed; he was found in this condition and was the most serious. The forty-minute ride by road from scene to door in either direction east or west would be his undoing.

Placing the folding cot on their rolling stretcher, I laid the plan out for the crew. We would get up as close as we could to the helicopter. One medic and I would load the patient leaving the other to stop the stretcher from blowing over. Big stuff can easily be knocked over and blown into the aircraft during scene call operations, creating an emergency within an emergency.

Getting within a few feet of the blade tips at the front of the helicopter, we stopped. Nate shook his head at our approach. We turned from the shoulder of the road to walk down into the ditch.

The blades, continuing to turn over the farmer's field, were fine. On the opposite side of the aircraft, the three-foot by twenty-four-foot swords swished in a threatening fashion. Overlapping the road's shoulder, they stretched out to the centerline of the eastbound lanes. They were barely above waist height, close to loose gravel.

As suspected, the stretcher mattress below the folding cot went sailing during the unloading. It tumbled down the shoulder of the road away from the spinning blades. A quick-thinking young volunteer firefighter grabbed it up before it stopped on its own.

With the patient loaded, I placed my hand on the medic's shoulder and yelled, "walk straight away from the aircraft bent over." He didn't need any more advice. While we were still stationary, the straps over the stretcher got an extra check. Closing the door, I crossed the front of the aircraft, one hand on the cowling to remain well clear of the danger overhead.

Entering from the aircraft's dangerous side, my shoulder seat belt combo went unfastened, swaying back and forth with the accelerating engine's vibrations and the blades. Its belt's security was not an option for this call.

It took a couple of minutes for the pilots to work out a game plan for our departure. I could use the time to have another look at the kid. Breathing in a shallow, irregular rhythm, the back of my hand was the indicator for the volume and rate. I had no electronic assistance to monitor the patient.

The simple oxygen mask was not enough for our patient now; he needed specialized care almost fifteen minutes away. Getting out a bag-valve-mask BVM kit, I hooked the oxygen to the tap on the back wall. The original mask stayed connected to a small cylinder until I checked again for a pulse in his neck. It was thready making it challenging to feel. The vibration in the aircraft threw me off. The kid's pupils told the story.

With a bump, our wheels came out of the dirt. We lifted a couple of feet off the ground setting up for a hover. This was the dodgy part. I had been in the helicopter when the pilots were prompted to set the machine down firmly from a couple of feet to check something. A temperature or pressure gauge reading, it didn't matter. Setting down heavy from this height, the blades could droop and hit the gravel. The kid's pupils were dilating.

With only a few seconds to realize I would be doing CPR in flight, the mask applied by the land medics was pulled off to the side. I gave the kid a couple of breaths to start from the BVM. The plastic airway already in place; it was a little big for the job. It would have to do for the trip. Now at treetop level, we transitioned into forward flight.

We had a primitive intercom on board. The medic did not have a switch to call the pilots. They called the cabin attendant. My call bell was a tap on the pilot's shoulder that wasn't flying that leg of the trip.

Standing in the cabin while in flight was usually limited to brief periods. The low ceiling and vibration made it difficult in the best of circumstances.

Nate got the tap. Looking over his shoulder, I made a chest compression-like motion pointing to the kid. He was already on the intercom with Scott, who turned when Nate's retort was "shit." I read his lips. Scott took the bull by the proverbial horns.

In the land ambulance business, there are code three calls. Urgent but not life-threatening; no lights or siren, a speed limit governed ride to the hospital. Then there are code four calls, life and or limb-threatening; use your lights and siren, go a few kilometres faster and cut some corners.

In a helicopter, there are a couple of navigation lights, no siren. The cruising speed was usually a constant. Up until now, there had never been a flying difference for code three or four. Who knew?

With a couple of seconds of lag time, Scott went into code four-mode. Giving the blades maximum lift, the nose dropped, and we pulled ahead. It was new to me. I could feel the "G" force increase slightly, right down to my feet. Our speed picked up quite a bit.

Nate came on the intercom and asked if there was anything I needed. I was busy doing compressions on a small chest. When it was time to ventilate our victim, I gathered my thoughts. "Tell dispatch to have a couple of security guards meet us on the pad with the stretcher and let the ER know we are doing CPR on a trauma" and gave the age.

I had not noticed we weren't heading straight into the hospital helipad. We were outside the control zone for the airport. Approaching the restricted airspace, the pilot could give a report of our inflight emergency as a medivac. It would provide us with priority over other aircraft. The tower would warn us of other aircraft in the area, doing their best to turn conflicting aircraft away until we passed. It is still the pilot's job to observe and avoid other aircraft in our path.

That all sounds good until you are a passenger, doing CPR standing up in the small cabin. There was more headroom in the chopper than the old SUV ambulances. A Suburban would have been perfect on this call; you could at least brace your back against the ceiling doing chest compressions.

My feet were spread apart, knees bent in a golf posture up against the metal edge of the pedestal holding the stretcher. That was until we turned. Making a sharper banked turn in an aircraft, the pilot can pull an extra "G" or two.

Starting a left turn over south London, I thought we were banking to avoid something. Scott was a smooth operator. I will never forget; my feet were glued to the floor, doing compressions in a left turn over the White Oaks Mall.

You might ask why I took the time to do some sightseeing out the window. The aircraft was now over on its side in a very tight maneuver. Looking up to see where we were, there was no horizon or landmark skyline to check. I was suspended parallel to the ground, feet stuck to the floor, looking straight into the mall through a skylight, doing chest compressions.

Pulling a tight enough turn to stick my feet to the floor beside the patient was a one-time experience. Well, there was that one time on the Twister at the Western Fair. I almost barfed in front of my kid. Flattening out of this turn, the wheels came down for landing.

The ride was over. Keeping up the CPR for the trip up the glass tube at the hospital's front, security ushered us into the elevator and to the children's ER. Staff were geared up for our kid in cardiac arrest. With their advanced care, including an airway and drugs, the pulse returned.

A couple of days later, the outcome was announced. The rollover got the best of the little fellow. I was hoping the rest of the family did well. The parent's other children would become the focus when they got past the high-speed crash tragedy. I can't imagine losing a child.

When a save is also a goal

It wasn't long before Aaron and Bernie had the good fortune of the first save with our original defibrillators. Medics talked it up, sharing the details. It was a hot topic. We were encouraged that we might get to the next step someday and officially be called Paramedics. Some might even get to the advanced care level running cardiac arrest calls with drugs and tubes, a long-held professional desire for medics.

On my first half a dozen calls with the 1000 model, the device's presence made no difference. Some patients received shocks that were advised by the electronic decision-maker. Most got the "no shock indicated" response to the analysis of their heart rhythm. It was a downer; this was not a miracle device. Nothing changed, or had it?

Medics are quick to see the downside of a situation rather than the positive. In retrospect, the doc in the box was a stepping stone. The same device is now in most arenas, schools and public buildings. Law offices place them in their front lobby, probably warding off liable suits. Oh, there I go, the negative side again.

The medical community known for its conservative approach was slow to advance pre-hospital care in the day. "Baby steps," we would hear. It was the right approach. We have not regressed over the years. Today the medical directive experts at the Base Hospital call it "Evidenced-based care." Baby steps have taken on a real swagger.

We checked the defibs every day at the start of the shift. The regimen included changing the battery out, checking the disposable pads that were peeled and stuck to the victim's chest and finally, a quick power-up. Like a fire drill, I was waiting for a blaze, no more practice.

Mom always said when I would dream out loud, "Be careful what you ask for, darling." Only a young medic dreams of cardiac arrests. Thankfully I kept my thoughts quietly to myself. In our business, it is never a matter of; if it will happen, just when.

On the evening shift, most medics preferred to watch television. Working with Art, we had some near misses, getting a pulse back with a shock. Soon after the shock, the patient's pulse would peter out. We had not experienced a real save yet. We didn't want calls tonight; there were some excellent TV shows on.

Stuck taking an ailing senior to St. Joseph's ER, we just cleared the hospital. Our dispatcher came on the air from their new center on York Street with the hail for a cardiac arrest. A sixties male who started with chest pain. The dispatcher advised that he initially told his wife to hold off on the ambulance. Men are stubborn, experts at denial.

The drive was a short five-minute run. Met and directed by an older man, our patient was upstairs in a bedroom. We were in for a carry down the stairs in a stair chair. For the time being, it was into the home and leave our rolling stretcher in a tight hallway at the bottom. Hands full, we carried the gear up to the small room.

Finding our victim spread across the foot end of his bed, his wife gave us the history, including a heart attack a year ago. The neighbour that let us in had been over to check on his friend. The patient was feeling unwell all day. That was telling.

Pulling the pulseless fellow off the bed, he accepted the airway. We started some CPR on the floor in the small room. It was time to give the portable doctor a shot at a save. Artie did the analysis that told us a shock was advised.

Standing clear, it was a simple push of the button to deliver the jolt of electricity to the patient. With a quick jerk, the patient pulled his arms off the floor in response to the current. Pulse check, no luck. It was back to the chest for more compressions and some breaths.

After a couple of minutes, it was time for another assessment by the machine, we followed the plan. With the shock advised and delivered by Art, we had a pulse back. That was an improvement.

Getting a pulse back, the victim still needed to be ventilated regularly. The bag was placed across his lap after loading him onto a folding chair designed to carry patients' on stairs. Artie gave a couple of quick puffs at the landing partway down the stairs. This was progress. Checking at the bottom of the stairs, the patient still had a pulse.

We were out of the house, loaded and ready to leave in good time. The patient's wife asked if she could ride with us to the hospital. Turning to the neighbour, he was no help. He lost his license with a recent stroke.

It was always a pain to transport a relative. Today it is a real exception to take a passenger with the patient. If the patient is not a young kid, relatives and friends make their own way to the ER. We have had too many complications with uncooperative passengers. This lady was no trouble at all; she even climbed into the cab on her own.

The radio patch to St. Joseph's was sort and sweet. In front of the patient's wife, I called ahead and spoke to a nurse. A witnessed cardiac arrest: the patient had suffered one previous heart attack. There were no surgeries; we gave two shocks, the patient's pulse returned. We had the medications in a bag. I was too busy to read them and drive.

Pulling up to the ER, I remembered a previous disaster when a passenger got out on the angle on the "downside" of the ramp. I asked the wife to hold on for a minute and ran around to help her out. We surely didn't need a fractured hip to add to the heart attack.

Once inside the waiting room of the ER, we sent the spouse to register her sick husband. It would be a distraction until we could get him into the resuscitation room to see if he really would be a save. The ER staff were happy to receive a patient that responded to a shock at home. Our last few weren't so lucky.

The doctor pulled Artie's hand and the mask away from the man's face. Incredibly, he was chewing on the plastic airway. Not gagging yet, he was regaining consciousness. Within minutes his eyes were open, the airway was popped out. This was a full-on save for the moment. I was impressed.

Led into the resuscitation room, our victim's distraught wife approached the gurney. A smile broke out when she looked through the green oxygen mask to see her husband puffing away and opening his eyes to her voice. Reaching out, she took his hand and called his name. I turned to open the door in a state of disbelief, leaving the patient and staff to carry on.

Stopped by the door, a tiny hand brushed mine. The patient's wife briefly stepped away from her husband's side. Quietly she asked why I had not recognized him. Turning back, I looked at the resting patient, drawing a complete blank. Remembering she just called out his name, there was still no light switching on.

In a brief conversation, I was reminded we played pool in a friend's basement a few years ago. Still a blank, she thanked me, asking me to pass her thanks to my partner as well for our kind care. I never crossed her path again and could not tell our mutual friend about the call. The Provincial regulations and our service policies prevented it. Passing the thanks on to Artie, we celebrated our first save with a hot cup of coffee.

How we do it

The "olden days" is a term used when referring to outdated practices in our childhood. In the seventies "EMS olden days," ambulance attendants were ruled by the "load and go" mandate. Responders received minimal training, possessed limited skill sets and willingly operated within choking patient care guidelines. Sometimes, the best we could do was to get our patients to the hospital quickly.

What a difference a few decades have made. Paramedics today operate under an ever-changing blanket of direction. It is often referred to as the "stay and play" program. We now bring the emergency room to your home or our scene.

Receiving a call for a cardiac arrest today, several systems are activated simultaneously. The closest paramedic crew is dispatched, sending an Advanced Care Paramedic ACP team if possible. When a Primary Care crew is nearby the patient, they are sent to initiate care until the Advanced medics back them up.

Dispatched at the same time, are our comrade's over at fire. With more stations and a lighter call volume, firefighters often arrive at the scene before the first EMS crew. Far be it for me to leave the underlying tension between some responders off the table. No matter which side of this outdated disagreement you reside on, we need each other. To the disgruntled responders from either service, Fire or EMS, get over your bad self. Our patient's come first.

Firefighters are trained to provide first aid and CPR. Pump crews are equipped with basic defibrillators. There is an ever-increasing number of paramedics switching to a fire career for many reasons. One that jumps off the page; the skills are transferrable.

An Advance Care Paramedic team at the scene of an "arrest" can be run off their feet, working independently. With additional responders to assist, the senior medic gets to zero in on the problem sooner. Anything to; eliminate distractions, treat the patient more efficiently, and reduce scene time. Focusing on delegated technical skills and the medical management of the patient, medics still follow the ABC's

Advanced Care Paramedics' comfort levels have come of age. Part of their relief is the result of working with the experienced assistance of other medics and firefighters. The EMS team can then direct their attention to the cardiac monitor and the vital sign values that the modern units display. After assessing the patient, the heart tracing gets the most attention. Is there a pulse with that blip on the screen?

Advanced medics often insert an endotracheal tube into the patient's airway. The paramedic inserting the tube crouches or lays on their stomach to look directly down the airway. A stainless-steel blade on a handle is placed into the throat of the victim, opening the airway.

The plastic airway goes between the vocal cords to get to the area where the airway branches off to your two lungs. This skill is learned on a mannequin then refined in a well-lit operating room under an anesthesiologist's direction.

Larry is one of my personal champions as an advanced care medic. I hope I am looking up at his face if I ever wake up on the highway following a collision. On a cardiac arrest call at a hoarder's residence one day, it was time to intubate the victim. Larry dropped to the floor, now lying on his chest amidst a small herd of cats and piles of stacked magazines and discarded belongings without hesitation.

What he missed was the cloud of fossilized cat feces that he displaced when he hit the filthy carpeted floor. Larry never missed a beat. Giving the best of care, his experience, professionalism and passion is the measure of a great medic. Following the successful procedure, he carried on with patient care as if this was the same as another day.

Not every call or challenge paramedics face is this extreme. Though the example is a testament to the determination of my friend and our colleagues in the profession. Back to work.

Critical patients require an intravenous line to provide a direct route for drugs, sometimes fluid. When the patient's veins don't cooperate, medics have a couple of options. First and the most immediate, they can squirt some drugs right down the airway. You would think that drowning a patient already in distress would be the last thing you should do. The lining in our lungs will absorb medications at an incredible rate.

The second and most recent intravenous skill offered to pre-hospital care is an IV start into a bone. Medics have a small cordless drill, you heard me correctly, a miniature boring device. The interosseous route, through a long bone like your shin, is a rapid option.

A special needle mounted on the drill acts as a boring tool "popping" through the outside of the bone. The newest method is an excellent route for drugs or fluids to be absorbed through the marrow found inside the bone.

With an airway and drug route in place, the patient's assessment continues to be interpreted then treated. Sometimes a single shock reverts the patient to a pulse-producing rhythm. From observing advanced care teams following their regimen, it usually takes a series of drugs, CPR and shocks to convert the patient to a heart rhythm that pumps blood.

Don't forget, CPR continues uninterrupted until there is a substantial pulse present. GO, TEAM!

Some drugs speed the heart up; others slow it down. There are also drugs to increase the pumping or squeezing effect of the heart muscle. The combination of these medications often kick starts the heart into a productive state.

Patients sometimes have a very rapid heart rate that can exceed 200 beats per minute. Called supraventricular tachycardia or SVT, the record rate may reach 300. Chest pain and that "fluttering or pounding" feeling often overwhelm the victim. When the heart beats that fast, it does not refill between beats, causing lots of problems.

Treated in the early stages, this condition can be resolved, heading off a cardiac arrest event. Medics can give a drug that stops the racing heart briefly and re-boots the heart's electrical side.

Like re-starting a corrupt computer program, the heart responds to the drug. Resuming a slower, hopefully, regular rhythm, it returns to a manageable rate and rhythm, refilling with each beat. Patients receiving the drug often react with an; "eyes wide open" response like a firecracker has exploded at point-blank range.

As cardiac arrest resuscitation progresses, the most significant physical demand for responders is CPR. With firefighters at the patient's side compressing the chest, they spell each other off, warding off fatigue and compromised performance. This well-choreographed process keeps someone on the chest, maintaining the temporary circulation efforts at maximum efficiency.

The team's work is routinely reviewed by looking at the heart tracing and reports later. London responders are world-class, with kudos pouring in from research groups following our studies. The quality assurance process keeps everyone informed of the success stories shared later between professionals.

As resuscitation continues, medics exhaust all their routines to return the patient's circulation. There are several avenues between drugs, shocks and fluids to help ailing patients recover. It is not unusual to leave a scene with all hands on deck, carrying a breathing patient to the ambulance for their quick ride to the hospital.

Standing at the edge of a room full of responders working on an unresponsive patient can be intimidating. Seeing CPR for the first time, a person's chest being compressed a couple of inches, is hard to process. A firefighter or police officer often holds up an IV bag when a close-by nail exposed by a picture frame snatched from a wall isn't an option.

Background sounds like a heart monitor beeping, or in some cases, not beeping away fills gaps between commands given by the paramedic crew. Other responders surround the victim waiting for coordinated requests from the medic directing the resuscitation. All in all, it is a daunting sight.

Now, for what you don't hear during a resuscitation. You have missed every lesson the medics have taken to build a collective repertoire for patient care. Each procedure has guidelines and exceptions. Previous experience on the road further strengthens their skills.

Choosing the correct device, size, quantity and medication dosage at the right time requires a conscious decision. Following the algorithms and protocols demands consideration and precision. Eliminating all the unrelated but treatable conditions that are not the cause of today's emergency remains equally essential.

Every drug or fluid a paramedic administers involves pre-approved permission from the Base Hospital, a group to be reckoned with. Standing orders learned and practiced in training scenarios are put to the test. Ontario has long surpassed the outdated "mother may I" American style of asking each procedure's permission on demand. Paramedics marching orders today often involve multiple layers of care before they exhaust their options on the scene.

Drugs and fluid given are selected because their intended effect will treat the patient's presenting heart rhythm and vital signs displayed on the monitor. These values, combined with the patient's past medical history, age and body weight, can vary the treatment. Medical math considering all the variables must be calculated on the spot to give the correct dosage. Something that is computed silently, without the aid of an electronic device.

And you thought the siren was the exciting part of a paramedic's career.

Here is where medics earn their money. Joining all the skills and treatments a paramedic can bring to bear is sometimes not enough. That's when a paramedic and physician get together on the phone. The "physician patch" allows them to review and share the patient's presenting condition, treatment and response.

Advice is received to try another round of drugs. In some cases, an order is given to transport. The receiving doctor can then reassess and provide care that is not possible or practical in the field. The physician will always have the final say. Younger victims often get a transporting order despite the crew's exhaustive efforts to reinstate the pulse.

Some patients just don't respond. Following a valiant effort by all, medics receive the order to stop resuscitation. The time of death is then pronounced by the physician. Crews bring the ER to your home. We would be delaying treatment, transporting a pulseless patient to the hospital before advanced treatment could start. Load and go is old news!

Cleaning up a scene following resuscitation is a job. The attending medic meets with the relatives and informs them of the death. Police are notified of the updated patient status if they have not arrived at the scene.

Paramedics must remain on the scene until relieved by police. Firefighters are released with thanks. EMS crews sometimes work with the same pump crews several times in one shift if the need arises.

Paper wrappers from the pre-packaged drugs and devices are bagged up; we make a mess. The attending medic begins to collect their thoughts and make crib notes. When the opportunity presents itself, a laptop computer is brought in to record the patient information.

The other silent component of patient care is paperwork. Truthfully, we are paperless today. Thanks to Bluetooth™ technology, some of the leg work is already captured for the medics. The heart monitor records a continuous tracing of the heart's activity. Each blood pressure, oxygen level, pulse and respiration are stored within its memory.

Transferred wirelessly on command to the laptop, the medic is left to document each procedure, drug and response encountered during patient contact. That is in addition to detailed patient history and assessment.

Some charts exceed ten pages. Paramedics are given a measly twenty minutes to complete the form. An allowance that is rarely underspent.

When the form is complete, abracadabra, it is blue toothed out to the ambulance! Each of our emergency vehicles is a wi-fi "hot spot." A copy of the completed form is sent to the hospital to be attached to the patient's record. The original is sent to our cloud in Toronto, giving Base Hospital access to the data.

The quality assurance process is then in play. Forms are reviewed in many cases at least twice. If the record is for a patient's death, the coroner is instantly sent an electronic copy. All patient information is encrypted to meet provincial privacy regulations.

When a patient was pronounced dead in the ER forty years ago, things were different. The deceased was covered up, and the room darkened after the family received time to begin their grieving process and say goodbye. It could take an hour.

That room was out of service until the coroner attended the hospital. There was paperwork, releasing the patient to a funeral home or issuing an order for an autopsy. A second overlapping cardiac arrest on route to the ER would cause a flurry of activity moving stretchers. Noses were often out of joint, prematurely moving the deceased.

With the volume of cardiac arrests today and their poor timing, the system could not support transporting every VSA patient to the hospital for a "look-see." There would be times when traffic jams would block resuscitation rooms. The resulting delay, affecting other critically ill patients.

Thankfully through training and progress, doctors have gained a healthy respect for paramedic skill sets. An earned trust factor is now the standard. Getting a pronouncement at the scene is an accepted and anticipated outcome for some patients. Responders and the police are then responsible for the "scene of death" when efforts are unsuccessful.

As a rule, paramedics do not flood the hospital with "dead people." Healthcare resources are too valuable and scarce to afford a barrier to care created by the unsalvageable.

Someone's foresight included increasing the skill sets and responsibilities of all the players. Nurses, Paramedics, Emergency Department Technicians and many other healthcare practitioners all take on more than their predecessors. Patients have grown to expect it. It is the face of healthcare today.

Cardiac history

Pre-hospital cardiac arrest patients have been studied, literally to death. Through research, there are care plans or algorithms that map out the most effective treatment order. Still at the top of the list are the original two, early CPR and early defibrillation. Hallelujah, some things never change.

Long before there was advanced care in our area, Dr. Smith and other local emergency doctors worked with a national action group. Their goal; raise the public's awareness of cardiac emergencies. To showcase the point, a competition between advanced care teams was proposed in the nation's capital.

Their mandate was accomplished by demonstrating skills that would reduce the cardiac patient's mortality and morbidity. The political thrust was to lobby politicians and pundits to legislate and fund advanced pre-hospital lifesaving care. Though ready for the education piece of the consequences of losing vital life signs, the public was under-informed.

When Dr. Smith approached a few of us to compete, we threw our hands up. We were primary care level Emergency Medical Care Attendants. Following his lead, the good doctor led us through several weeks of practice to prove a point. Four of us were drawn in with a reward.

Paramedics usually like food as a bonus. In this case, an all-expenses-paid trip to Ottawa for a couple of days sounded like a deal. Train, we did. We held up our end with the basics and learned the resuscitation routine's rudiments when you threw in the tubes, drugs, and a defibrillator.

Arriving at the competition, teams represented major Canadian centers from coast to coast. We were outgunned, or so we thought. As the match unfolded, we performed better than a lot of teams on the basics. We didn't know any better, the old stick to what you know.

As it turns out, we were not smooth enough to make our mark with the best. Teams familiar with the drug choices when a curve was thrown at them exercised that medic instinct. Bravo. We did place third from the bottom of about eighteen teams. Competing as the only pseudo-paramedic squad, we were happy with our finish.

It would be three more years before we saw our first SAED on the streets of London. Individuals that pursue a career as a medic seem to be drawn to a life of service. It is a silent personality trait. Some might deny it; there is life beyond public service. But the quality is there.

What else would keep you coming back for more and more training? Skills are added regularly to our repertoire as research identifies the benefits. Other treatments are removed when the lack of evidence proves them ineffective. Medics are reviewed regularly, the pressure at times is excessive.

Working shifts taxes you physically. Entering a call scene that can routinely push your senses to the limit is just part of the job. Cleaning up the mess and writing reports following a call is the least liked aspect of the profession. It is the drill. The person that completes the details and comes back for their next shift now that is a paramedic.

Celebrate

With the number of poor patient outcomes, one would think you would lose hope. Paramedics will tell you: it is difficult at times. The stress can be overwhelming. To provide some relief after each long year of these calls, there is a celebration.

Statistics are researched from a mountain of patient records. Lists are drawn up of our County's cardiac arrest survivors. In honour of the patient's "close call," they are invited to a luncheon to meet their rescuers. "Survivors Day" brings a surprising number of patients, their families and the responders together to celebrate life!

Introduced to the paramedics, firefighters, police and dispatchers that came together as a team to care for them, patients often get very emotional. Pictures are taken, hugs and handshakes exchanged. Tears are often shed by patients and responders alike. The ages of the survivors range from their teens on up.

While focusing on the survivors, responders often report the event heals them as well. What began as someone's last day has become a turnaround for more than just the patients.

Families are relieved to meet their loved one's rescuers. The event helps close the loop since most missed the life-changing incident.

Some responders leave the celebration to return to their shifts within the hour. Remember; see a paramedic; thank a paramedic!

6

Strictly Crashes Act I

What is it that fuels our innate fascination with accidents and the resulting carnage? Curiosity has earned its place in my heart as the sixth human sense. The peculiar faculty explains away morbidly inquisitive spectators at boxing matches and car races. A lot of ticketholders are not there to see a winner. Many onlookers attend the event anticipating blood and guts.

Passers-by, any accident or incident are referred to by the police as "rubberneckers." They slow to a crawl to take in the sights. Sometimes causing secondary collisions, the gawkers hate to miss a detail. Modern-day observers bring out camera phones, snapping pictures and videos of responders working at a scene. Amateurs post images on social media and media outlets, all before you can say tow truck.

We often watch the news to see and hear the details of that crash we passed earlier, including the casualty count. All bets will be taken that it is impossible to find a paramedic that has not been asked, "what's the worst accident you have ever seen?"

Each emergency group seeks answers to a battery of questions during their initial size up at a collision. Medics assess the speed involved and look for deployed airbags. From the position they find the victims, determine; was anyone ejected from the vehicle? Police probe for; did you smell alcohol on the driver's breath, was there a cell phone near the driver, which victim did you see behind the wheel? Firefighters focus on the presence of trapped victims, flammable fluids or electrical wires on the ground or near the vehicles.

Responders are good at painting the picture of crash scenes after the fact. Using their senses recalling the features, the specifics will be graphic. Depending on the severity of the incident, some items become etched in memory. The lingering thoughts are a testimonial to the stress shouldered by emergency workers.

Drawing on the five basic senses, seasoned responders recall unusual incidents. The facts as they relate them tend to be specific to their profession. All bets are off once you ask the question. Be careful what you ask. The cat will be out of the bag, as dad used to say.

Professionals arrive quickly and observe victims in a broad range of conditions and injuries. Some are dead, sometimes dismembered. Who do you think covers them up? Late arrivers or observers, fortunately, miss the bloodbath, only seeing blankets covering the departed.

Sounds fill the air around a scene, with victims expressing their pain and other approaching emergency responder's sirens. The noise of metal giving way to a straining hydraulic rescue tool. A droning gas-powered generator providing light at a darkened scene. Sounds overlap, adding to an emergency worker's mental and sometimes emotional record. Responders talk aloud to coordinate their efforts in a dynamic environment. Communications are often vivid to enable exact intentions.

You would think that taste would be limited to food. Responders get to experience the grittiness or taste of talcum powder lingering around the interior of a vehicle following airbag deployment. Sulphuric acid and hydrogen sulphide are responsible for that rotten egg taste. Often the result of a smashed battery, the flavour sticks in the back of your throat.

The odour of gasoline sends fear into responders committed to working within arms reach of injured and trapped victims. Most would never consider leaving until the patient is freed, packaged and on the medic's stretcher. Exposed human tissue, especially in a wet environment or when burned, leaves an olfactory marker. When others walk away, paramedics and firefighters tough it out.

Finally, the feel of an injured extremity as you support it, helping a flailing victim into an awaiting splint. Holding a patient's head with blood-soaked hair during a rescue while hiding under a heavy rescue blanket to avoid metal shards or flying glass. Your knee on a car seat as windshield glass shreds uniform pants leaving your blood on the victim's already blood-stained car. Responders take their licks.

In four decades, crashes have come in all forms; cars, trucks, bicycles, motorcycles even helicopters. They have been on our streets, roads, off-road, in fields, creeks and airports. Some incidents are dramatic; others have brought an accompanying "why would you do that" moment.

Some calls left me wondering; why do people at the scene say the things they say. Not every poor choice is alcohol-related, though there have been a few. Sometimes there are genuine "accidents." However, there are so many preventable incidents, it begs the question: Will people ever learn?

After the scene is cleared, notes are compared. Most seasoned responders return to their stations, and with a minimum of interruption from their recent experience, be able to eat a meal or snack. Senses are put to rest; it is time to recoil. To ready yourself for your next response. You tell yourself; it was just a call.

A fatal head-on crash was my initiation on the second shift following two weeks of initial training. No paramedic is guaranteed a gentle start to this profession.

Trapped

Serving as a volunteer firefighter for years, you are outside the car most of the time. While medics toil inside to assess, treat and immobilize injured victims, the fire folks open the crumpled wrecks and prevent a fire from starting for everyone's safety. Sometimes my boundary lines were blurred. In the early days, ambulances carried light rescue and extrication equipment.

Starting in the ambulance business, I tried to wear both hats. It wasn't always pretty. A London crew responded to the highway for a transport collision resulting in a driver trapped in his cab. The eighteen-wheeler rolled over a small car, killing one of the occupants.

Excited drivers deserted their trucks and cars to assist the injured victims. The highway was unofficially closed in seconds. A Provincial commercial vehicle weigh scale station nearby made the call for responders. Years before cell phones streamed along the route, drivers used citizen's band radios or "drove for help."

Two closer ambulances, including one from an adjoining county, initially responded. Following a brief assessment, one patient in the car was rescued, the second was presumed deceased. Some refer to it as DRT (dead right there). In addition to an obviously fatal injury, the patient was hopelessly scrunched inside the now "super" sub-compact auto.

Covered by police with yellow blankets, the car was left on the roadway abandoned for a higher priority. There was nothing more to be done at the time. Following the incident, the vehicle would be moved to an enclosed facility where it was painstakingly dismantled to release the victim.

As devastating as the loss was, the focus changed to the trapped truck driver. This stretch of the highway did not have fire coverage with rescue capability. As luck would have it, my community's volunteer squad was the closest rescue available and responded.

The driver was trapped by two obstructions; first, the mangled cab was bent around his lower legs and chest. The aluminum rig collapsed, enveloping him like an oversized ball of tinfoil. Unfortunately, the remaining cab did not protect him from the second hazard.

The tractor-trailer combination was hauling an extended aluminum dump trailer filled with granular fertilizer. Losing control after blowing a front tire on the cab, the rig rolled, crushing the car. The impact sent the truck and trailer rolling over again, onto its passenger's side.

With the weight and speed behind the transport, it slid down into a steep ditch next to a concrete culvert. The second threat to our patient was imposed by tons of tiny grains of this agricultural product released by the impact and rollover.

Back at our office in downtown London, the action attracted me from an inviting lounge chair. I stood next to the dispatch console with a cup of coffee in hand as the scene unfolded. Our radio scanner chirped out the request for Lambeth Rescue. At work, I was paralyzed; I had the ambulance hat on. Disappointed at missing the action, be careful what you ask for.

The first crew on the scene, in a unique move, asked to speak to a doctor on the Provincial common radio channel. It was a one-time request that would not be necessary today. Paramedics are trained with skill sets to cope with extended times at the scene. Today, rescue crews are better educated and equipped to attack the metal and plastic that entangle victims at crash sites.

Listening to a familiar voice on the hospital end, the crew painted the picture of the deceased victim that was a matter of fact. It was the opener for a heartfelt request for a physician to attend the scene. Describing a male trapped in his cab, the injuries could not be confirmed. The cab was repeatedly being filled with moving particulate. Crews were expecting rescue on the scene shortly.

In a casual response, the doctor advised the request could not have come at a better time. It was approaching a shift change in the department. One of the day shift doctors and a nurse could be sent to the scene. Advising they would be several minutes packing for the extraordinary appeal, they asked how they would get to the location.

The call attracted the attention of our Operations and Communications supervisor. Standing next to me, Donald laughed as I shifted from foot to foot, itching to go to the scene with the rescue crew. He knew how keen I was to get into the fray.

Dan, my partner for the shift, stuck his head in the door. Hearing all the hubbub, he was curious to see what Donald would do with the request. The suspense was squelched in an instant. Donald turned, laughing and pointed to the door.

Tapping the transmit button across from me, Jimmy parted the airwaves to respond that a crew would pick them up in a few minutes. The assignment; pick up the doc and nurse and transport them from the downtown ER to the scene. The severity of the incident cried out for a helicopter medivac scene response. It was years too early for trauma hawks in our region.

Arriving at the emergency room doors, a doctor and nurse in their scrubs carrying a plastic box stood anxiously awaiting our arrival. A couple of faces behind the glass separating the department from the ramp emphasized the department's reaction to the unusual request. The downside to the mission; both hospital staffers were underdressed for the call, including their footwear. Oh well!

There were questions on the way out to the highway; we did not have all the details, just crew reports. The drive was not unusual for the doc and nurse. Our guests regularly escorted patients on high-priority transfers. They were excited at the prospect of going to a scene and volunteered.

Advising that other ER staff passed on the adventure, I was hoping there were no surprises. Helpful as specialized caregivers, they lacked the everyday situational awareness that experienced responders take for granted. Our added task now was to watch out for our angels of mercy. All eyes would be on the staff, looking like a couple of fish out of water.

Police re-routing vehicles around the incident received a warning. They were expecting our arrival and knew its purpose. A waiting cruiser ran ahead of us along the highway's shoulder to get frustrated drivers out of our path. It was slow going on the soft gravel. Stranded drivers stood on the roadway in small groups talking, smoking, sharing their frustrations with the inconvenience. Leaving our sirens on continuously helped.

Stopping on a slightly wider area on the gravel shoulder, Dan warned our helpers to watch their step. The ground dropped off to a nasty grass-covered ditch a couple of feet away. The thought of a doctor in scrubs and a nurse in an old "hoover" style ER wrap around one-piece dress doing the "rag doll" down an embankment would spoil the moment.

We were still a hundred feet from the mess. Approaching, you could see a car cocked crookedly on the roadway. Surrounding the vehicle in a protective cloak, two ambulances and as many police cruisers. The thin slits between the lowered roofline, doors and rear windshield opening revealed yellow plastic emergency blankets covering a victim.

Volunteer firefighters in a pumper approached from the now-closed side of the incident. Driving the wrong way down the un-obstructed lanes, they enjoyed a clear path to the scene. They were used to highway runs.

Spread over the lined highway were car and truck parts. The trail stretched from the first impact, shunting the metal coffin ahead to where the shuddering truck crushed it during its rolling evolution. Passing the wreck, the hulk of a vehicle sailed onto the awaiting shoulder and partially down the hill.

Starting behind the car wreckage and showering, the aggressor's route in the collision was a broken, then widening stream of granular fertilizer. The once agricultural product was now a hazardous material. Spread around the scene, it was nearly impossible to approach the truck without crossing the ankle-deep grit.

In the day, most medics wore a version of a military boot; police wore the same. Our hospital-bound staff walked the last few feet through the powdery product, bits now trapped in their institutional footwear. Distracted from the contamination, it would only be the beginning for our guests.

Climbing down the hill, it was easier to see into the cab through the missing windshield. The glass was long gone; the void left behind allowed rescuers to reach into the cab. Ahead was a familiar voice, a quick "Brad" validated recognition of the back of the medic's head.

The accident and rescue were now active for over one hour. Compounding the problem, it was cold today, then the rain began to fall. A brisk wind on the highway made it worse for responders away from the truck; we were sheltered. There were many helping hands for the doctor and nurse making their way down the hill from a couple of truck drivers and firefighters behind me. Dust and diesel ruined their shoes.

The fertilizer spilling into the cab had already been cleaned out at least once. Rescuers cleared the way for the patient's head to remain above the dusty granules. A truck tarp being held outside acted as a dam preventing fertilizer from overtaking the space again. The driver's face expressed a grimace that spelled "get me out."

Part of the initial rescue was to stop the flow of powdered nitrates. Compounding the problem now was a small rupture in the saddle tank holding gallons of diesel fuel. Some leaked and mixed with the fertilizer. Shovelled away by firefighters, it posed no immediate threat.

Years later, in Oklahoma, the world would see deadly results when the two products are combined and detonated.

Getting a report from Brad, the doctor could only get to the victim's chest and arms. He was trapped from the waist down by the wheel and dash of the cab. Initially, it was difficult to see the trucker from his belly down. Fertilizer kept coming from everywhere. Fortunately, the critical end of the patient was above the powder.

A gauze dressing covered the nasty laceration across his forehead; the driver was amazingly calm. I would find out the calmness was a disguise. Medics learn never to take things at face value.

Thinking he might have to do a field amputation of a limb, the doctor came prepared. I could see instruments as the nurse opened the plastic toolbox, carried by a police officer as if made of gold. The doc backed out for the moment, deferring to the nurse.

The ER nurse was covered to her shins standing next to the truck when she announced she needed to keep the trucker motionless to start an intravenous line. Attaching the line to the bag and then priming it with the fluid, I handed it to a nearby truck driver. Our nurse leaned into the cab to poke the vein on the back of the driver's hand. The IV started as if she was in a well-lit room in the ER.

The hospital crew stood a few feet back to witness the victim's release, handing off patient care to the rescuers. The doc was concerned that he might have internal injuries. A large steering wheel still pressed against the trucker's belly.

Stuff flew around the cab in the rollover. A sleeping bag came forward and propped the driver up. It was as if he was still behind the wheel in the hopeless attempt to regain the long-lost control of his rig. Like someone was whispering in my ear, I heard a singular voice and a couple of taps.

Less than politely, I shouted, "shut up!" Earning several startled looks, I turned to the driver and asked if he had been alone on the trip or was he doing a team run with another driver. Behind the driver was a sleeper cabin mangled from the crash, slightly smaller inside but there.

It was like a time delay. A puzzled look came over the man's face; the area was silent now except for the tapping. "My nephew" was all he could muster, the disguised calmness making perfect sense now. Turning to one of the captains from our rescue unit, I announced we had a victim in the sleeper, possibly a kid.

Where the hell did he come from? Was he sleeping in the back when the accident happened or thrown back there in all the commotion? The rescuer's calls to the voice got an undeniable response; this kid was wide awake and scared. That's always a good sign. There were two rescues in play now, the second emergency taking almost an hour and a half to get off the ground.

In our area, the fire fighting world was just coming of age with their assignment to rescue accident victims. Most departments, including our squad, were still working with hand tools and some air-powered shears. The good old abrasive saw that spat out a shower of sparks as it cut metal was on its way out. Keeping the sparks from flammable substances was difficult and distracting.

The driver was in a confined space. Making my way to the cab was not a problem. Butting in was an exception. The initial ambulance crew remained in place with the patient until the rescue crew decided to cut the wheel away from him. Ideally, the move would offer enough space to drag the victim, shoulders first, free of the cab.

When our rescue crew stepped up, the saw was offered to me. The captain thought I could also keep an eye on our patient while cutting. I jumped in at the chance. We did not have a powered hack saw yet; it was an old arm strong hand saw.

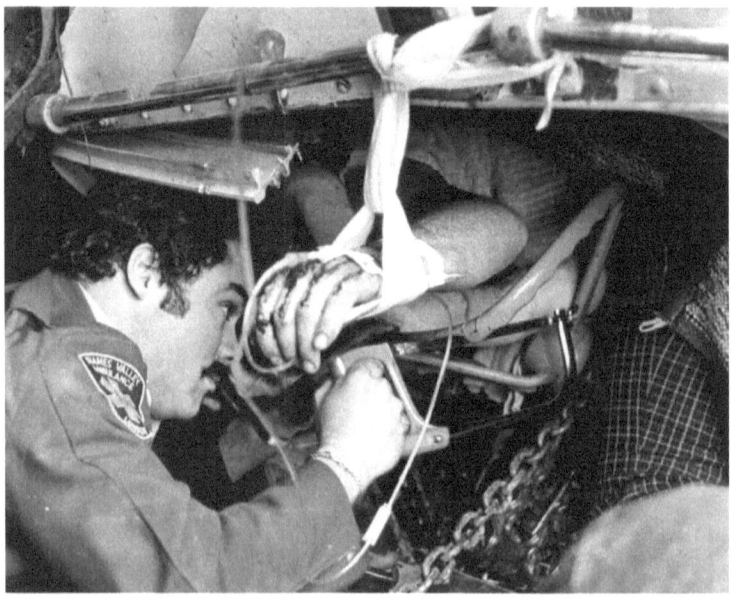

I could hear the air chisel above me and behind my head now. The rattling on the aluminum, cutting into the sleeper compartment, was like a deafening drum beat. Stopping to make sure the kid was lying down away from the sharp chisel, the pauses were not long enough to recover and appreciate the silence.

Cutting the steel steering wheel in two places did not release the fellow. It gave him some breathing space to lean towards the dash and away from the seat pushing at his back. The driver complained of back pain now. Hearing the symptom, the doctor dove in hands first and had a second look at our patient. The mandate was repeated that we needed to get the fellow out, and soon.

It had been nearly three hours since the crash occurred; the patient was cold. Wrapped in a blanket like a shawl was not keeping up with his core temperature loss. The shivering was the cold, and pain was from all the jiggling caused by the rescue.

Finally, the crews outside cheered, signalling the young fellow was out. I could hear the hubbub as he was being carried out of the ditch. He wound up being transported as a precaution, a good move, considering the scene around us. Seeing his uncle now would push a bad experience over the top.

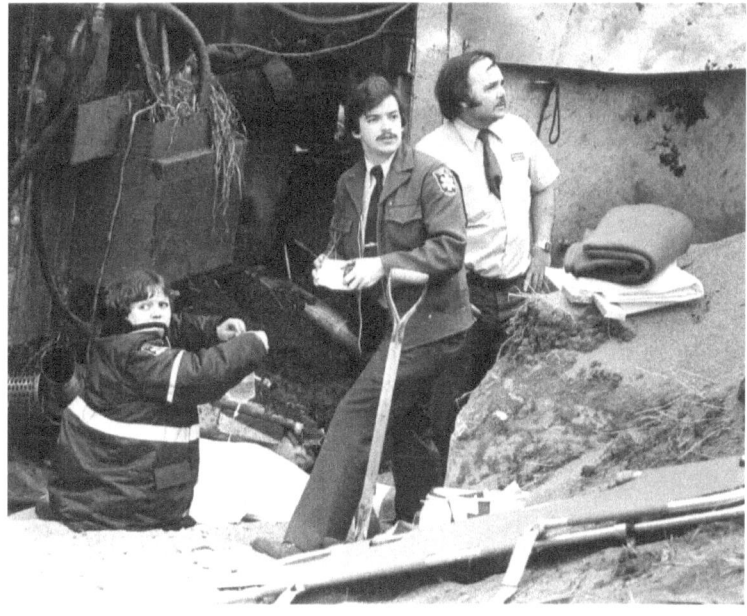

Another firefighter from our squad, a new guy to me, was able to burrow down through the fertilizer around the victim's lower body. Headfirst into the cab without his heavy coat, the firefighter found the driver's feet. His heavy insulated boots were stuck under large brake and clutch pedals.

With the victim's feet still trapped, we could see an opportunity to take a shortcut. The heavy boots were the linchpin to his entrapment now. I had cut one of the three arms out of the steering column. Our driver could lean to the side when his feet were free.

Sliding in headfirst to finish pulling the section out of the steering wheel, the volunteer retreated. That got me within reach of the victim's boot laces. It took minutes, working upside down and with one hand. Even our handy dandy paramedic shears were too wide to get under the laces.

Unlacing the boots and enlisting some help, rescuers pulled the man out from behind the wheel. Our fella was disconnected from the truck. The steering wheel's missing part made some space, allowing a wooden backboard to be pushed up against the patient.

Sliding the man out on his belly wasn't pretty, but he was clear now. About to roll him over onto his back, the doctor interrupted and suggested leaving him as is for the ride. It was a sight to see our driver hours after the fact lying on the stretcher, clear of the truck and load.

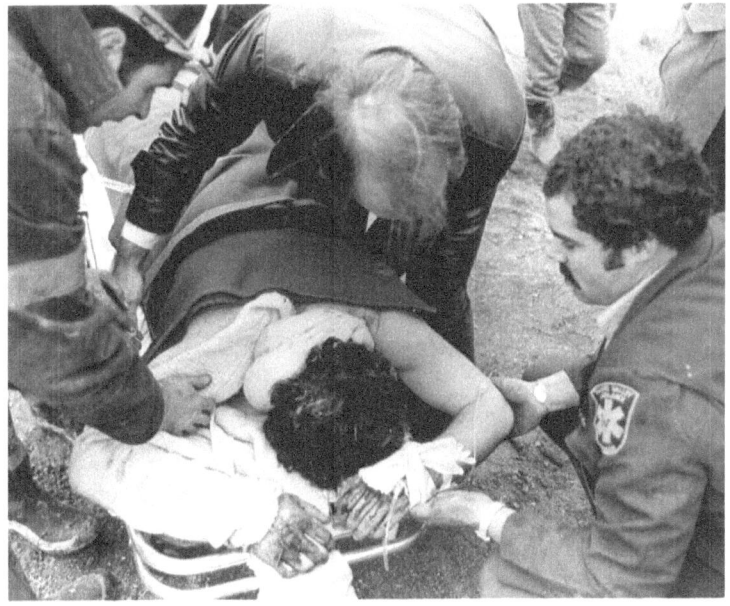

The rest of the call was routine; we did not transport. The doc and nurse rode in the other ambulance with the patient. The kid made it to the ER ahead of him, an hour earlier, where they were reunited. We cleared the scene and returned to the office. Diesel fuel and fertilizer dust behind us on the highway, we were finished for our shift.

Crush That Bug

Did you ever see the cartoon from the circus show where the small car pulls into the middle ring? Clowns just keep climbing out. When will they stop? How many are in the car? So, imagine a VW beetle full of kids smelling of alcohol trapped up against a tree. Well, some smelled of alcohol. The space was so small you couldn't tell which did and which didn't.

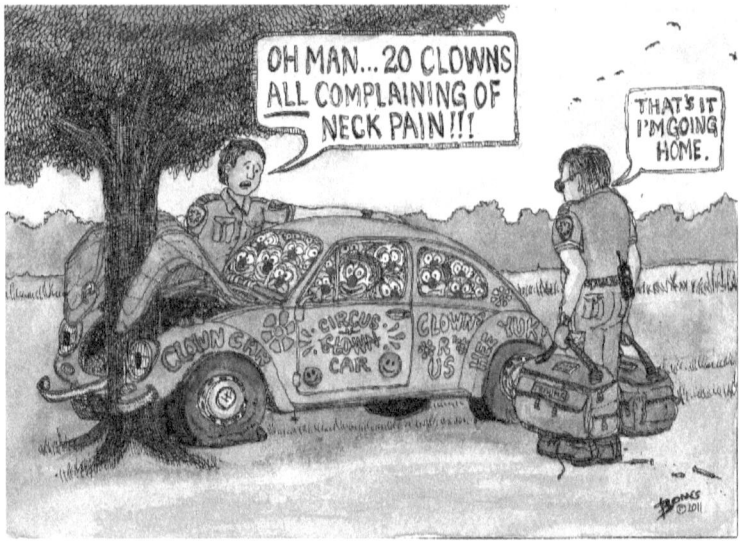

Credit: Chris "Bones" Skelton

Arriving at a single-vehicle accident in the day, there was no backup. One vehicle involved, one ambulance responded until you called for help. There was also no fire rescue response until you called. Ahhh, progress, Fire/Rescue and a second ambulance are a regular routine now. Hugh made the call tonight.

Arriving to see a car head-on against a tree was not a first. Seeing eight more hands waving through the windows and screaming for help past the driver's left arm waving out his window was a surprise and a first. Five kids stuck inside; everyone had similar injuries.

Thrust forward with the impact and sudden stop, the front seat occupants were crushed. The situation was compounded by the backseat passengers flying ahead against the seatbacks. Knees first into the unpadded metal dash, both front seat occupants dislocated a hip joint strained beyond its limit.

Three rear-seat riders slid into and started under the front seats; two had dislocated hips. Separate left and right legs against the outside of the car went around the obstructions ahead of them. The victim's other knees stopped abruptly, hitting each seatback.

The center rear seat passenger straddled the hump in the floor. Riding with a foot under each seat, she fractured a single shin. Her one outstretched leg could not bend backwards. The bone collapsed when it could not yield and slid under the older vehicle's exposed tubular metal seat frame.

The early sixties bug was not equipped with seat belts. Hugh and I witnessed a miracle that there were no dead kids in this; tiny steel egg-shaped horseless carriage, pending coffin. Smashing the "trunk" end of the car into the tree, a "U" shaped hollow made its way almost to the dash.

Calling for more help took seconds. Getting the two remaining ambulances on night shift to the same crash, leaving the city with zero units, took minutes and minutes. It was quiet and lonely out there.

The silence was broken with moans and shrieks from the trapped teens. Leaving the kids in the car turned out to be our best bet. Keeping a patient with a dislocated hip as still as possible until it was time to package and transport deferred the pain and held it to a minimum.

The four outside victims were screaming to get out. The patient's legs were all at an angle, spread apart when the thigh bone exited its socket in the pelvis. A sure sign the actual discomfort had not started yet. Some noise started when I went to open the door. Bound shut, the impact into the tree temporarily fastened the driver's door.

Our first reinforcements to arrive was a crew with some experience. Rob and Mike were clearing St. Joseph's and closer than the car at the office. It was as fascinating to watch my coworkers as the victims. Inaudibly asking the same question we did minutes ago, I yelled out "five" to Mike as he approached, carrying the tin first aid kit and oxygen bag.

We were at a standstill until fire arrived to help with an extrication. Rolling up behind Rob as he parked behind us was Engine 8 from Western Road. First, on the scene from the fire department, there was no friendly exchange between services. Tensions were up and down between the ambulance and the fire service in the day.

The pumper crew had a few hand tools and water at their disposal. Firefighters spent the initial minutes on their "size up," a necessary step to direct the rescue crew, still rushing to the scene. At least there was water available, less risk if a fire started from leaking gasoline. I couldn't smell any yet.

Arriving together, Tommy, our supervisor and Leon, came from our downtown office, arriving just behind the rescue unit. The shiny new yellow box-style truck was the pride of their fleet. It must have pissed off the fire guys to be chased by a Suburban SUV ambulance.

Reaching into the passenger's door, the front passenger was gently lifted out of the car and placed on a backboard. Six hands from medics kept the misplaced hip joint as still as possible. A neck collar was taped around the male patient's large neck during his assessment before the lift. Even without neck pain, with this impact, everyone got collars tonight.

Small movements caused the victim's dislocated thigh bone to rub against his pelvis. There was no pain control in the middle of the night at this scene. Screams startled the other intoxicated and injured friends; it started all over again. The temporary calm was interrupted before starting to immobilize the remaining patients, one down four to go.

Setting up beside the car, the rescuers brought their tools up to the mangled vehicle. Having heard the "size up" from the first captain on the scene, the job sounded easy. Open the driver's door and remove both seats after the driver was safely out of the way.

The driver was the most seriously injured. With facial injuries from the steering wheel, he was also a candidate for abdominal and chest trauma. The semi-circular metal ring on the wheel for the horn was broken off, lying on the floor. The unpadded wheel was unforgiving to the patient with the impromptu stop.

Hugh started some oxygen on the driver through the window earlier. Unable to get him out, we were still in the assessment and first aid mode. The driver also got a pressure dressing applied to his forehead. We finished all the easy stuff. It was like the bases were loaded, and no one was able to hit. We were as stuck as the patients', though not trapped.

Hearing the gasoline engine start raised goosebumps on the back of my neck and arms. The "K12" rescue saw carried on the rescue unit pre-dated the "Jaws of Life."

Designed for releasing doors and removing the roof sections of cars after accidents, it had its place. Goosebumps should be reserved for loud air shows and meeting celebrities. The saw could also start fires.

It only took a couple of minutes to cut around the door skin and shear off the driver's door external hinges. The firefighter guarding the scene against a flash fire leaned in with the nozzle in his hands. Emitting a slow but steady stream, he was at the ready.

There was another scene where the saw scared the crap scared out of a couple of our medics. Cutting the door hinges at that accident, the shower of sparks leaving the side of the whirling blade hit their mark. Leaking gasoline ran under a thick blanket of snow next to the car. The explosion sent our ambulance crew into the ditch face first.

The plastic mattress on their ambulance stretcher was burned on the underside. It was the first place flames leapt to from the flaming gravel beneath. One medic had the coattails on his parka shrivel from the instant heat. The patient was not so lucky, already critically injured from the impact, inhalation burns to the lungs contributed to his death.

Everyone working the ambulance side is at a disadvantage. We wear polyester uniforms, a material that's sure to "shrink-wrap" us if a flash fire sparks to life. A fire never happened again to any of our medics, fingers crossed. The singular incident left a mark etched in our memories. For that reason, we are still slightly jealous of our comrade's fire-retardant coats.

Tonight, the door hung by its latch. It was a quick cut to release the rusty panel giving us access to the bleeding driver. Blessed with some screaming and an uninjured hand, he reached out to grab at ours. We quickly slid our victim onto the plywood board.

Hugh left me to tend to the patient back in the ambulance while returning to help Tommy with the next patient being released. I kept up the oxygen and had a better look at this fellow's hip in the light. We were in a holding pattern until the other patients were "packaged."

A few minutes later, Hugh returned. We had the worst patient in the group. Using their folding cots, the other crews were left to take two patients each. It was a task no one envied. Caring for two victims was distracting.

It was a short ride to London's newest emergency room. There was a sour note in the nurse's voice during the radio patch. News of receiving five patients, all suffering orthopedic injuries, was the warning from hell. No ER deserves all the patients.

Rules were rules, I reminded our greeter. In the day, the closest hospital got the patients; this was not a disaster. I should have kept my mouth shut. The "stink eye" from the nurse carried over for a couple of shifts. It was a couple of months before I could talk her into a date.

Suspended

Randy was a humorous fellow, always a chuckle, as he told a joke or purposely misused a word in a sentence. We enjoyed working together over the years. He had a tiny stature, something we all made jokes about. Working a Sunday night shift, we both thought it would be a good time for a "shut out," no calls. Starting at midnight, you would think everyone would be tucked in and readying themselves to return to the grind Monday morning. Nursing homes never close.

The dispatcher got two falls out of us from facilities on either side of our would-be station in the ER at St. Joseph's Hospital. The institution was surrounded by gold mines of potential patients in long-term care homes: the first emergency tonight, a fractured hip, the mainstay of every medic.

The second run was for a dislocated shoulder, not so typical. After the injury was treated, the ER would summon EMS to return the patients to their respective starting places if the findings were minor. In the day, we did low-priority transfers too. Do the math; two calls could multiply to four in a heartbeat.

Clearing our plate with no returns was the unfortunate result of positive findings for both elderly victims. Our station at the hospital had no bricks and mortar. We parked outside on the ramp and sat behind the ER's desk on stools trying to stay awake and look official.

Hard on the back, we tired of getting up in a brief fit of guilt to answer inquiries at the window. The questions were best suited for a nurse; we were bored. On a quiet night, the nurses sat in the office behind our stools, smoking cigarettes and knitting. That was healthcare in the seventies.

I would have walked to the coffee shop in pursuit of a hot drink, like a desert-bound soul looking for water. Randy could care less about coffee. It took the promise of a cold soft drink and a doughnut at my expense to get him to pick up the phone to call the dispatcher.

Telling Jimmie that we were going to; "get some air in a low tire" was a code for food or coffee pickup. Using an ambulance for non-ambulance purposes was a no-no, though we all used the lame excuse.

A few blocks away was a coffee shop, a budding Canadian icon. With a coffee, a can of pop and two glazed chocolate treats, I was out of the door in a flash. The less time spent in the parking lot reduced our chance of being reported by someone.

Sitting on the ramp back at the hospital, the radio was silent as we sipped on the drinks. A few laughs were the result of licking the sugar off our fingers. Still bored, the shift was heading to the midpoint when Jimmy belted out our car number.

"One-five-seven London." Randy had a slight case of nerves. He always acted startled, muttering "jeez" when our unit number was called out of the blue. This was no exception. I laughed as the clip for the radio microphone hesitated to release the speaker, delaying the response. "One-five-seven," the abrupt reply.

"One-five-seven, code four to Abram Street at Brixell Avenue. A single-vehicle MVC, a van into an abutment at the creek". "The caller passed the accident a few minutes ago on their way home but didn't stop." Of course, it was before cell phones.

Leaving the almost empty coffee on the ledge of the ramp, I jumped back into the rear of the ambulance. Randy was ready with the van shifted into drive. Another disgusted "jeez" roared through the window dividing the cab from the patient compartment. The old-style van provided no front seat for a passenger.

It was a short enough ride to the scene; the streets were quiet now, people finally retired for the night. The worst part of this section of Abram Street was the absence of streetlights. It went pitch black when you got a few blocks east of Adelaide. Good thing there were no deer in the city; it was more like a country road.

Sitting cockeyed on the south side of the street was an old sixties Dodge panel van. You remember the style where it looked like the driver was sitting over the wheels. The dark-coloured vehicle created a shadowy scene. Its lights were likely extinguished by a smashed battery under the hood.

As we approached, the truck's damage looked to be mainly from hitting the shin-high concrete wall. The barrier protected vehicles from falling off the edge of the road into a sometimes-dry creek bed. The stream came and went with rain and melting snow. Years later, it would be replaced with storm drains safely hidden below the roadway.

Exiting the ambulance's rear with the blue metal first aid kit in hand, I missed a minor detail. Some unexplained damage would soon change the odds of having a simple call. One of the rear doors in the van was bulging slightly. It looked like someone closed the door on a ladder, too long to fit in a painter's truck. Not so lucky tonight.

Closer now, the thought crossed my mind that the van struck, then rode over the end of the wall. Ending up on an angle, the cab stuck out above the creek. It had not toppled to the ground below yet, though the driver's door and front wheels were hanging in mid-air. You could see the marshy ground, almost five feet under the door.

I wondered, approaching the driver's door, would I find the quiet vehicle empty? The result of an impaired driver's misadventure, maybe an abandoned stolen vehicle? That was until I climbed onto the concrete pier then leaned out to the door a couple of feet ahead. A bloodied hand was weaving red streaks back and forth across the closed window in a waving motion.

Sitting in the seat, the man was groaning, his distress muffled. Opening the door when he did not respond to my request, the sight inside was ghastly, a first for me. Looking in at the driver, my gaze panned past the fellow's face. Both hands were bloodied, grasping the steering wheel in pain. The blood was drying.

Looking down at his legs, one was partially hidden by a dark pipe. My cheap flashlight caught the green metal tube starting at the floor, turning under his right arm and passing behind him. For a moment, I thought it was thrown forward in the crash, narrowly missing his torso.

The engine in the sixties vintage truck stuck up between the front seats, looking past the driver's seat. Covered in a metal cowling with a lip around the top, it was an ideal place for a coffee. The truck was a beater; the interior was worn and dirty. Was he a welder with some steel tubing in the back on the way home from a job?

Asking where he was hurt, I was the recipient of a frustrated expletive. When the fellow sat back briefly in his seat, it was not to show me the injury. He was pushing back with his one good leg, a response to some incredible pain.

His right leg lay next to the engine cowl. The denim pants were torn away. A little bit late, the light bulb came on in my head. The van hit the end of the abutment. Sticking out of the concrete was a tubular guard rail made of steel.

The tube pierced the floor, missing his foot on the gas pedal. Passing between the guy's legs under his right arm, the steel continued through to the back. Peering into the rear of the van over his left shoulder, my small light barely reached the doors. The weak orange beam revealed the reason for the bulging door.

Our victim was flying when he hit the concrete. I noticed the oily smoke now. The engine took a hit when the oil pan rode over the concrete wall. Pushed against the rear of the van was a thick green pipe.

Randy's voice spooked me; standing on the road, he climbed onto the short concrete wall and used my back as a steadying point to try to look around at our patient. Without a thought, I yelled, "fuck, Randy, don't push me in." Where did that come from? Great way to address a seriously injured patient.

Using my left hand with the light to hold the door open, I had the other braced on the side of the van to avoid a fall. It was a near miss. I pushed to get my weight back over my feet.

The plunge would have placed me neck-deep in the stream bed and mud. That's when I caught a glimpse of the driver's right leg. Aiming the light again at the hole in the jeans, it was a bloody mess.

The patient's right thigh bone, the femur, was exposed and obviously broken. The inside portion of his leg was torn apart from the pipe passing by. The force split the tissue and muscle wide open.

Looking more like a piece of red meat glistening at a butcher's counter, the bleeding was incredible. Smaller nutrient arteries fed the muscle; no blood was spraying about. He was in luck tonight; the largest vessel in the leg, the femoral artery, had been spared by the transiting pipe.

If the femoral was lacerated, gushing blood could have easily hit the ceiling. Leaning forward to get a better look, the van rocked forward. Our victim cursed again. I could not detect alcohol on his breath. That was a plus though there might be less pain with a couple under his belt.

Asking Randy to open the kit and get me all the large dressings. A hand passed under my right arm with four paper packages. Despite his angry outbursts, our patient was up for helping himself when I asked.

Opening the large cotton dressings, I made them into a bulky four-ply bandage. Telling him to push the cotton into the centre of the wound, he quickly helped himself. Another expletive erupted from the victim.

It became obvious. We could not get the victim out of the van ourselves. We also couldn't wait for help to start. Sending Randy back to call for rescue, I reached out and placed my hand on the patient's arm.

Speaking to the man calmly, I asked him to hold on while we secured the truck. I felt terrible leaving the victim in the van alone, but we needed some insurance that we wouldn't get banged up in the process of helping him.

Returning to the ambulance, I hopped into the back and opened the crew bench. Stored under the attendant's seat were some hand tools, splints and light-duty rescue equipment. Coiled up in a corner was a piece of old sisal rope. It took a few seconds to untangle. Throwing it out ahead of me on the road made it easier to find the snags.

Yelling at Randy now, he rolled his window down. Asking him to line the ambulance up with the van and park ten feet behind left my partner in the dark in the planning department. He probably thought the headlights would help when we took the patient out.

I don't think Randy expected me to throw myself onto the ground in front of his front left wheel. Parking the ambulance, he jumped out and asked, "what the dickens are you doing?" Explaining that I was tying the ambulance to the van to steady it, went over his head.

After tying the rope to our vehicle, I jumped up, grabbing the other end and shimmied under the rear of the rocking van. Without the line, the engine's weight plus the two of us up front hanging over the wall would have the rear axle bouncing.

Our weight in the van's cab helping the patient could send it nose-first several feet down into the weeds. The rope stretched around the axle twice. With a few knots for good measure, there were no Boy Scout manoeuvres here!

In disbelief when I asked, Randy put the ambulance into reverse to tighten up the rope between the vehicles. It still might rock a bit but would not fall into the ditch below. I could hear the Colborne Street pumper crew's siren in the distance but no police; where the heck were they?

Randy was the lottery winner. He was smaller and lighter, but it didn't take a short straw to drive my point home. The green tube's jagged end met us when the bulging door popped open on the first try. Randy climbed into the van through the rear doors. His job was to see how we could get our victim out of the driver's seat and onto a backboard.

Squatting just inside the rear doors, there were boxes and bags to shove out of the way to make room. Posing as a two-hundred-pound counterweight, the cheesy flashlight now in my right hand shone past Randy towards the groaning driver. The floor of the van was littered with junk. It was not the tradesman's mobile workshop that I envisioned.

A bloodied left hand waved over the victim's right shoulder as if to reach for help to escape. Giving him something to do, I reminded him to keep both hands on the bulky bandage on his gaping leg wound to stop the bleeding. The hand retreated with another groan. Engine 4 rolled up, steering around our van to leave room for the approaching rescue.

Yelling the plan ahead to Randy, I returned to our truck and loaded a backboard along with a neck collar and a splint on the stretcher. An eager firefighter struggled to help lower the stretcher from the ambulance, unfamiliar with the contraption. Looking to my right, the yellow rescue unit was coming straight at me. In the middle of the night, its siren grinding out its advance. We could use the help right about now.

Randy stood behind the seat, holding up our victim. Leaning to the side, he was on one foot behind the driver's left shoulder. I asked if the van's seat could be moved backwards? Randy and I stopped moving. I made it to the rear of the driver's seat when we felt the rear wheels coming off the ground. This was a reminder to push the plate away and lose a couple. It wouldn't tip, just rock in place with the sisal tether.

From the rear doors, an authoritative voice piped up. A red helmeted captain from the rescue spoke up, asking what his crew could do. I pointed out we needed to keep the van from rocking while we removed the victim.

The captain probably laughed at the amateurish attempt to secure the van. It's not like it was going to plunge down a hillside and burst into flames. That's movie lore.

Leaning against the rear of the front seat, I could see a simple metal frame with a small backrest. Our volunteers practiced some rescue techniques with a similar vehicle behind our fire hall during training. We could work around that. Hearing a few voices outside the back door, I asked if the rear wheels were off the ground. A "no, we're tying the truck off too, go slowly" drifted in.

I leaned over the patient's right shoulder, flashlight in hand. Following the beam of light to his leg, the dressing was soaked. Reminding him again to press on the wound, he was entirely aware of the situation, now crying to climb out under his own power. Our victim was several months and some surgeries away from using the injured leg again.

A firefighter behind me asked again what we needed, finally, lots of helping hands. I asked for more bulky dressings and the yellow splint on the stretcher. Seconds later, the canvas splint and bandages were poked at my back.

The firefighter behind me let me know his friends were not sitting on the threshold at the rear doors, taking a break. They were a counterweight. The whispered thank you was an underpayment for our appreciation at the moment.

Leaning around the patient, I hung the flashlight's handle on the gear selector and braced it, so a narrow beam of light pointed at the bloodied leg. Placing the splint on the engine cover to my right, I opened several dressings, positioning them over the driver's hands. The quiet command to pull his hands off the bloodied bandage and replace them over the fresh gauze worked.

Congratulations, I was now the second bloodiest person at the scene, though not in pain. This mishap was before medics were graced with the protective gloves you see them wearing today. Barehanded I reached down to see how far the gaping wound extended. Through torn pants, the back of our patient's knee looked intact.

The jeans gave way around the bulky sopping bandages using bandage scissors, providing a better look at what had to be splinted. The van jiggled as the rear wheels went light from our weight. Firefighters shifted as they secured the vehicle. We were safe now; no one was going to let us go into the creek.

The leg suffered an obvious fracture that needed support; shattered white bone ends were partly covered by tissue and fresh blood. The limb had to be splinted before we moved the patient. There was no room for the yellow canvas support ahead of the seat.

Reaching past the fellow down beside the engine, cowling to release the seat, finding the small lever on the seat's frame was challenging. Warning our victim it might hurt, the caution was an understatement. He was all in for anything that would get him out of his predicament.

The vinyl upholstered driver's seat was overflowing in blood. Cold and exposed to the open air, the blood clotted into a dark red jelly, pooled between his legs dripping over the edge. The lever clicked, moving the seat rearward about four inches. The change brought out a bloodcurdling scream. Randy supported him by reaching under his arms.

Our yellow canvas splints were a local adaptation to an old military piece of kit. There were strips of wood sewn lengthwise into the canvas cover with a thick string across one end. The principle was to cradle the extremity, wrapping two-thirds of the way around.

Using the small hooks along the two parallel edges, you laced it closed like a shoe. The design was simple, but it worked, and you could throw it on the garage floor and clean it with car wash wax and bleach after the call. This was before the disposable age.

With each movement, the fractured thigh risked pinching the nearby artery sending our victims bleeding into overdrive. The long yellow splint wouldn't fit. There was the matter of a green steel tube in our way. The obstruction needed to be removed first.

Calling back to the crew behind us, they thought the guard rail was still attached to the concrete below the driver. I had the advantage of a ringside seat. This would take some finesse. The tubing appeared broken off with the motion of the van's undercarriage scraping along the concrete abutment. The van must have provided a wild ride to admit the tube through the floor, then past the driver keeping the final bend before settling down, trapping him.

The curved rail was hanging through a nasty hole in the floor to the left of the gas pedal. Wobbling, I trusted the tube could be lifted out and around the injured leg if it was free of the concrete below. We needed some karma to lift it clear and miss the wound.

Explaining to our friends what we needed, I turned to Randy, who whispered, "good luck with this one." He was still supporting the patient, who was now wincing from the pain. Moving the pipe was a gamble. More delays and a shower of sparks from a saw below wasn't my idea of a fun night on the road.

There were four hands at the ready behind me. With a slight resistance from the bent tubing on the floor and a hint to the rescuers to lift the other end, the pipe cleared the injured leg. Letting go, I heard it hit the road outside with a clang seconds later.

I was in for a clean-up after this one. Randy was covered in blood up to his elbows too. Reaching down with the opened splint, the right side of my chest pushed against the engine. My left shoulder was under the patient's right armpit against his side.

Getting the splint down to catch the patient's heel would have been a bonus. This wasn't even the correct splint for a femur fracture. The best substitute was something to support the splintered limb until we had some real space to work. The clock had been ticking for too long already.

With the heel of the victim's shoe hanging over the canvas's end, the splint's laces hit about half the hooks. Good enough for now. Calling over my shoulder, I asked for some help and our plywood backboard.

Moving over to the passenger's side of the cab now, my heels were off the floor as I stretched over the engine cowl from behind the seatback. The front of my light blue shirt was covered in a generous mix of blood, dust and grime from waist to neck.

Tying the bad leg to the good one with a couple of reliable triangular bandages supported the injury. Holding the legs and moving them over to the door to the left only worked when Randy, who was shorter than I, did his version of standing on his toes.

My back was hurting now, with one arm stretched under the steering wheel to support the splinted legs. Randy had to be running low on steam too. Happy for the help, the fire crew were on the mark, offering hands to take over the extrication.

Our firefighting rescuers pushed the foot end of the board onto the engine's cowl as Randy and I maneuvered the victim to the side of the seat. Telling the patient to stiffen his intact leg to help support the bad one was a good distraction, the diversion, stopping his screams after a couple of volleys.

My hands were slimy with jellied blood trapped on the seat as Randy and I slid our new friend bum first onto the board. The cowl provided the support we needed in our small workspace with all the junk and the crowd we had invited in for the event. With the patient safely on the board, the worst was past.

Randy handed off the top end of his patient to another set of waiting hands behind him. He was stuck behind the driver's seat and took the board's foot end for the final move out of the crowded vehicle.

The patient exited the rear doors as if levitating. Lots of hands kept our victim level. A missed step would have sent him off the board. Not a chance! On the stretcher, it took three straps to secure him, leg and all.

There was one snag left. Asking the fire crew to untie the rope, Randy shook his head as he announced, "someone tied our ambulance to the van." The comment drew a couple of quiet snickers.

The last laugh was on him. The rescue crew used the steel cable from their bumper-mounted winch to replace my rescue improvisation.

As I sat in the brightly lit ambulance, I realized my goosebumps responded to the heated air coming from the small fan on the floor. Our guy, happy to be out of his teetering plight, also welcomed the warmth. There was blood running out of the splint.

Finishing what medics refer to as their secondary survey, this fellow was lucky. Missing his torso, the jagged end of the tube ripped his nylon jacket on the way by his right side. Another hit to his belly or chest, in addition to the leg, would have changed everything. Most likely busy trying to steer out of the collision, the gap provided an escape route under his arm.

Our victim suffered a critical injury but weathered the insult and delay in releasing him from the van. Some oxygen to help his breathing went unnoticed; the moaning and screaming returned. Moving the splint's laces aside, I packed the last of our bulky dressings into the divot in his leg. It seemed the screaming was a reaction to the event; applying a third handful of pressure dressings did not elicit a scream this time.

The short drive to the ER was a blessing. There was no time to belabour the injury and answer his questions; "what happened" and "where was the accident." He remained conscious; there was no head injury here. There were likely a few nightmares slated for this fellow's future.

Leaving the trauma-resuscitation room after Randy and I slid the board onto the hospital gurney, we took stock of each other. Both covered in blood and grime, there was no hope of a simple cleanup. It took a drive to our homes in the middle of the night with the supervisor's blessing to do a quick change. Other than a graphic story to tell some sleepy medics back at the office after cleaning the ambulance, the rest of the night was a welcome shutout back up at St. Joseph's.

Don't Move

Did you ever look at someone as they blurted out something totally ridiculous and have your little voice beg to offer up, "if you could only see yourself now, buddy"? When you are the calm, sober observer and caregiver in these situations, the temptation is overwhelming. Having made some mistakes in my day, I held my innermost thoughts to myself tonight.

Responding to a rollover collision in a sixty-mile-per-hour zone, the possibilities for complex multi-system injuries are boundless. As Donny and I raced along to the scene, I enjoyed the "zoom." He was a driver through and through. Cautious but aggressive, my chauffeur tonight competed as a rally racer a few years back, placing in the Shell 4000. Oh, and throw in a decade-plus on the city fire department driving red rigs before ambulances.

Working this shift in a new Dodge van with an extended roof, you could stand to move around while doing patient care. I could also ride up front in the cab; the experience was still a novelty, finally, a purpose-built vehicle for EMS in our province.

The location for our call was commonplace for crashes. It was in the city but still offered the opportunity to do highway speeds. Donny revisited his last call on this stretch. He responded to the report of a motorcyclist that lost control, striking a steel roadside sign.

Arriving, the first thing he and his partner noticed was the contents of their patient's leather jacket. Spilling out onto the gravel shoulder were shards of brown glass beer bottles, the old "stubby" style for the beer historians out there. His last call was his last call.

Clipping the NO PARKING ON THE SHOULDER sign, it bent over, travelling between the biker's leg and the gas tank. The rectangular placard acted as a scalpel opening his thigh. It didn't sever the rider's leg; Donny still wonders why. The torn jeans left nothing to the observer's imagination that day. Something was missing.

Wincing, he offered an indifferent snicker. Donny described some pink tissue nearby. There, glistening on the gravel, freshly levelled by the passing rear wheel of the out-of-control motorcycle, were the rider's testicles.

A sad sight for anyone, frightening for others even if you could not identify the pink bits. Horrifying for the guys that responded that night. Phantom pain was shared or imagined by several at the roadside if Donny's recollection was any measure.

As we pulled up on the scene tonight, a badly damaged Ford Bronco sport utility vehicle sat upright in the distance. You remember the older boxy body styles. From our view, there was not a side or corner that missed the impact. It sat well beyond the gaggle of police and citizens as they stood guard over the patient.

Donny cocked the ambulance across both lanes, lights flashing. We were protected if anyone decided they would go around the two black cruisers. Their flashing lights marking the opposite edge of the scene down the road. People do stupid things.

Getting out of our ambulance, I was met by a nurse who stated she thought the patient suffered internal injuries. Thinking to myself, what are you chasing me for. Stay with the patient. First aiders can really help in an emergency. A lot of samaritans believe that reporting their findings is their reward for helping.

Staying with your patient is the priority; we will listen to you. Really. A good medic will take the helper's report, filtering out the irrelevant parts. A great paramedic will take the information at face value and not unnecessarily critique the volunteer's content. The public doesn't do this stuff for a living.

Although it might appear dismissive, the attending medic is mostly listening as they are taking over. The patient and responder benefit from voluntary help. Then the paramedic gets down to business, building a patient assessment and treatment plan. We don't always have time to thank first aiders, sorry.

The nurse was standing by for another assignment; she would get her chance. Our victim was lucky, relatively speaking. Ejected out through a whirling SUV window, he tumbled to a stop in the middle of the lane, coming to rest on the white hash marks. You could see the fellow trying to focus his eyes; he had been out for a while. Lots of lacerations earmarked him for the potential pointed out earlier by the first aider.

His extremities were surprisingly intact, torn clothing and bleeding but still in one piece. Starting at his head and neck, he was aware that we were there, he responded to my first question. "Where do you hurt?" "Fuck off" was not the response from a multi-system trauma patient that I was anticipating.

The puff of his exhaled breath that propelled the expletive told a story. One that I relayed to the constable standing a few feet away. "You smell the beer?" The simple nod of his black forage cap sporting the chrome police shield in the darkness was all I needed. The officer arrived before us and smelled the same evidence I did. With any luck, I might even avoid court!

Donny rolled up behind me with the stretcher, a backboard and collar. I had enough hands to carry the oxygen kit, first aid box and a flashlight for a start. Asking for the collar, I turned to our good Samaritan and told her we could use some help in a minute. That impressed her.

And it started. "Don't touch me, asshole," was the response to explaining that I would be placing a collar around the victim's neck. Offering to help him get to the hospital was obviously not good enough. The patient informed us that he would kick the crap out of us if we touched him again. It was time to level the playing field.

Having been with him for a few minutes, I had not seen a muscle move except his eyes and mouth. Touching both hands and feet during my assessment, pinching each, there was no response. I suspected a neck injury well up the spine. The interruption to his motor and sensory nerves might be temporary. I reasoned with the highway's speed and the scene around us; our victim was facing the worst.

Getting right down in his face, I intercepted the next blast of defensive bravado. Explaining that I would gladly help him up, I asked the patient to lift his hand up to shake mine as a peace treaty. Unable to offer his hand as a settlement to our disagreement, I directed him to move his other hand and, in turn, raise his legs. The silence was deafening.

It still was not clear enough for our victim. "Listen, I think your neck is broken; if you lay still and let us help, the injury won't get any worse." "If you try to move, it may be your last; lay still." Well, the tear ducts were working. There was no apology in response, but I am a big boy.

Placing the collar on tightly, it was time to use the volunteer again. Donny and the nurse took the patient's torso and feet while I stayed at the head and supported his neck. Just like the books tell you, we did our "one, two, three" count. Rolling the patient onto his side, the helpful police officer beside us slid the spinal board behind the fellow, now silent. I noticed that the back of his jeans were wet during the roll, adding to my suspicion of a head and neck injury.

The previously cursing fellow lay quietly on his back for the moment. Barely an inch off the road surface while we strapped him onto the ageing plywood board, the mood changed. Thanking the nurse and releasing her from her service, she looked pleased with the gratuity. It was time to get this fellow into the ER.

The drive to the hospital was quiet. I reached through the window to take the microphone for the radio patch to the nurse. Time and reality had their way with our victim. The alcohol's effects were driven away. Realizing our collective concern, the fellow's senses picked up on his unresponsive limbs.

A Message

Not every collision is catastrophic. Paramedics respond to various incidents, ranging from "fender benders" to long entrapments with injuries and fatalities. For the participants in an "accident," it can be the worst day of their lives; just ask them. Plans are interrupted; receiving injuries or seeing friends and loved ones in your car that are injured is unsettling.

In an urban service, some medics might see nearly one hundred collisions a year. The numbers are staggering over a career. When a friend pipes up with "I saw you at the accident the other day," you are expected to recall every detail to validate their rubbernecking version of the incident.

Unless it was a pink corvette upside down over a ruptured fire hydrant, many accidents blended together over the years. That is until someone brings up an irrefutable point. I was stopped in my tracks the other day when a woman recognized me in the hospital. Imagine this; I was the patient.

I was on the receiving side of the questions. "Do you work for the ambulance service?" I asked how she knew me since I was not in a uniform and drawing a complete blank. Offering up the fact that she had been a patient of mine almost twenty-five years ago, the incident escaped my memory. This lady reminded me she was the driver involved in a collision in her new car.

Assessing her at the scene of the accident, she reminded me she was very distraught. When she could not acknowledge a physical injury that was urgent, I turned to her emotional state. She was concerned about her friend beside her, but again there were no serious issues.

Getting to the heart of the matter, it was her badly damaged shiny new auto. The incident drove her to this state of frayed nerves, nearing tears. A thought that dad shared with me the day I got my driver's licence came to mind. I enjoyed the privilege of driving his car; the phrase privilege stuck with me.

Expressing it as a dad moment, she smiled as I spoke, "Curly, it's just a car. If you are ok, you know they built one a minute in a factory somewhere. They can always build another one." In the circumstance, these words calmed the anxious woman.

She reminded me that she has never forgotten the message and has used it since. So, have I. She thanked me for the care I gave, and when I shared the ongoing project of writing this story, she was more than happy to see it put to paper.

Wired

You think of physical danger in the public service when you hear of the police responding to violent calls, robberies and the like. Who thinks of a paramedic being at risk of violence when responding to an accident? I must attract folks who are underwhelmed by our service.

Responding to the report of a serious collision at dusk one summer evening, there was lots of time for Leon and me to talk on the way. Leon served in the military, and with my volunteer fire experience, we exchanged stories regularly. This evening was no exception.

With the report of a car in a ravine, talk of asking for rescue was bounced around. Back in the day, the provincial police often made it to the scene before the other emergency services. Our luck petered out on this call.

Waved over between several abandoned cars along the roadside, passers-by were frantic in their insistence that we go down into the ravine to help their friend. Fresh tracks through the grass on the road's shoulder pointed out the car's path before veering off into the void ahead.

It was easy to see why the "friends" did not go to their pal's assistance with all their enthusiasm. A car rested on its roof at the bottom of a steep slope. The wreck was challenging to see in the dwindling light.

Someone left the scene to go for help then returned. That side story was being shared behind me. Recounting how the police dispatcher was interested in knowing if the caller thought alcohol was involved, the call taker backed off before offending the caller. Good question, though.

With more pressing matters at hand, Leon and I came up with a game plan. It was not much of an arrangement; he would stay on the roadway and call for rescue. You know who was going down the hill. Did I get handed the short straw or what?

One thing in our favour, the responding rescue crew, were allies. Friends from the department in the community that I served were coming. It was a ten-minute drive. Who knew how long the police would be?

Taking a rope from the back of the ambulance, I tied off on the driver's side of the rear bumper and tossed the end over the bank. It was for safety only and to aid in the return to the roadway. Tying a neck collar around my arm, I could hear the patient calling from within the overturned vehicle below.

Equipment would have to be lowered to the car. There were not enough hands to carry everything down while using both hands on the rope.

The dust on the grass and loose dirt on the way down would pave the way to a uniform change later. Hearing the group above, more friends called down the incline. Where were they for their friend, trapped in the car? It was only thirty feet down.

Reaching a small dirt ledge, the car was just below me. Hailing the driver, there was a loud reply of "ok" when I called out to inquire. What looked like a simple rollover from above should have been fatal to the driver. The car flipped in mid-air, at least once. The sight of the fall and landing contradicted what I found when I reached the car.

Thrown into the ravine over the years by local agricultural enthusiasts were dozens of rolls of rusty brown farm fence and balls of barbed wire. Coming to rest well down the hill, who would have guessed their presence would save a life and threaten an ambulance attendant in a single moment.

Acting like a corroded airbag, the rolls compressed on impact. Trapped inside the inverted car was a young fellow who should have been pale from the fright alone if it weren't for the flying dust and rust coating him. Not much worse for wear, he was more intent on escaping than waiting for help. It was lucky his friends were around.

Checking on his condition at arm's reach, I peered through strands of old wire to make eye contact. This fellow was all out stoic. He was mad at the thought of being in a predicament. Explaining that I was waiting for help from firefighters, the tale unfolded.

Several friends were out for a lark this evening when someone suggested they go to a well-known stretch of straight road and have a race. Seems simple enough. That is until someone says the race was in reverse. The odds were remote that the contest would end well.

Luckily the wire thinned out as it rusted. The brown threads flattened when I stepped on them, bracing myself against the car. A fall into the mesh without the protection of a car around me would be nasty. I really don't like the sight of my own blood and could not recall the date of my last tetanus booster shot at the moment.

Standing on the old fencing, it compressed below the upper frame of the inverted door that opened with a stiff pull. A few springy strands returned when I swung the metal frame over them. Knee first on the upside-down cloth liner on the car's ceiling, I leaned in. Barbs of rusted wire snagged the lower end of my dusty pant legs.

With a small scream now, I had something to work with, a sore shoulder. Simple enough, the victim's collar bone poked up against skin when the fellow pulled his shirt back. The bone looked fractured; you didn't need an x-ray. From above came an edict that is clear to this day; "if he dies, you die." It wasn't Leon's voice.

Where the heck did that come from. Repeated, the threat sounded like several friends above were feeling guilty. Likely a combination of alcohol and the most featherbrained idea by young drivers in my career.

Calling out to Leon, I postponed the need for any other emergency equipment. A few triangular bandages would support our patient's arm taking his collar bone out of play. The dressing made of stiff cotton is also used for rigging a sling to cradle a fractured arm or wrist. In fact, a triangular bandage is the Jack of all trades in pre-hospital care.

The approaching siren was a welcome sound. Despite replying that their friend's injuries were minor, it provided no relief to the gang above. They heard him scream then call out again. The vocal group sounded convinced their friend would come out of the ditch in a body bag.

Leon's voice rose above the madding crowd to advise that my buddies had arrived. In a split second, he announced the triangulars were on their way down. Looking up, the faint fluttering of two near white, once folded dressings sailed through the darkened air. Landing a few feet above, I mustered a; "Thanks, Leon!" Some help.

Reaching further into the car, the victim had not taken the simple advice of "stay still." The victim righted himself and was sitting on the cloth roof liner above where his head had been earlier. Cradling the affected arm, he was silent.

The neck collar was a formality. This fellow was mobile and would have climbed out on his own if I moved out of the doorway. A quiet but firm warning to not climb out gave me the chance to slip the support around his neck. At best, it might remind him to stay still. Two triangular bandages tied tightly were only a suggestion not to move the injured shoulder.

A familiar voice echoed down the hill. "Whaddya need?" Gary, a neighbour and captain serving on the volunteer department, was a welcome addition. After hearing the police were still not here yet, it was time to get down to business.

Our patient could not climb up the hill. Despite his impatience, the last warning stuck. "You can't climb a rope with only one hand. You might fall and really get banged up."

Calling back up, I asked for a Stokes rescue basket, a better rope and two firefighters. It was dark as friends arrived at the side of the car, small flashlights in hand. You could hear the portable generator start-up; artificial light began to flood over the hill.

"Holy crap" was the victim's response to the car surrounded by the rusting wire. Our patient was lucky; his injuries were not worse. There were a few minor cuts that we would look after later.

We needed to get our patient out of the ditch and prove to the naysayers above that he would live to race another day. Though I hoped it was a forward-facing contest.

Assisting the young fellow out of the door, he was in a rush to leave the topsy-turvy ride he just experienced. Luckily there were no fuel leaks, and that he was not ejected from the vehicle. I was surprised he had not suffered more injuries.

Two firefighters arrived with the basket. Offering no resistance, the fellow lay back with some help. We explained he would have to trust us to get him up topside. Leon called out again, asking if there was anything we needed. Lots of help this guy was tonight.

Strapped into the orange plastic basket, the patient was finally on a backboard secured inside. There were lots of helping hands from above. The three of us shared a side, and the foot end, steading the basket.

A stronger rope was tied through a hole at the head end of the Stokes. We were yanked up the hill in no time. Arriving at the top, our patient's friends crowded around the basket to check on their fellow racer.

Standing off to the side, the officer I hoped for earlier. Explaining I wanted to talk to him before we left, I gave Leon the running report as we transferred the patient. Strapped to the backboard, it would keep him flat while moving him over to our stretcher.

The fall alone was worth the price of admission to the ER for a check-up. He wanted to jump off now that we were on level ground on the dark gravel road. Closing the rear doors of the ambulance behind Leon, I looked for the officer.

Friends were innocently giving their deceptive version of how the mishap occurred. The officer walked away and back over to his black and white cruiser several yards away, where we spoke. Explaining how the crash happened, I suggested he check out the fenders of his friend's cars. The fellow was tapped by another car in the reverse race when it began to sway back and forth while using the now "rear wheels" to steer.

All is well that ends well; there were no serious injuries. This was a race that no one finished with a trophy. Unless there is a stupid cup.

Needless

Leonardo Da Vinci's concept drawing of the helicopter from the fifteenth century never got off the ground. Igor Sikorski's flyable model in the 1940s still looked like it should never fly. So, interested in rotary-winged flight, I snooped around a flight training school.

I came close to leaving the ambulance business to pursue a career as a "chopper" pilot. Following a few introductory flights, the pursuit never got off the ground. My affection for rotary-wing flight was partially satisfied when I was hired as a cabin attendant on the local medivac helicopter. It was a part-time gig lasting nine years.

The high school bus servicing our village took a route on the way home each day that passed a driveway storing a treasure. There beside a house were the undeniable remains of a couple of small helicopters. It would be years before our paths would cross.

Donnie and I stood in the garage bay at the office on a breezy Sunday day shift, sipping hot coffee. The morning was all but a shutout. We serviced a "we can't wake grandpa up for Church" call. The outcome was well predicted before we were halfway to the residence.

Returning to the base, there was the regular assignment to deep clean an ambulance, ours. The "weekly" so aptly labelled was an intervention aimed at catching all the "goobers" substitute, blood, vomit etc., that escaped the clean-up following a specific call. Stuff just fell into the cracks.

Pulling the equipment and supplies out, counting, repacking, and cleaning the ambulance's interior before reorganizing was a ritual completed on the Sabbath. Most dreaded the process. All lying aside, the rig looked and smelled better when it was done.

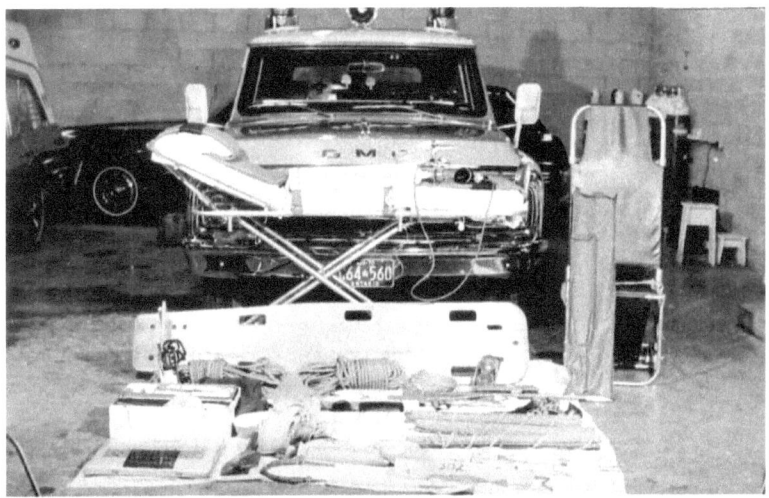

With the "scut work" behind us for another week, the sky was blue for the moment. Afternoon breezes settled in for the kite flyers out there. My second coffee caught up; it was time to give myself breathing room before the next run. It didn't take long before Donnie hammered the bathroom door open. His salutation; "Holy shit, there's a helicopter crash!"

Now, for a guy who spent several years in the Canadian Air Force's pararescue division, you would think this was a routine call for him. Donnie's stories of parachuting into crash sites around Canada after military aircraft "augered in" sounded exciting. He spent many a night with injured and sometimes dead flyers waiting for help at the crash site serving as an airborne first responder.

Leaving the office, there were more details. At the edge of the city, in a cornfield, witnesses observed a small helicopter crash. There were reports of two injured. A second ambulance to back us up was delayed clearing the hospital; we were on our own for a few minutes.

The blue sky disappeared, replaced with low boiling clouds; the substitute spelled wet medics. Heavy rain started with a cruel vengeance before we got to the edge of the city. On a gravel road for the last couple of miles, this was my territory for volunteer firefighting. We had a greeter.

A fellow stood on the side of the road in the last burst of a brief but all-out summer rainstorm. Donnie stopped to speak to the witness, waving us onto the gravel path over a culvert at the edge of a standing cornfield.

Pointing out ahead of us, the man cried as he spoke. The last bit of rain rinsed away his tears. A helicopter was somewhere in the middle of the field; a small plume of smoke marked the location. The six-foot mature corn crop blocked our view.

In his usual decree, Donnie drove away, green corn stalks and heavy cobs breaking over the hood of our Ford; "God hates a coward!" Clumps of mud spun off the tires; we would be in shit later. Dents in the hood would earmark the damage for our fleet guy Monty. With some luck, Donny might survive; the fleet guy also served in the air force.

It seemed like forever; the distance was hard to judge. Corn dropped away to a wheat field with a bump caused by a furrow separating the two crops. A man and woman stood off to the side of the wheat field on a gravel path. Sitting in pieces was the remains of a small helicopter.

Blades bent; it was everything you have seen in a movie. The aircraft's outer skin was in wrinkled pieces wrapped around aluminum tubing that had once been the frame. A control console was driven into the ground, flames curling out of pieces of wreckage nearby.

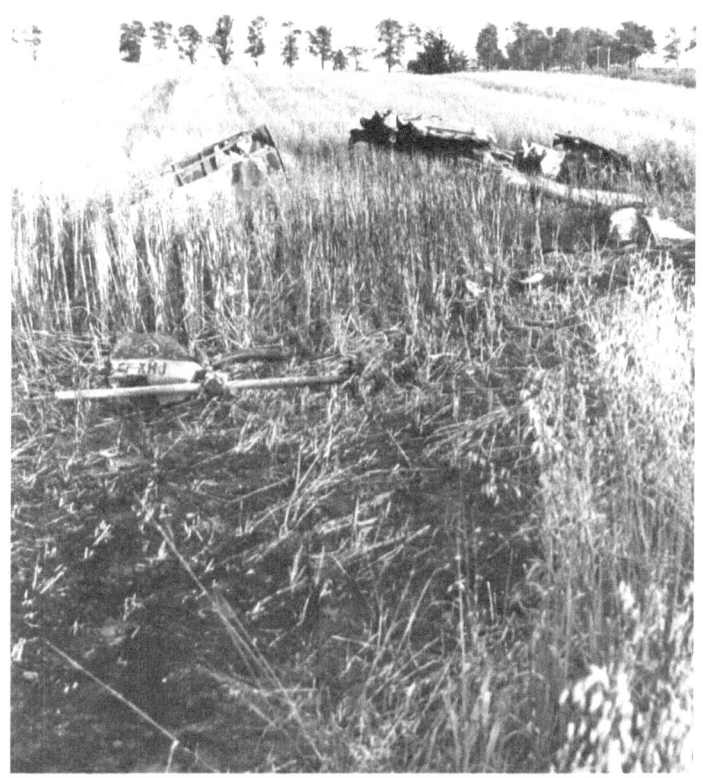

Climbing out of the ambulance's rear, now on autopilot, I carried the oxygen kit and first aid bag. It would be a futile gesture. The woman was being consoled by the fellow who resumed speaking to her when we dismounted the ambulance.

Lying on their sides beside each other was an adult man and a smaller child. Both were obviously dead. Clothes burned off; the only remnants to prove they had been dressed were shoes, belts and the zippers from their missing trousers. Extremities pulled into a fetal stance from the extreme heat, the bodies showed signs of severe injuries caused by the impact.

Eyelids missing, the two looked like angels. The soft tissue of the lips withered away as darkened teeth now ringed the opening. It was a variation on gruesome; unlike a straightforward vehicle accident, the burns were dramatic.

The smell of tissue splashed in "Jet A" fuel then instantly ignited was a first. A fire in a helicopter crash is unavoidable. Fuel is stored in tanks behind the rear seats in the cabin. In an aircraft accident, everything comes forward, tanks rupture.

Speaking now to the man who came forward to offer some information. The woman was the wife and mother of the occupants of the helicopter. His story should remain sealed. It would suffice to say that I had seen the aircraft under re-construction years earlier.

The Provincial Police showed up following our path into the wet cornfield. There was nothing we could do here; it was a helpless feeling knowing the story. I have been to a few aircraft incidents in my time, witnessing one. This topped the list.

STOP means STOP

As a kid, I learned how to ride a bicycle, starting out with one hand on the porch's railing at our house. It began back in the days when there was little perceived risk riding a two-wheeler. As much as it was entertainment, it was transportation around our neighbourhood in Lambeth.

Cycling couldn't be risky; mom and dad didn't give my sister and me helmets. Hockey cards packaged with chewing gum were clothes pinned to our bikes. The tapping noise on the spokes gave a kid that "Harley" feeling!

Bikes weren't dangerous until ambulance calls changed all that nonsense. Riding a bicycle in the city is a departure from the small village streets around my childhood home. Add lots of speeding cars and stir in some bound and bent drivers with a "me first" attitude. All bicycle riders are second-rate citizens, and besides, "I have a driver's license," think some motorists.

Now, toss in that "bulletproof" mindset held by some teens that have grown up in the big city. Surrounded by speeding autos, the combination can be deadly. Warm weather and the rush to get home can make any car driver or bicycle rider careless for a moment. Or hazardous.

Screaming down a side street, the young female in her teens was weighed down with a backpack. It was only a few blocks to home and supper time. Maybe it was the risk of being late for the evening meal again or the pressing homework slung behind her.

Approaching a four-lane thoroughfare, was there a memory of successfully crossing the wide street like a rocket at a quieter time. Because you got away with it once without stopping does not guarantee a pass on repeating foolhardy behaviour. Some cyclists exercise their perceived highway right of way blindly, hoping other motorists will yield. It was an innocence to be reckoned with tonight.

Do you remember the original minivans? They had that sliding side door with a rectangular window. Geeze that would hurt. Artie and I just cleared the hospital and were headed for a coffee. It was early on into an evening shift.

Assigned to a call for a car versus a bicycle, I recounted to Art how a recent cyclist fatality this month was scaring me away from ever driving a bike in the city. The poor victim badly under the influence of alcohol was my age. He turned a corner, cutting inside a large truck. The rear wheels went right over the victim's abdomen and pelvis.

It was a learning experience. Knowing the coroner who officiated at my call, I attended the post mortem an excellent anatomy lesson. I hadn't ridden in years. The lights and siren only lasted for a minute; we were right on top of the scene.

Seeing the mangled bike ahead on the ground, I was surprised that there wasn't a body stretched out on the road or the nearby boulevard. The bicycle was scrap metal now, the front tire bent over sideways to the hub. Handlebars designed to go straight out to the side were bent forward from the deceleration caused by the impact.

Was our victim under the van? It would not be a surprise; after seeing several over the years. Severely injured victims sometimes end up trapped under a vehicle. A few victim's injury lists would be crowned with the ongoing burns inflicted by a screaming hot muffler or catalytic converter.

The sound of a shrieking victim is terrible; the smell of burning flesh is worse. You are helpless until rescue can swoop in and execute their specialized craft.

We came up behind the van, so it was impossible to see the damage that the rider caused to the front of the vehicle. Pulling our stretcher up onto the grassy strip, gawkers ahead of us were looking at someone on the curb.

Sitting on the grass with her feet on the road inches below was a sobbing teenager. Still strapped on her back was a bulging satchel, full of homework intended for this evening's post-dinner assignment. Our victim, blood streaming from her face, held her head upright with both hands. She was not slouched over; her head was facing straight ahead. It would be an essential clue.

There were deep cuts across her forehead where she hit headfirst. Thrown forward when the bike folded up, the victim was using her hands to pull her blood-soaked hair back out of her face. Her wrists were sore but not deformed. It was a miracle with the sudden stop that she escaped fractures. The neck was higher on the priority list for now.

Coming alongside the van, it became apparent how the bicycle ended up with a bent wheel. The young lady broadsided the vehicle. She was breathing, crying and responding to a citizen's questions as we arrived at her side, all great signs.

Missing was the rectangular tinted window in the sliding side door. Small bits of dark glass lay along the curb behind the vehicle. The family-oriented limousine was now equipped with a gaping hole on the passenger's side. The vehicle's low profile lined up perfectly with the patient's head and torso, another inkling of trouble.

Removing the backpack was the first order of the day. The driver of the minivan was squatting at her side. Offering up that the rider came from nowhere, the lady managed to slow her vehicle to a crawl. The driver sensed that the student rider was not about to stop. Despite the red octagonal traffic sign posted at the intersection, the cyclist approached at full speed.

In fact, the van's emergency stop had thrown the anticipated timing for the patient way off. I would bet she thought that the traffic would pass, offering her the necessary clearance to sail across four busy lanes. The buildings on this thoroughfare were well back from the corner. The unexpected response by the van changed everything.

The van's driver described how the patient flew headfirst through the window up to her waist. Carried a few yards to her right, the rider fell backwards and off to the side of her mangled bicycle. From the gutter, she crawled or hobbled to the curb.

The fact that the window gave way seemed to have saved her from more blunt trauma. The young lady was not wearing a helmet, suffering the wrath of shattering glass. This was before the days of the public conscience for safety.

It seemed that our victim's most obvious complaints were; the bleeding lacerations on her face and sprained wrists from forcing the handlebars forward. With a leading question, the first two injuries were painless compared to her response to, "what hurts?"

From her seated position on the curb, the most significant complaint was validated by the tone of her voice and tears; "sore neck." Time to step up to prevent our victim's emergency from growing into a disability.

Our backboard for suspected spinal injuries was already on our stretcher beside us. Getting the girl onto the cot from her seated position would be a variation from a simple immobilization. The first order was to get her to stay still; the verbal warning was overkill. She was scared to death to move.

Applying the collar was a cinch. The patient held her chin in her hands; the sore neck was wide open and waiting for the foam ring. Artie laid the board beside her.

With a quick warning to continue to hold her neck, I reached under her arms. Art cradled her behind the knees as we slowly lifted her onto the waiting plywood slab. Some success when working with traumatized patients comes from narrating your intended actions and moving slowly. We managed both.

Supporting the girl with our hands, we got her flat onto the board and strapped down. During the assessment, the victim confirmed she felt her hands and feet though there was some tingling. While that sensation is never good, there was no numbness, and she was wide awake and responded to our questions.

With her head and neck secure, the cuts got some attention. The bleeding slowed; some dressings laid over the cuts helped. The teen held her hands out in front of her now and cried at the blood. Some sterile water and a towel reddened from cleaning the bloody hands calmed her.

The lift into the ambulance was a little unsettling. Again, the warning before the move was reinforced with "we won't drop you." The brief ride to the hospital was spent giving more emotional first aid than physical care.

The teen's neck was the injury with the most potential. As it turns out, there were structural problems with an un-displaced fracture. The girl continued to have symptoms in the ER. The good news: following some surgery, then immobilized on her back with a strange-looking piece of hardware around her neck and shoulders, the outlook was favourable.

Once there was time to reflect, vanity kicked in, followed by more tears. It was not a surprise for our patient to hear from the ER doc she would need stitches. Going forward, the referral to a plastic surgeon for the right stitches would be a surprisingly small price to pay for such a daredevil move.

Ok, I think it's time for a breather. The balance of the anecdotes on collisions is waiting for you further on in the book. With the highlights of literally a few thousand accident responses to call on, treat the change of pace like a coffee break. Paramedics may see a couple of crashes a shift; this is not the time to ramble.

You will smile when the second installment opens. The author bares his soul, sharing firsthand the description of accidents involving my ambulance. Remember, I never said it wasn't partly my doing.

7

Oh Babies, Cute Babies

As a small child, when parents introduce you to siblings, most of us are instantly indoctrinated with loving and caring customs for that sister or brother. Parental attention that was once exclusively yours, that rite of passage is taken, you move on. When you're an older kid, babies hold little intrigue. They are more of a nuisance, competing for attention, your toys, a sandwich... They can be a real pain.

Moving through adolescence and into adulthood, babies take on added meaning. When you become an aunt, uncle or cousin, there is a value-added proposition. Assumed to be mature and seeking responsibility, you are entrusted with their care when you babysit (why do they still refer to it as babysitting when the kid is twelve years old? One of life's mysteries).

Finally, becoming a mother or father, you are propelled to hyperspace. Pulled in all directions, the responsibility is undeniable: protecting your child becomes a natural quality.

In true Rod Serling fashion, decelerating from hyperspace, you return to a single dimension. As a paramedic, you are belted into the front seat of a van hurtling along a street, responding to the report of imminent childbirth. Welcome to the world of EMS. Many of us in the industry delivered our first baby before being admitted to the league of parenthood.

On the topic of childbirth, I have often asked myself the question: Moms, why would you leave such an important event to a couple of strangers? You plan with precision, attend prenatal appointments accompanied by your spouse. Some families take the mid-wife route, another option open to the qualified and mostly uncomplicated cases.

Time is spent preparing your home for the arrival of that little bundle of joy. Mothers to be, attend showers. Future dads hold guy showers, diaper parties; a new age is born. One thing remains constant. Paramedics earn that stork pin each year delivering babies through some misunderstanding, sketchy planning, or a rank surprise.

Thankfully, almost all out-of-hospital births go off without a hitch. Through training, medics learn the childbirth basics, adding to their understanding of the region's anatomy and physiology. Today, paramedic students practice with lifelike mannequins in the classroom, studying variations on the theme of a "normal presentation." In the beginning, we did the bookwork and watched a 16mm movie depicting childbirth. It was a flickering glimpse into the sheer terror involved with your first delivery.

I attended to the patient(s) on eight childbirth calls; each encounter sent my heart fluttering. The adage, "the mom does all the work - just don't drop junior," was instilled in me en route to a couple of near misses in the early years. It isn't quite that simple. Being in the right place at the right time is another line to remember.

Quadfecta (Yes, it's a real word)

In the early '80s, my career drew me to Northern Ontario, where I worked for six months on one of our fixed-wing Provincial air ambulances. The town was a dividing point in the northwest corner of the province, taking off daily from Sioux Lookout. We covered many First Nations settlements and smaller isolated communities.

Instead of the back of a van, our patient compartment was the rear of a Beechcraft Super King Air 200. What once served as a business aircraft had been modified, repurposing its small restroom. The precious and limited space was converted to an equipment rack. Who would have the nerve to poop in a tiny room at 30,000 feet with a curtain your only privacy, less than a foot from your nearest cabin mate? Only a medic would think like that!

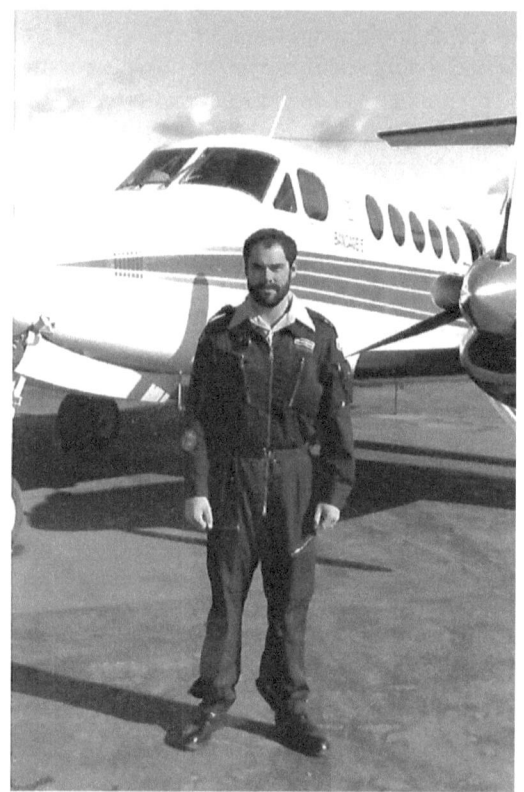

Bandage 5 – 1982

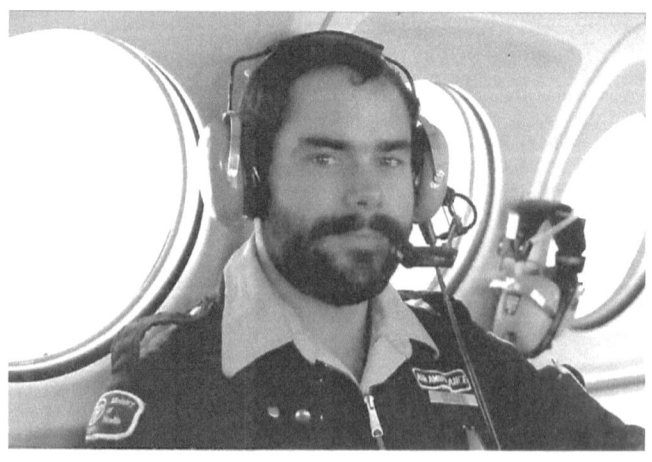

The cabin was more modest than the standard ambulance interior, modified to carry two patients on small folding stretchers. We held the radio designation "Bandage 5", named by a young patient at Sick Children's Hospital in Toronto, during a contest. We rose each morning with the prospect of picking up patients anywhere in the north, transporting them to Sioux Lookout, Winnipeg or Thunder Bay.

One cool summer evening, we were sent off to a small community piloted by Ray, a seasoned bush pilot, Dan, a college aviation program graduate. Both were evenly tempered fellows; they seemed to enjoy every flight.

Our pick-up location tonight was an unusual little airport. Not adorned with standard runway lights, instead "smudge pots." The small kerosene-filled balls were set out along the runway's sides and ignited for each night flight. The airstrip was a World War II base operated by our southern neighbours as an early warning radar station. Decommissioned in the seventies, it was now primarily for private aircraft and the Provincial air ambulance system.

Our dispatcher's quick call to the local Ontario Provincial Police detachment activated the airport staff who maintained and lit the runway. I had flown in before, but only on daylight flights, a simple assignment. Tonight, landing long after sunset, we touched down and taxied between two rows of smoking, flickering markers. We waited patiently for the ambulance to arrive with our full-term mother.

Smaller hospitals provide a fantastic service to expectant patients, delivering then caring for newborns "in-house." That is until there is a hitch. Through experience and good judgement, local doctors choose to hand off patients that could present a threat to mom or babe in a remote setting. They send patients at a higher risk to larger regional centres with specialized resources before the going gets tough, a welcome relief to nervous moms and dads.

It was more than good fortune to be paired up with a seasoned medic for this call. It was to be my scheduled night off. The other cabin attendant asked for a favour. Avoiding the night alone in a motel room was a plus for me, and the exchange would be redeemed for extended days off. Tonight's shift was shared with Vern. He was a registered nurse with obstetrical experience and a casualty care attendant from southwestern Ontario. His mentorship would prove invaluable.

Each air ambulance base was equipped with a transport incubator. We employed it for transporting neonates from hospital to hospital. Alternatively, they were also used to house newborns after liberating them from the safe confines of a relieved mom. When carrying a newborn, the plastic and aluminum capsule is quickly transferred into an awaiting ambulance guarding its priceless consignment. The safe and secure chamber has see-through sides to monitor all the excitement while providing a warmed environment.

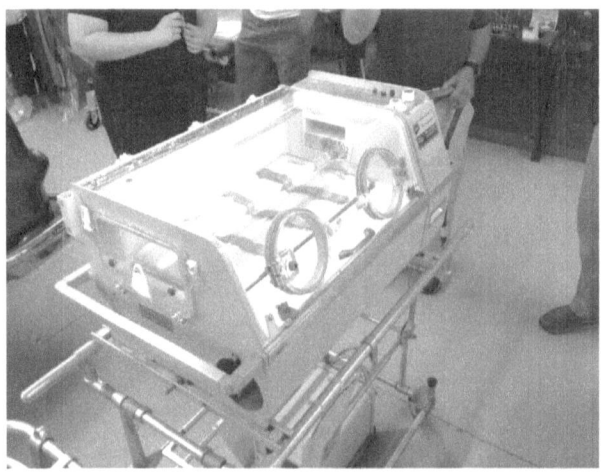

Transport incubator

After a few minutes of sitting in the quiet darkness, we could see our comrade's approaching headlights. Having worked land ambulance for eight years in a receiving centre for everything from trauma to neurosurgery and obstetrics, I had a sense of how the plan should unfold.

We respond to airport calls arriving daily in London. Some aircraft are simple to load and unload, then others pose a challenge due to the size and height of the cargo door. In our industry, medics are regularly called upon to adapt to tricky challenges and overcome them for the patient's sake. A successful transfer takes cooperation, which, on the face of it, sounds so simple. This should have been the case for a small-town ambulance crew who, as it turns out, was a working husband and wife team.

From the moment they arrived at the rear doors of their ambulance, the husband who had been driving had something to say. There were a couple of shots taken for insecure items that fell to the floor of their rig. Then it was how the stretcher was unloaded with the uncomfortable mom slouched low with knees drawn up and out to find a comfortable position.

I had seen this maternal pose before. The position was reserved for a task more complicated than walking a tight rope if I were any judge of the grimaces and sometimes horrible noises moms could make. If the patient is not centred on the cot, it tends to tip without a lot of compensating. More adapting is required on the part of the paramedics. There was no time to whine and moan.

I took the lead tonight, attending the patient following a discussion with Vern during the thirty-five-minute flight in. More than willing to defer to his vast experience, he reassured me I would be fine. My mentor would be there to coach if necessary. Besides, he might get the more challenging part of the bargain if there were any complications with the baby, fingers crossed.

Paramedics are used to changing conditions, trained to expect the unexpected. Experienced medics master almost anything. The bantering between the locals was building to a fever pitch, testing my logic. Now disruptive, it was beyond obvious.

With a quick glance at my co-worker, it was time for Vern and me to coach our way out of this pickle before there was a genuine mishap. As our crew approached the door, we offered a suggestion to our earthbound comrades. The direction was given to stop short of the door and lower their wheeled stretcher. The patient was loaded on a "number nine" folding cot for the trip to the airport. If the land crew stopped too close to the door, tilting the folding cot up to our cabin floor would risk catching the foot end on their stretcher. The resulting imbalance would only compound the difficulty the crew was having.

Our advice was declined, and of course, the inevitable unfolded. In a struggle to steady the tipping cot that hit the rolling stretcher below, mom started to tip. The resulting scream distracted our flight crew, Ray and Dan, nearly banging their heads together while leaning through the flight deck door at the same time.

Until now, they had been concentrating on their flight plan to take us safely to our destination. I looked ahead to the pilots and just shook my head in a "what can you do" fashion. Mom, secured to the stretcher, was saved well short of a disaster by ten hands. Four paramedics and the patient clung to the cot as it was lifted into the aircraft. Though not before bringing about a change in her condition.

Mom was in the local medical facility in active labour when all went calm, no more contractions. Waiting and monitoring, the doctor decided enough was enough and called for the air ambulance. The lift into our aircraft turned out to be a pivotal moment. The jolt frightened mom, jump-starting her own labour. It was a relief that she was now strapped to the bench in our cabin.

With the pre-flight business concluded, our engines started, the pressurized cabin door closed, and thoughts of waving goodbye to the ambulance crew ended abruptly. The patient was into a full-on contraction, screaming, sweating and holding on for dear life.

It will never be clear whether mom's death grip on the aluminum frame was a safety move or some small comfort to the overwhelming pain. I would have gladly given her my brand-new Walkman, small recompense had she suggested switching places.

Only thirty minutes out from our destination, we were kept busy monitoring vital signs. The balance of our duties included calming mom down following her harrowing introduction to the Provincial transfer system. Several contractions into the flight, the rate increased to two-minute intervals.

A luxury afforded to an urban paramedic is the often short transport distance from pick up to the destination. In many cases, if mom isn't pushing, there is time, and there is no need for looking. We should have been so lucky. There was a whole lot of thought going into the pushing now, so the inevitable was required.

 Our patient was very amenable to us examining her during the last few minutes of the journey's airborne portion. We were facing an additional twenty minutes following unloading at the airport then on to our destination. A lot can happen in twenty minutes.

Vern and I were surprised that the baby who had so recently gone into hiding was now in a rush to look out the cabin window at the approaching Thunder Bay airport. A calmer environment that lasted for several minutes vanished; I turned to look at Vern. It was apparent we were going to be a part of this happening. The mom's screams erupting were on instant replay. Dan looked back at us. It seemed that tonight's call was as close as the flight crew had ever come to a mid-air delivery.

Within a minute, the baby was crowning; we were staring at the top of a head. Oh Lord, we had arrived at ground zero. Simultaneously, sliding off my seat and kneeling on the cabin floor, I could hear a familiar sound, the accompanying vibration coming up through my knees.

The landing gear doors were opening, wheels travelling down in preparation for our arrival. Passing us now off to the side, the locally famous Candy Mountain, a ski resort. Looking ahead through the flight deck's windscreen, parallel rows of landing lights appeared, defining our destination.

Forget the airline safety rules of "Return your seats and tables to their upright position and obey the seat belt signs." I wasn't about to be thrown down the aisle holding a slippery newborn for the pilots to adore! I called ahead to our captain Ray to get his attention.

Ray wasn't the baby type. He was a stickler for safety and procedure. Dan and Ray turned, knowing we were interfering with their final approach, annoyed but curious to see what was up. My edict didn't require much of a sales pitch. "Put the wheels up and go around; I'm busy for a minute."

Within a second, I could hear the engines spool up. Ray called the tower with a message, followed by the landing gear's corresponding sound cycling up into the plane's belly. Looking at Vern for approval, his grin was reassuring. He could see my excitement, experiencing a first in my career. Mom wasn't grinning, no wonder.

With her prenatal preparation kicking in, our patient's breathing was rhythmic. She began her final push after two hard contractions. We would now change the official flight plan from five souls on board to six. Pride doesn't begin to describe holding a newborn for the first time, at 5,000 feet to boot! Adrenalin had kicked in - I was probably shaking from the thrill, and having been on my knees in a moving environment for several minutes didn't help.

Turning our tiny girl around for mom to have her first glance, the ordeal was over. Mom was covered in sweat, the screaming done. Over the cabin noise, I called ahead with the hail, "Hey, boys." Both pilots turned around; they were as excited as we were.

The baby was quickly wrapped up to conserve her body heat. The crew responded to Vern's earlier request to turn up the cabin temperature, something I had not thought of. In a second first-time experience, I completed the task of clamping and cutting the umbilical cord before handing mom her first child.

Vern quickly placed the babe in the incubator. It was plugged in and warming from the moment we took off for Thunder Bay. In many urban deliveries, land medics simply place babe on mom's stomach, arriving at the hospital in a couple of minutes. There's no time for a wriggling, screaming projectile in an airplane, however. The brief rides often deny medics and moms of another experience.

Once around the airport in a holding circuit, the belts were re-fastened. The flight crew dropped the gear down again, this time for real. It took a couple of minutes with everyone prepared for the landing, and we were taxing up to the apron in front of two waiting ambulances (more experience and planning on Vern's part).

With one unit for mom, the other for the baby, separating the two patients presented less confusion en route and only a minute separated mom and babe, a decision that avoided the task of having to pack everyone into one ambulance. With the baby doing fine, screaming like a freight train, Vern departed with the isolette in the first unit. My crew loaded up mom, and off we went to the hospital, a brief but dark ride into the city. Mom was uncomfortable before we were halfway, the ETA provided by the medic driving.

With the training kicking in, I began some massage of mom's abdomen. A few minutes later, I achieved another first, seldom repeated in future urban deliveries. The placental delivery was simple and a total success. Really, it was nothing; mom did all the work for a second time; thank you very much.

Our arrival in the delivery room was uneventful, almost anticlimactic. Hospital staff were unimpressed with their two new patients. I guess being in the business, it was old hat to them. I was still amped up with adrenalin from the experience tonight.

One procedure did strike me as strange until the delivery room nurse answered my question. It seems that an out of hospital delivery must be tracked. Since we were about to disappear into the midnight air, nurses' stopped us wanting to know who to give credit to. Remember, this was not supposed to be my shift. The other medic that asked me to cover for him wailed away when he heard about the delivery. The reward for working; to be a part of the first delivery on Bandage 5, another first!

About two weeks later, we were out flying late one evening and ran out of service time in Winnipeg, Manitoba. We were "time X'd," a Transport Canada term for a regulation prohibiting a flight crew from becoming fatigued. They capped air time and specified minimums for "prone rest." Let's face it, who would want their pilot falling asleep at the stick?

We delivered our patient tonight to the downtown hospital. Now, slouching on chairs in the lounge at the fuel service provider, the crew line from the tower rang. Dan answered with his name and the aircraft registration, followed by a simple "yes, we are." I assumed he was acknowledging we would be overnighting in town.

Hanging up the phone, he informed us we were being summoned to the control center. Mr. doom and gloom, I figured that the boys buzzed the tower on our way in, and we were heading to the principal's office. We entered the Winnipeg centre to find a large room full of consoles and radar screens. There were several controllers and a supervisor. Our arrival was announced by phone to one last person.

Coming out of a long narrow room protected by sliding glass patio doors was an air traffic controller. The woman introduced herself as having worked the shift the night we delivered the baby over Thunder Bay. Her comment was followed by a round of applause from the remaining controllers sitting nearby.

I was at a loss, announcing my ignorance. Dan shared the introductions and asked the controller working tonight in the glass room to share her wisdom. It seems that after midnight, Thunder Bay hands off their control zone to Winnipeg centre, which conducts business long distance. Our tour guide informed us that we were far enough north to briefly be in an area controlled by the civilian air traffic control for NORAD (North American Air Defence).

We passed through an area and above the altitude being monitored to provide an official warning for unauthorized aircraft, a friendly service extension for our neighbours to the south. When we delayed our landing due to the imminent birth, it was noted in their shift log as unusual, prompting curiosity that evening. All's well that ends well. We enjoyed a coffee and were on our way. Who doesn't like a dramatic entrance? Although it would have been a blast to buzz the tower.

Years later, I was at home out in the back yard when the telephone was handed to me after another "yes, it is" moment. Totally out of context, the female caller identified herself as the mother of the little girl born over

Thunder Bay. Mom tracked me down through the Ministry of Health. It was the young lady's birthday that very day. The teenager wanted to talk to the second person that held her. The loop was officially closed.

There you have it, a Quadfecta: working in an airplane, childbirth, cutting and clamping the cord, and delivering the placenta!

Surprise, surprise

Details, life is always about the details. When it's time to share a moment of "full disclosure," the truth is still your best bet. A personal favourite line comes to mind: "The truth shall set you free."

Surprises should be reserved for packages wrapped in festive paper, decorated with curly ribbon. It would also be nice to have a cake and candles. That's a little difficult when the surprise is your full-term baby being introduced to you from the floor of your basement apartment.

Who would harbour that secret for 40 weeks, then scream and ask their spouse to call the ambulance? This one still escapes me after decades.

On a quiet day shift, Randy and I left the downtown ER, stopping at the variety store around the corner. Back in the day, we were not graced with portable radios. Usually, the driver was delegated to wait it out in the ambulance and honk the horn if a call landed in our laps.

Hearing the horn toot several times, a minor panic ensued as I fished fifty cents out to pay for two cold drinks. Randy was to blame, wanting a brand not available back at the office in the pop machine.

Thinking I missed the first hail, delaying the run, I asked, "so, where are we going?" as I hopped into the seat. "Got a kid call," he responded. Now for a guy who prefers details, that proclamation carries several possibilities. The emergency could range from a kid trapped under the wheel of a car to a tyke with his finger stuck up the chute on a gumball machine. I should probably tell you about that one sometime, but not now; we have a call.

Randy prided himself as the owner of a corny sense of humour. "Somebody in labour," he spat out, a note of disdain in his voice. My driver wanted no part of kids; Randy and his wife were mutually bound for a life of childlessness. Randy was as kind a person as you could meet, but he wouldn't risk the Maverick's upholstery by serving ice cream.

As we arrived in front of the older home, a fellow stood on the front walk and waved wildly, long before we came to a stop. Yes, we can see you, I thought. Had the baby already arrived, usurping our assignment? Getting to the rear doors of our ambulance, he met us doing a two-step, narrating the impending scene in disbelief.

This fellow was not a conspicuous member of the proud expectant dad's group. You know, that clique that voluntarily attended a prenatal class to prepare for the experience. We heard later, the dispatcher who'd received the call details from the excited man tried asking a couple of questions.

First, the caller described, "terrible pain that comes and goes." The clincher followed this reply; "the pain is so bad she couldn't hold it anymore. She lost control of herself all over the floor." In his defence, he was engaged; he didn't run away!

The call taker's suspicions peaked following the caller's denial of an obstetrical history. With the unabated screaming in the background, the dispatcher asked to speak to the patient crying out in pain. This was not the routine for dispatching an ambulance. The initial caller was not making any sense. The distraught woman responded, acknowledging she might be pregnant with the phone to her ear, something she was guarding given the brief responses.

The dispatcher's sixth sense kicked in, saving us the surprise, a big thumb's up for him. The conversation back at the base later proved to be as entertaining as the call when we exchanged details. We got the Reader's Digest version on the air. The bombshell of a revelation was delayed for the moment, following our guide to the basement.

Obstetrical and oxygen kits in hand, we left the stretcher at the back door and headed down the small steps to an apartment. More of a cave, protected by a low overhanging wall in the stairwell. Something worth ducking for if you value your sense of humour.

Opening into a small one-bedroom suite with a shallow ceiling, our patient was lying on the floor. Consumed with pain, it looked an awful lot like the patient was having a hard contraction. She was a generously proportioned woman to start, which likely aided her unsuccessful effort to conceal her now obvious condition.

Diving in with a conservative question, I asked how far along she was. Over my shoulder in a ventriloquial manner, the question prompted dad's response, "what? She's not pregnant." It was a defining moment for mom when she shared her secret with her duped co-conspirator. There was a brief gasp followed by a "what the fuck?"

Now it was time to get down to business. It turns out mom was not being followed by a doctor, so she was stumped for an accurate gestation estimate. We were at the point where we had to expose mom to examine her. The baby was delivered to the ears. There was no secret here, no need to whisper. Opening the obstetrical kit, I pulled out the sad submission for gloves. Within a couple of minutes, I had a bouncing baby boy in my hands. Looking at this little fellow with hair and fingernails, he was tired of sitting around and chose to break the news today.

It was time to move mom up and out to the vehicle for the ride to Children's Hospital - the old one with the ramp facing Colborne Street at South Street (It was a long time ago). This was one of my few city deliveries that warranted cutting and clamping the cord before moving mom and baby.

It would be tough to carry mom up the stairs backwards in a stair chair. The delay in sending Randy back to the truck for the collapsible wheelchair gave me time to clean up the baby and wrap him. The new dad could lend a hand while we were lifting. This, of course, after presenting him to mom briefly for a cuddle. It was a step at a time leaving the basement. You could not stand up straight with the low clearance and the weight of the lift. It was not the time nor place for a slip-up.

The hospital trip was interspersed with cheerful commentary from a happy dad riding up front with Randy, having had a few minutes to get used to the news. He was probably buying cigars before the end of the day. It was still early.

The baby arrived at Children's safe and sound on mom's tummy, something you would not get away with now. Today, we would be held to the standard of using a car seat or our specialized baby restraint. Oh, but for the good old days.

Dad shook both our hands before we left the delivery room, the destination a formality since the baby had already arrived in more ways than one. There was a time in the basement where I was convinced that we were in for a punch, not a handshake. All's well that ends well.

Sad, just sad

Paramedic's memories from one call to the next often vary. Sometimes you only retain a sampling of the original details. Some medics tell of themes, like cardiac arrests, burns, or kids. For others, it is the vision of a similar injury, a smell or sound resurrecting the past. It seems that trivial details are a personal specialty. That's before you even get to the reason for the memory popping up; just ask a psychologist.

This sad tale comes to mind when I pass a familiar coffee franchise. Years ago, the same plot of land contained a white clapboard house, two doors in from the intersection. The modest home was sitting apart from surrounding structures on a poorly lit street in its day. Today, the area is built up, filled in with stores and a strip mall with the home long gone.

It was always slightly awkward working with Alf. He was the quiet type who wouldn't say shit if he had a mouthful. A fellow long retired from the military, he found a second career. Alf could have been my father; the gap was so vast in our ages. We would ride silently for half a shift if I was not working him over.

He was a great guy, but the exact opposite of my youthful extroversive tendencies. In our industry, you are constantly adapting to changing priorities and challenges. The first thing that derails a paramedic crew is poor communication. It doesn't have to be verbal. Eye contact or another silent signal work well. The fundamental principle is to learn to communicate before you are on a call. Alf presented a challenge.

We were assigned to work out of a small satellite station from four until midnight in the east end. The place looked more like a dingy sitting room at a call scene than a workplace lounge. Escaping the worn, uncomfortable recliners and the dry air from hot-water radiators lining the walls, calls were a bonus. Your entertainment was watching a 12" black and white television perched on a table next to a tea kettle with a frayed cord.

An old black dial phone sat next to a paper pad on the small desk inside the door. This was before the era that introduced radio dispatching with pagers, overhead speakers and direct lines.

With only three rings, Paul, the dispatcher this evening, issued the call details. A frantic mother of a teenage girl reported that her daughter just delivered a baby. The newborn was in a toilet for some reason.

Alf could not recall a situation like this from his past when I asked. It left me with an empty feeling in the pit of my stomach. What do you do in this circumstance? The reading I had done did not include this scenario.

Pulling out through the hospital grounds, you had to cross railroad tracks to get to Dundas Street. Taking this route with Alf for the first time, I grabbed the sides of my seat, hanging on for dear life. Last month, Rob had taken the same way out, driving code 4 with our four-wheel-drive SUV ambulance.

Hoping to thrill me with a Ferris wheel-style ride, he sped over the raised crossing. The move tossed me straight up into a zero-gravity collision with the ceiling. I ailed with a sore neck for a couple of days. All fears were unfounded tonight. Alf's driving was as tame as his conversation. For the remainder of the ride to the scene, not a word was spoken. I was getting nervous.

The mother of our patient waved us down. Her house was not marked with a front porch light. It was a typical alert issued by the waiting resident. Our rolling stretcher made it to the front hall; the small bungalow was tiny and unkempt.

I carried a disposable obstetrical (OB) kit under my arm, and with the oxygen bag in hand, we were led to the back of the home. The short route passed through a hall littered with bits of garbage and discarded items, a telling sign of indifference.

The tension was evident when mom and daughter were reunited in the bedroom. Our patient was lying sideways across the bed. There were bloodstains on the wrinkled linen around her. A corner of the bottom sheet pulled clear of its hold on the mattress.

The surrounding room was a disaster; there were layers of abandoned clothes on the floor, flattened by the regular traffic. Some books and paper, evidence of attending school, were also caught under what could best be described as; an abandoned elf-like black Halloween costume. The goblins had come and gone months ago, so had Christmas.

Our patient, lying quietly on the bed, remained silent when asked questions about tonight's summons to assist her. The sidelong looks at mom highlighted the continuing strain between them. Asking the concerned parent to retreat to the living room, she left. The flood gates opened in mom's absence.

The teenager revealed her guilt with the early response that she did not know who the father was. I promised her that it was not a problem. The questions were posed, reinforcing their importance. We needed the facts to assist the hospital staff and us in helping her. It was enough of a distraction to get to the issue at hand.

With a fast pulse and some obvious bleeding to contend with, the young girl cried, relieved that she finally shared her guarded tale. We settled into some information gathering, her history, including the timeline. The girl missed her period for five months. Having some pain earlier this evening, she went to the bathroom, believing this would relieve the problem.

After sitting on the toilet, she described several sharp pains, enough to make her sweat. That was when it happened. When I asked, "what happened," she replied, "the baby came out in the toilet." Looking patiently over my shoulder, Alf was getting anxious, shifting from one foot to the other. I could tell he just wanted to get out of here; my agenda differed.

Attempting to calm the teen and get the real story, I gave Alf an assignment. Go back to the truck for a clean pillowcase. While he went on a linen hunt, I asked the leading question, "where is the baby now?" The question brought the patient's emotions to a peak. She looked tortured, crying, head buried in her hands. Rolling to her side, I could see more blood on the bed.

The patient explained that she did not want to tell her mom. Sitting in the bathroom until found by the concerned parent, there was a confrontation. The elder was thinking some pot was being smoked behind the door until the crying suggested another problem. There was one final detail, the baby was in the toilet for almost an hour and still there.

Hearing footsteps behind me, I turned and headed to the bathroom. Passing Alf, I grabbed the folded white hospital pillow cover on the way. The small bathroom was a mess from months of cleaning up and doing their make-up. The ladies-only place was a shamble. Open and expended tubes and other toiletries littered the toilet's top and a small shelf under the window.

The open toilet lid said it all. Floating in pink-tinged water was a well-formed fetus, easily recognizable. A tiny pale umbilical cord dangled from the long-departed baby. It was probably the most saddening sight I had seen. The innocence of this death, unequalled in my career.

It is one thing to see someone lying dead on the highway or a "garden variety" cardiac arrest. To know that a baby died before its time was a novel experience. Our patient was holding it together, considering this sight.

With no gloves for ambulance attendants in the day, I did what so many of us did. Reaching into the toilet, I scooped the abandoned, lifeless neonate out of the dirty porcelain vessel. Wrapping it tightly in the linen, I handed it to an awaiting Alf, stationed at the door. I took the time to wash my hands and then dry them on my shirt, not trusting the wrinkled towel offered to visitors.

Returning to the patient, I assisted her to the bedroom door. We met Alf, having already deposited the second patient somewhere out of our sight. Taking a few steps stationed on either side of the teen, we arrived back in the living room. The mother of the patient stood motionless, preparing herself for a repeat of the previous encounter.

With little, if any emotion, our patient turned away from her mother to sit on the clean white linen-covered cot. That's when I noticed the small rolled package sitting where our patient's knees would rest shortly. With a free hand, in one motion, the tiny bundle was snatched from the stretcher. Depositing the dampened cloth silently into my coat pocket, I covered it with the flap.

The patient showed a lighter mood and agreed to have her mother ride up front in the ambulance with Alf. That was welcome news; the rift was showing the first signs of healing. The two, separated for the ride, would have time to forgive and accept, a positive sign; it helped me. I hoped it was helping them.

The ride in was uneventful. Our patient let me assess her vital signs again. In a brief radio patch to the ER nurse relaying the details, I recognized the voice at the other end. This grad would add a calming effect when we arrived. Alternatively, she would be a great professional referee if things went south. Always have a plan "B."

After being triaged by the charge nurse, our patient was sent to a private room reserved for gynecology and obstetrical cases. The examination lights were off to start with. This detail offered a softening effect, less intimidating. The patient wanted her mom now, likely due to the foreign environment, another reassuring sign.

We pushed the stretcher back to the waiting room door. Alf shuffled out to the entrance to change the linen and ready the ambulance for the next run. Sitting in the writing room, our patient report form was fundamental. It left little space for the details. Instead, excelling in an early version of "tic boxes." The record was computer-read in the big smoke of Toronto; the government was forever gathering statistics.

Surprising me, approaching from behind, Alf and my favourite nurse stood silently. She was recently relieved of the assignment to act as a referee for mom and daughter when the mood calmed. The nurse and Alf filled the writing room door. The cubbyhole, unable to hold the three of us and the desk, was a repurposed closet. There were no secrets kept from the curious public now positioned behind me with the room's recently installed window facing the waiting room.

The nurse, sporting a puzzled look, spoke up, asking, "where is it?" Alf, with his "huh" face, appeared equally bewildered. At the moment, I must have resembled Alf's brother. "Oh, the baby," and without losing a beat, I reached into my right pocket, retrieving the now pink stained linen bundle. The attempt to protect the young mother's fragile emotions revealed my impromptu effort to hide the small mummy-like packaged child.

In an incredulous reaction, both were temporarily silenced. The nurse, realizing she was on stage to waiting patients and relatives, squelched her belly laugh and smiled. Quickly expressing an acknowledging near-silent snicker instead. Alf was truly mortified, never breaking his military poker face carrying the moment.

I never did see him smile after leaving the hospital. There wasn't even a sarcastic comment on my innocent blunder. I am sure the nurse told the story at coffee later, behind closed doors. Rest assured, it was the best the author could come up with in the circumstance.

The next afternoon arriving at the base, I stood for a moment at the lounge door punching the time clock. Oblivious to some dwindling snickers, I crossed the room to place my lunch in the fridge.

Returning to the lounge in the hopes of taking the last seat, my move was interrupted when Kelly stuck his head out of the radio room. "Hey Darbs, is that a fetus in your pocket or your toque and gloves?" As God is my witness, I went as red as the rotor lights on the fleet in the garage. Alf sat to the side, breaking into a smile and snicker. It had to be a delayed reaction, contradicting his disbelief from last evening.

I received two offers that night to swap co-worker's coats for my legendary parka. Others wanting boasting rights for the hiding place for that poor kid. I guess there must be some light in such a regularly dark place that we find ourselves in.

Not so fragile

When it's your call, it's your call. No one likes a call stealer. Especially when it comes to childbirth. Paramedics are proud professionals, up to the task. There was a day when the industry employed medics temporarily with a minimum of training, specifically for summer vacation coverage. Something I thought was reserved for isolated northern services. These issues were to collide shortly.

Like many others, I did not approach the career looking at it as a summer job before pursuing a university education. Decades ago, the government allowed students to work after only first aid and CPR training and a couple of "in-house" orientation days.

Without hesitation, the temps were tossed head-first into the abyss of pre-hospital care. It was intended as a method to pay your way through school, a brief career at best. The spinoff was cost-cutting. Some experiences were better than others.

The danger was that you could walk into the worst call of your career on your first day. Thankfully the risky situations were mostly averted with some good luck and seasoned caregivers attending over shoulders and through the rear-view mirror guiding the temporary staff. I had my moments and some close calls until additional training and experience smoothed it out. It was time to pay it forward.

Karen, a young university student, going into her second year of a health-related career path, was bubbly and quick to tell me about herself. A trait I could appreciate and relate to. I hoped we could communicate when the time and situation demanded it. For her first day on the road, Karen was surprisingly composed. The brief training time must have been intense, I thought.

In my case, initially finishing two weeks in the classroom, I still fretted, living in fear of attending a critical call too early in my career to process and act on what I was seeing. Instinct left me feeling too green to possess the confidence to do the right thing at the right time in the right circumstance, an understatement when it came to childbirth. Good co-workers, patience, and perseverance, but mostly training reinforced with experience helped me through the early years. Those times are challenging for any medic to this day.

Sometimes innocence is a safety net preventing the fear that many of us lived through. For summer students, the role of their driver was all-encompassing. Students were never extended driving privileges for many reasons, a successful measure to make the best of the worst. With strict direction to drive the students, full-time medics attempted to narrate what they were likely to see and what they should do for patients, all before arriving at the scene.

The ambulance Gods were kind to Karen for her first morning and graced us with a couple of routine transfers. The round trips to and from the cancer treatment centre eased Karen into her summer experience. For her, some simple lifting then chatting en route. Karen was surprisingly intuitive and seemed to connect with the ailing patients we transported daily for cobalt treatments. This was a good start.

We made it back for a brief lunch at the office, and then the pace picked up. There were only five units on the day shift until noon. You hoped the clock would roll around and add the extra crew to cover lunch breaks. Today was not our day; the noon car was shuffled off to the Toronto airport with a foreign visitor recovering from a medical emergency.

When the city was reduced to one unit, the last available crew was sent to the city's centre, aptly referred to as "central standby." Located at Colborne and Pall Mall Streets, it was thought that the crew could get to any corner of the Forest City with equal response times.

Sitting on a side street would be the perfect time to continue our conversation interrupted earlier, filling in some blanks on emergency care. We had barely opened chapter one before the radio crackled to life. Dispatched to the south end of the city, we responded to a patient that called in her own emergency.

According to our dispatcher Steve, there was a language barrier with the caller. Steve would know; he had an English flavour of his own. Through the thick accent, he picked up that no one was home and "baby is coming."

Off we went on a "zoom," the term a close ally in the business, Matt had given to "code 4" driving. Karen became silent, seeing the world from the other side. It's all fun and games until you cross that intersection against the red. You hope that everyone has seen the lights and heard the siren. Despite stopping first, there is always a risk. We talked about emergency driving earlier. Karen agreed she was happy riding shotgun.

Our approach had been rather noisy, with the pick-up location on a busy street. In the best of times, the attendant would be calling out street address numbers. They were often hidden this time of year with tree branches and other obstructions.

Arriving at the patient's residence, the two-car garage door was open. There were no vehicles home, so it was easy backing into the driveway. I was getting nervous now, our first scene call together, Karen's inaugural emergency run, what a theme for the opener!

What faced us next can best be described as one of those shock value moments. A sight that should have been reserved for a seasoned team. The luck of the draw thrust this unprepared kid into the line of fire, retreat impossible. Standing in the doorway inside the back of the garage was our patient. She was wearing a colourful pleated dress, probably below the knee length.

I say probably because the dress wasn't hanging naturally, covering her knees. Mom to be had a look of horror in her eyes. She was holding the front hem of the dress up around her neck. Wearing no undergarments, her exposed body told the story. I thought Karen was going to stop breathing. It was a toss-up as to who had a better facial expression now, mom or Karen!

Mom, speaking in broken English and Portuguese, communicated the unmistakable news, "Baby here!" Leaving our stretcher in the rear of the ambulance, we ran up to steady our patient. Her feet spread apart, she was balanced on the threshold at the kitchen door. It was a couple of feet above the garage floor.

A glistening baby's head was protruding generously out of mom. In a second, we were informed that this was her third child; the first two were delivered at the hospital. Looking at a green partner on a challenging call, my first thought was to assume control and swap roles, but we were under strict guidelines with the summer students to handle the call from the driver's seat. This was it.

Karen and I each held the patient's hands. I asked the now tottering woman to come down to the first step and sit back on her kitchen floor while I went for the stretcher. Turning to Karen, I offered her some firm but polite direction.

Lay mom down on the floor. Place two of your fingers, one on each side of the baby's head, at the base of the neck. Position the other hand in front of the soon-to-be delivered chest. The baby was turned sideways now; more fluid was leaking out around the head and neck. The child sliding out almost to the shoulders before I turned away to retreat to the truck for our equipment.

There is a lot to be said about training and experience. Hoping – no, praying that nothing would happen with the few feet I had to cover on the round trip with the stretcher. I still needed to grab the obstetrical kit out of the cabinet. Plans change. I heard mom scream behind me, Karen following with some muted reply.

For the life of me, the EMS Gods could not have been nastier. Mom pushed again in my brief absence. The slipperiest little girl on the block that day slid right through Karen's waiting but inexperienced hands. Remember the earlier reference to "don't drop junior"?

Thankfully mom was lying down, her feet planted on the first step. As I came around to Karen's side, she lifted the little girl off the first step. The baby's shoulder was lightly salted with gravel from the wooden tread. The baby had not actually fallen, rather more of an assisted slide to her resting place.

Opening the OB kit, we put the disposable cloths to good use, drying off the tiny patient. Mom, oblivious to the faux pas, was glad to see her baby after a quick clamp and cut to the baby's umbilical cord. Karen tightly wrapped the little girl in the small sterile flannel blanket. We all exchanged smiles.

Mom was more than stoic, sitting bolt upright to hold her third child. The protective mother bear instinct kicked in. She took little urging to accept our assistance onto the stretcher for the brief ride to the hospital.

The hospital staff received their report more from the driver than the attendant. Not wanting to miss the details, I relayed the truth and nothing but the truth. In a surprise, the receiving nurse was not shocked by the "gravelly" description of the brief trip down the stairs.

I believed she had seen worse after hearing her rendition of greeting a couple one evening at the hospital entrance. It had been a home delivery. The dad drove mom to the hospital with the child still connected. I suspect the upholstery needed a good cleaning.

Sometime later, at a round table with some work friends, the discussion turned to weird turns of events on calls. The conversation made its way around to childbirths, and the gravel story surfaced. It bubbled to the top after a few drinks, an industry culture familiar to most public service responders.

The story morphed to; can you imagine if she had stood up and bolted for the ambulance. The kid would have been bouncing there like a Yo-yo? As impossible as it seems, I have had that thought recur a couple of times. Karen did save the day. She was there for the catch, sort of.

You know what they say about assuming…

During that same round table conversation, a medic broke into a belly laugh and shared a moment from a childbirth run. It had taken place approximately a year before I began in the industry. I'd only heard the third-hand version until this occasion. Donny and his partner were on their first childbirth call. They were presented with a mom in what still seems like the worst pain I have ever heard described. You know, the kind where the guy tells you he hit his thumb with a hammer splitting it wide open. Incredibly it did not hurt for a few seconds. This sounded 10 times worse.

Donny and Ben arrived in the bedroom of a couple's home to see mom holding what they thought was the baby's protruding head. In the medic's rush to get the patient on their stretcher before the delivery, they dashed off to the hospital, committing the ultimate sin: not completing a primary survey.

Making their way to the hospital's delivery room, code 4, an ER nurse took the radio call and relayed it to the labour and delivery room, based on their description. Ben, the attending medic, God love him, interpreted the gaping chasm under his riveted supervision as a - and I quote, "fractured skull." Baffled staff hearing the report could not figure out how an unborn child had sustained a fractured skull.

Preparing for the worst, the receiving nurse in the delivery room pulled out all the stops. Calling out the troops, she assembled them in a well equipped and lit delivery room. Highly trained nurses and doctors were expecting the challenge of their careers. In what likely turned out to be the hospital's funniest story at their Christmas dinner, Donny and Ben burst through the doors and could hardly contain themselves when the doctors removed the red wool Hudson's Bay blanket.

The mother, who was well informed of her arriving baby's condition, had neglected to mention that her obstetrician warned her of the impending breech birth. For the uninformed, that is when a baby does not drop into a head-first position in the pregnancy's final stage. You always keep your fingers crossed for a head-first presentation or delivery. Babies showing up bum first will always be a shocker for paramedics.

A harrowing experience filled with feelings of helplessness in the pre-hospital environment, breach births top the list. Until recently, there were few procedures paramedics' had been trained in to resolve the problematic presentation. Sometimes, a hasty ride to the hospital is the treatment that we are ultimately forced to provide.

There is no substitution for the experts waiting in a well-lit delivery room. Thankfully the hospital staff see a lot of things through their careers. We never heard any stories of them making fun of arriving medics, though it must have been tempting.

8

Regulars I have known and loved, sometimes

Professionals in the public service will relate to the term; "regulars." Retail and service sector workers enjoy similar relationships in a more relaxed setting. Like marriage vows, it's "for better or worse." In a less formal instance, customers can be challenging when their needs are not met.

Unhappy patrons are consistently held to the standard of being "right," a mantra often expressed by successful businesses. Contact with civil servants often empowers the consumer with the presumption they are right. It has been my experience as a supervisor over the years to hear: "I pay your wages; don't you forget it."

Imagine the same faces that just keep showing up, and there is nothing you can do about it! Regulars are part of the job for those that serve: DON'T YOU FORGET IT!

As sad as it can get, some of our frequent flyers are life's less fortunate. They need help and turn to responders and not always in an emergency. We temporarily relieve our patient's distress, often distracting them by default, sometimes providing an escape.

Police and paramedics see a generous overlap of these individuals, contributing to each other's profession's mutual respect. As an emergency responder, maintaining your professional candour can be a test. It is said that the very people challenging our patience contribute to an even temperament in a career. The journey from start to finish will always be an ordeal.

Burnout along the way, including incidents of less than an exemplary performance by responders, is not unheard of. The tales below offer a cross-section of the souls we meet. The humour expressed is not intended to malign those in need. Instead, the focus is on exposing the coping skills of those serving the public.

A professional responder must always provide the best service. Going forward, we sometimes share the humour with other responders to cope and come back able to face the next shift. We often refer to it as dark humour; understanding the rhetoric reveals the human side of a first responder.

Willie

Willie, the whistler, was a fella who loved his drink. Willie could be regularly seen tipping a paper-wrapped libation in my early ambulance days while sitting on a front step adjacent to King Street's market building. Later in the day, sleeping on a bench or in an alley harming no one. He was the kind type, still exuding pride in himself, unconcerned he had less than others.

Who knows what his story was? He could have been an executive before his social realignment. Our first meeting was at the bus terminal, the location, a red herring. Willie was a continuous resident of the city's core for as long as I knew him. Arriving at the scene with an arm slung out of the passenger's window, I enjoyed the warm day at hand.

Our summons was for someone down on the sidewalk in front of the terminal. It had to be a bonified emergency. A gaggle of curious onlookers blocked my initial view of the victim. Although there were no tears, my brief service to the sick and injured cleared up that misconception. The public often does not react to terrible sights until later. Cardiac arrest victims are a perfect example.

Dismounting the old SUV-style ambulance, Hugh, my partner today, a five-year veteran of the industry, spoke right up. In a low voice, as we wheeled our stretcher and oxygen kit to the patient, he provided the introduction; "you're going to love this guy. It's Willie, the whistler."

That's when it struck me. There are no trees around here. Why do I hear a bird chirping? The streets in our Forest City are always a luscious green in the summer. There was no green here, just concrete, glass and steel.

Admission to the patient was the swing of an arm as we approached. The reaction to our arrival today was the smiles from parting onlookers as we made eye contact with our would-be victim. Sitting on the ground with his legs crossed was a smiling middle-aged man sporting lots of whitening whiskers, the fellow's tanned complexion, likely from his appreciation for the outdoors.

Although Hugh was driving, he initially addressed the patient, "Willie," he said, "this is my friend Chris." For the moment, I was taken aback. Willie never skipped a note continuing to croon out this bird call, validating the crowd's behaviour.

When Willie stopped, I connected with him by asking what type of bird the chirp was mimicking. I knew the tune, but my ill-spent youth had been more aligned with high school football, weightlifting and hunting groundhogs than bird watching. With the proclamation that it was a Cardinal, I was ready to conduct business and addressed why we were hailed. "Want to hear a Blue Jay," he replied?

I think I was the only one not laughing at my unsuccessful attempt to control the situation. For the moment, that power was not within reach. The next call had you wanting to buy a bird feeder if you were a homeowner. In an earnest attempt, I addressed Willie as "Sir," asking the leading question: "how are you feeling?"

Now with a stomach full of "come alive for a dollar five" (That was the current cost of the cheapest wine at the LCBO). The evidence was shrouded in a brown paper bag on the sidewalk; how would you feel. The flawed question drew more laughs from the gallery. "What can we do for you?" I asked this time. We obliged the request to help him stand up, a reasonable one since he was blocking the sidewalk.

The appeal made more sense once I followed the patient's eyes and acknowledged the approaching London police officer who left his idling black Chevrolet in the street. Willie was heading off a ride to the "tank," as he referred to the police station cells.

Roy, a seasoned officer, spoke right up to Willie, not having to prove who was in authority. "Well, is it going to be me, or them," his decree? Willie found a new admirer or, at least someone, who had not heard his playlist.

On the way to the hospital with no specific complaints, the talented fellow entertained me with several melodic impressions of local birds. There was a short chat before handing him off to an unimpressed ER nurse.

I discovered one of the rarely shared trade secrets of Willie's truly amusing talent; a set of broken and discoloured dentures. Gaps between the false teeth allowed him to force air through the irregular space, adding to his range and sharpness of the calls.

Honestly, he didn't need to pull the dental appliance out to show me the cracked acrylic tooth, nor the debris from meals long past. Leaving the department a few minutes later, I could hear staff laughing as he offered to entertain roommates in the ER. Willie shared several seasonal bird calls over the years until his migration south.

The Bickerson's

Who wrote: Love is full of many splendored things? Marriage is another "thing" for some people. My favourite married regulars would cross my path for years, eventually succumbing to age and poor lifestyle choices. Often arguing, the couple would exchange slobbering kisses as if to make up before one left the other for the hospital, the first of many rituals to brand them with their distinctive trademark.

The couple really were harmless, often calling for one patient, then finding both needing our help when we arrived. Ralph and Darlene were a sight; both led hard lives, not only with drinking but in tandem with financial hardships.

They added some spice to their behaviour, attracting a host of anti-social habits along the way. Our love birds challenged responders and caregiver's patience every time they were in my presence. Most medics had a story.

Despite this behaviour, their antics garnered a following of all those they met. I often wondered if Mr. and Mrs. were the retired couple, stars of the 40's radio show "The Battling Bickerson's." I am not quite that old; my parents often spoke of the "olden days" when radios preceded television on a Saturday night. Ask a kid to look it up; they will likely stream an episode before you could say MP3.

Ralph

Ralph and I met shortly after I started in the industry. As the new guy, I was limited to attending to the patients, not yet receiving the nod to drive. John and I were working the day shift. We were sitting at the office downtown when a call landed in the radio room for a VSA.

A three-letter-moniker, it is the acronym for vital signs absent. Simply put, an industry term to describe a pulseless, breathless patient in cardiac arrest. This and serious car collisions were the pinnacles of calls early in my career, testing the training given to all as a baseline.

Steve leaned out of the radio room with a smile after hanging up the direct 911 police line. In his familiar thick English accent, he announced, "here's a dead one for you, mate." As a dispatcher, he would often be the only one left at the office to do call-ins. Needing replacement staff for the balance of an open shift or the next tour, dispatchers would call medics at odd hours.

Still living at home, mom would answer the phone. When Steve called, he would ask, "can Chris come out to play?" When mom and Steve finally met, she took a step back and said later he was the old English comedic actor Terry Thomas's spitting image. Steve must have heard this before; he was always using the radio as his stage. I think he realized we thought he was a blast.

John chuckled as we pulled out of the bay. He was so laid back; it was probably my enthusiasm that gave him his laugh for the day. The call was to the central fire station downtown at York and Waterloo. It was the building that, years later, would become London's EMS headquarters.

In the business for several years, John was a quiet but humorous fellow with his dry wit. He knew more of the history back in the day when we had our issues with Fire. Thankfully, it was a relationship that has improved drastically over the years.

I was still innocent, offering service as a volunteer firefighter and working for the ambulance service. Did it show that I was an over-eager responder? Little did I know at the time, the professionals held us, fire hobbyists, in poor regard.

This call would leave a sting; what an understatement. Pulling up to an open bay door facing Waterloo Street, a fire crew surrounded a man on the ground. Working diligently on the collapsed victim, a lone firefighter was performing CPR. I recognized him as Terry, having met previously on a call where I assisted the fire service. An experienced rescuer, he had the situation in hand.

Our job now was simple; assume care, and transport to the hospital. There's always a catch. John and I got to the victim's side, stretcher and ventilator in hand and were pleased when our rescuer gave a good report. Terry stated that the incident was witnessed, and resuscitation began immediately. This rescuer was full-on heroic, doing mouth to mouth, never losing a beat.

Our patient was heavy set, putting us to the task of safely loading him on the stretcher then into the vehicle. Stopping only to add a simple plastic airway to aid in ventilating the victim, we dashed back to the ambulance to load. Comparing my limited ambulance service experience to this seasoned rescuer was an error. I made the mother of all mistakes.

I chose to "load and go," an outdated principle of patient care when we could only offer the basics in a pre-hospital setting. Hindsight will always be 20/20; complete your assessment. This was a glowing example.

With less than three minutes on the scene, this poor fellow was now well on his way to the expert help awaiting in the ER. In a dash around the second corner, I stopped compressions and braced myself. Something caught my eye. Did I see him move his arm or not?

The chances of seeing a patient in cardiac arrest be successfully resuscitated before receiving some specialized drugs and a resounding jolt of electricity through his chest was a mere million to one. Did I have a save, my first? Had the initial rescuer and I redeemed this fellow? Is life ever that simple?

The same principle applies to ambulance work that applies to that deal you just negotiated when buying a used car; if it looks too good to be true, then it's likely not true!

Looking over his shoulder through a well-aimed mirror, John saw the hand the second time, as did I. In a grinding halt, while bouncing over the railroad tracks, we came to a stop. Turning in his seat, John yelled: "Ralph, get up!"

Crap was I surprised when our deceased victim propped himself up on one elbow. Ralph promptly pulled the airway out, issuing a belly laugh that propelled the odour of an inferior vintage wine into my face.

It was a move that pushed me back on the crew bench, wondering what my next maneuver should be. Only then did I stop to look. I spotted the crust of wine and spittle around Ralph's mouth camouflaged by the long whiskers, a positive reminder to double-check the basics.

It wasn't enough that Ralph let a two-hundred-pound firefighter thrust his full weight down on his chest, threatening to fracture ribs. This character admitted a four-inch plastic tube into his throat, then more compressions from me, something that would see most of us gag. To boot, he now dared to sit up and laugh at us.

John informed me later that he became wise to the prank while leaving the fire station. There is no substitute for road experience when it comes to this job. Finishing my patient assessment now; this fellow had no complaints.

Staff waiting for our patient at the hospital quickly resumed normal operation, abandoning the resuscitation room when Ralph arrived in tow. He was laughing at all the fuss.

Roll the calendar ahead two seasons. Cleared for driving duties, I was just getting comfortable operating an emergency vehicle in the city. It sounds simple enough until you realize that the medic driving was also responsible for assisting junior attendants through the rearview mirror. The multi-tasking assignment was as distracting as texting and driving, especially with less than two years under my belt.

The job was enjoyable, being paired with a medic with some experience. Dan came from a smaller service, though all EMS road time is valuable. We hung out together, learning from each other's past calls.

After a double patient transfer from University Hospital down to the cancer treatment clinic then returning, it was time for a break. We checked in with our dispatcher before leaving University ER; we could not get a break. A family delivered their sick child to an adult-only hospital. He now needed transport to the original Children's Hospital downtown.

Our hearts were in the right place. There is nothing like a sick kid to curb a whine before the first peep. The little guy was a joy to meet and transfer; Dan kept him amused with the gadgets around him in the ambulance. A brief blast from our siren doubled his laughter and startled his accompanying nurse. It was confusing for the few people out strolling through the University grounds, hearing the siren without the lights flashing.

With a quick change of linen at Children's hospital, we were a block from the office when Jimmy's voice popped out of the old tube-style 2-way radio mounted under the dash. The only dispatcher to snicker at me on the radio, you knew he was preening his handlebar moustache, giving us this call. He favoured the senior crews having their coffee, probably their second break!

They say truth is stranger than fiction. This is worse than a case of déjà vu. We were off to the central station, London Fire headquarters, for a VSA. I had not met enough pulseless people yet to forget.

With half a dozen or so dead people under my belt, I could remember each one. The previous cardiac arrest at the fire hall was covered in my next sentence to Dan after acknowledging Jimmy's call. We both roared at my description of Ralph up on one elbow at a complete stop on the tracks. We couldn't be so lucky today. I was crossing my fingers that it wasn't a firefighter in distress.

What do you know? A different bay this time on the Waterloo side, there were three to choose from? Here it was, the same sight, a fire crew, bent over observing, hands on their knees surrounding a person on the ground in front of a pumper. Kneeling beside the victim, the good Samaritan was in full CPR mode. No one looked upset at the ghastly sight before them.

Approaching behind the rescuer, I walked around to look at the patient and size up the situation. In an unbelievable set of circumstances, it was Terry. My heroic rescuer from the first VSA call here. This unconscious patient was in for a detailed assessment, a lesson learned six months ago.

Although I was driving for the shift, I was better positioned to assess the patient's airway standing by his head. Dressed in a wrinkled and noticeably soiled suit jacket, cleaner shaven this time, was Ralph.

He had been sweating; salty perspiration stained his dark jacket. Was it the warm weather? Maybe he did have a heart attack this time? A small trickle of vomit ran from the corner of his mouth.

The rescuer was back on the mouth to mouth again for two breaths after a quick fifteen compressions. I was about to do a pulse check when I saw it; an eyelid flickered. Flabbergasted, I did a pulse check for the requisite time.

There it was, a carotid pulse, regular and strong. Giving a less than professional "shake and shout" manoeuvre, the term for checking a victim's responsiveness, I yelled in his ear. "Ralph, get up." Like raising the dead, Ralph sat up, almost striking Terry in the motion.

Standing up and walking around to address him from the front, I accused Ralph of playing a sick prank on the firefighters. I stopped short of demanding he apologize to the rescuer.

Turning to Terry, I did not have the tenure to dress him down. I politely informed him that this was the second time I had seen him doing CPR on the same victim with identical outcomes.

His coworkers could hardly hold it in. I left thinking that doing mouth-to-mouth on Ralph was enough punishment for his actions. I venture a guess his crew took care of the rest. Over my career, I have done mouth-to-mouth three times on adults and another three babies. Bonified dead people.

We resorted to mouth to mouth in "the old days" when faced with a breathless patient's dilemma and no equipment within reach. Paramedics did not have small ventilator bags for neonates or infants in the early days. Of the six, only one infant vomited in my mouth. Thank God!

Ralph and I met several times before he finally died. Years after, his wife Darlene was placed in a nursing home and came to the same end. He called for minor issues, except when a roommate in his boarding house robbed him one evening, striking him squarely on the head. He got the best of care, never offering any trouble. Ralph was in his eighties the last time I responded to care for him.

Darlene

Now, Darlene, she was a real case. She could turn vicious in a heartbeat; there was a mean streak brewing inside her for sure. She and Ralph lived in the east end of our city, on the second floor of a 4-unit building. We would be faced with lugging her down a set of stairs fit for an athlete. Very narrow, the handrail was long gone. The only saving grace was that you could lean against a wall on the way down to steady yourself.

She would get on that old green plastic rotary dial phone and call up the ambulance service, mostly when she had been drinking. I seldom treated her during a real medical emergency, though she faced a few.

Darlene was the unfortunate recipient of a below-the-knee amputation. Her sentence came at a time when there was less assistance offered to patients to cope with the activities of daily living. I am unsure if it was through a traumatic incident or a medical condition where she parted with her leg.

At our first meeting, she called us for a fall. The emergency today, the result of a fascination with sherry, Darlene's favourite drink. It was "sherry, made right here in London," she was quick to tell you when you asked what she had to drink.

In tandem with imbibing, Darlene liked to take regular breaks from lugging around her prosthetic leg. This was the most significant single contributing factor to her habitual falls.

Crutches were still necessary to help with both legs under her and an unsteady gait. In her case, the wooden sticks were not the perfect substitute when she abandoned the replacement limb either. Using them demanded that she hop-forward using the single remaining foot.

Darlene would want some food or another bottle of her sherry, hopping to the other room to retrieve her sustenance. She was no spring chicken, in her sixties and built like a pear, she struggled to stay upright. An athlete would have to be on her game to hop around with the imbalance caused by the missing appendage.

Often, Darlene's calls for help were accomplished by pulling yards of cord across the floor to retrieve the phone. Our assignment; simply respond and pick her up, returning her to her chair. The lounge chair, badly soiled, flattened cushions, was a green cornerstone in the living room.

The only upholstered furniture there, it was her roosting place day in and day out. If that chair could talk. After just a couple of calls to the apartment, you could tell she was sitting in that chair when she bellowed down the stairs on your arrival; "come on up, boys," like an audible GPS.

You were her friend when; you were attending to her, paying homage, fetching a glass of water or a tissue. Often Ralph would be out and about the city, so she was fending for herself.

On one such occasion, we had done our thing; she had no medical complaints. She was settled in with her water, so we gave her our parting message. "Don't call us again tonight unless there really is an emergency." The statement, conveyed in a softer, friendlier tone if you were there to hear it!

Offended and without warning, Darlene hoisted her pseudo leg turned non-lethal weapon by its strap. From its idle position leaning on the chair and in a swinging motion, the fake gam caught me at the wrist.

The pink plastic leg with the black shoe, no sock, took me by surprise. My ego, the only victim of a sucker swing!

Second, only to the locally made sherry, Darlene's other vice was her love of cigarettes. There was that overflowing brown glass ashtray on the small table next to her chair. It was an offensive testament to their relationship. Over the years, there were several close calls with the glass receptacle. It was always in our way to get her onto our stair chair and down to the street.

On past visits, evidence of Darlene's missed attempts to hit the ashtray left their mark. Butts littered the already dirty and stained hardwood floor below. It came as no surprise to be assigned one evening to a fire standby call, the task to support our firefighters and potential victims for a reported fire at her address.

No apartment was given on the initial call, though it was a kicker to see Ralph sitting on the front lawn. Rescued by firefighters, Ralph was coughing and spitting soot on the sidewalk. His once white sleeveless undershirt and face were now covered in dark carbon stains.

With a second unit requested in the event that there were two victims, I began caring for Ralph. My partner, Colin, brought the stretcher up to join us. I approached Ralph with the oxygen kit and first aid bag, unsure what I would find.

Ralph descended the long narrow stairs in sock feet. Surprisingly he wasn't burnt, just smoked out of his place. Despite hacking away, he was doing well. Fighting the oxygen, some gentle persuasion and my firm grip on his wrist, he relinquished his control leaving the mask in place.

In this circumstance, you never knew just how long he had been in the smoky environment. Ralph needed the hospital trip to follow up with blood work to reveal just what got into his system.

Fooled before, experience teaches you that you can never tell from arms-length what was inhaled. Some patients that express the most displeasure at the thought of a hospital visit wind up on a ventilator admitted to the intensive care unit.

With an elbow from Colin, I turned to the front door of the four-plex to see a couple of firefighting friends exiting with a writhing, screaming Darlene in tow. Too generously proportioned to lift using the "fireman's carry," Darlene was lifted fore and aft (a medics approach); one rescuer lifting under the arms, the other attempting to cradle the lower half behind the victim's knees.

Making the process more challenging was the imbalance of missing one leg below the knee. For safety's sake, patients need to cooperate. Darlene couldn't be further from the mark! With a fresh "F" bomb to greet us, we turned to welcome her, now lying on the lawn beside Ralph.

Remaining in the smoky apartment several minutes longer than Ralph, she was in a foul mood. Obviously, short of breath from the smoke inhalation, it was difficult to tell just how bad it was.

Medics usually judge a patient's distress comparing to the task of speaking in complete sentences. Using full sentences demonstrates the least affected breathing. A patient's malaise will present in sentences shortened to three, two, then one-word passages.

With her persistent use of the same one and two-word expletives, we assessed Darlene in moderate distress. Adding to the difficulty was her history of being a heavy smoker. I could relate, although I had never smoked a cigarette. A few years of fighting fires as a volunteer had me puffing a couple of times, too stubborn to wear a breathing mask and tank.

More concerning was the burn to Darlene's intact leg. It was the one closest to the table with the ashtray in her living room. We exposed the burn, covered by a loose-fitting dress. Now darkened and wrinkled, the rayon-like fabric shrunk, reacting to the heat.

It wasn't a deep burn but very painful. There were bits of the fabric stuck in the seared flesh. The smoke's odour, some burned flesh and hair added to the normal fragrance present during previous patient assessments.

Offering their oxygen, firefighters stayed close by to keep an eye on her. I asked the crew to set up a mask and give it to Darlene as Colin ran back to our unit to check on an ETA for the second ambulance. The team pulled up with a silent arrival, lights-no siren, just as Colin walked back to our impromptu triage area.

Hailing a fire captain, I asked what happened inside. He was close by on the lawn, taking a rest. The air tank was still on his back, face mask dangling from the regulator strapped to his waist. He explained that a fire started in a chair, likely careless smoking. I described our history with the patient and centred her out as the suspect from our prior experience.

The Florence Street station captain stated they found Darlene lying on the floor close by the chair. That was after they passed Ralph at the top of the stairs exiting the smoke-filled apartment. I asked the fire officer if he had seen her prosthetic leg and received a negative response; it was worth a shot. Telling him just how important the leg was to her, he waved a colleague over, giving his crew a command to check upstairs.

Moments later, two firefighters exited, removing their helmets and air masks. The second fellow out of the door held the fake leg by the ankle. The last time I saw the fibreglass appendage being held instead of attached, I caught it on the wrist. Luck was on my side tonight.

Following the crew were two other firefighters carrying Darlene's badly charred chair. The exiting firefighters threw it out on the lawn to be doused again by an awaiting team assigned to protect the exterior.

It turns out both Ralph and Darlene were drinking tonight. Surprise. Darlene likely fell asleep and dropped her cigarette into the chair alongside the cushion. As responders, we had all dealt with this scenario before.

The second crew transported Ralph, laughing and happy to be outside in the fresh air. He pulled his oxygen mask off to talk to neighbours as he was wheeled away. Darlene got the lights and sirens approach on route to the hospital. At the time, we were not sure she fared as well with the additional smoke and the burn.

Darlene wasn't in a life-threatening condition, though with the combination of injuries and the constant cursing, it was worth the emergency approach to transport. The siren partially drowned out the noise she was creating. The trip was shortened by a couple of minutes.

Darlene recovered, suffering a minor burn and getting over the smoky experience. They never lived there again; she wound up in a nursing home. Ralph declined the opportunity to share a room with her, outliving her, probably a conscious decision.

Big

In the past, most paramedics considered someone to be morbidly obese, with a starting weight of 400 pounds. Oh yes, approximately 180 kilograms. We transitioned from imperial measurement to metric during my career. Today the medical community has assigned the clinical term "bariatric" to describe obese patients.

Fortunately for paramedics, only a few patients in our community met this criterion in the early days. Our wheeled aluminum stretchers were old school. Rated for a maximum of 550 pounds. This included the 80-pound stretcher itself. Today, following decades of horrible lifting injuries suffered by medics, technology has graced the industry with powered ambulance stretchers and a hydraulic lift on a specialized vehicle. How times have changed!

In my early years, there was this six-hundred-pound, six-foot-six-inch tall woman with a house full of kids; they were her caretakers. She was lucky; we were more fortunate. In all our encounters, she always wanted to walk to the ambulance.

Not suffering from any other physical ailments, she was plagued with mental health issues. I escorted her to the ER several times. The woman would climb out of the depths of depression and walk away from follow-up care. Our last meeting would be to remove her deceased body and transport her to the morgue. Now there was a sad story and not a pretty one.

Lock the door

Then there was the fellow living with his wife in the one-bedroom apartment; thankfully, there was an elevator. The fellow was able to walk, but we still needed to get him up from his waterbed. He was a whopping six hundred pounds and shorter than your five-foot ten-inch author!

We would arrive more than once to find the patient on his back on the jiggling mattress. The vinyl bladder bulged along its sides; the man was unable to get out of bed. You would think, so just roll him over to the side of the bed and sit him up. The saga only starts here.

Some disconnected health care providers suggested the water bed for comfort. A home visit would have been in order before the decree. The bedroom was barely large enough to hold the kingsize bedframe within its walls. There were no tables, dressers or other furniture within.

The double bi-fold closet doors at the foot of the bed were removed so you could still access the clothing. You needed to stand on the watery surface to view the contents of the compartment. The door to the bedroom was opened when the bed frame was assembled. Long trapped along the side rail, the damaged mahogany door offered no further privacy.

This call marked the first occasion that I called upon our firefighting friends for some help to lift. There were no more EMS crews left at the time to assist. The other four teams faced their own predicaments.

In a conversation with the patient's wife, she was out of options getting him to a local family doctor's office for care. House calls had long since vanished. Remember the good old days? I can remember my doctor visiting the house when I was a kid. This fellow's distress began during his efforts to climb off the bed.

With help from the arriving firefighters, two of us climbed onto the mattress, now a taut plastic vessel. If this bladder burst, we would all surely be drenched. The residents in the four apartments below in the building would follow suit. Standing with one foot on the side rails, my water walking friend and I pulled, then pushed up on the patient's shoulders from the head end of the bed. This maneuver was accomplished as the patient gripped a re-purposed aluminum tube from our portable stretcher held in front of him.

Four more helpers stood on the bed's foot rail holding the tube. Backing down into the closet opening for leverage, they finally pulled the fellow into a sitting position. With a few well-placed hands on the metal tube, we assisted in turning our patient towards the bedroom doorway. This scene would be repeated several times over a couple of years.

On a subsequent response, his wife invited me to the kitchen to discuss his current predicament. I never varied off the direct route from the front door to the bedroom during previous calls.

In concert with the family doctor, his wife, a calm soul, attempted to control the patient's food intake. She installed a sturdy metal hasp on the fridge door, secured with a padlock. On a later visit, a second hasp and lock had been added.

For most bariatric patients, caloric intake is only part of the overall problem. I wondered for years if he found the hiding place for the original key. Or did he learn to pick the lock? It was a sad case; his wife deserved a medal. I never heard the outcome for this fellow.

A test of our empathy

Another bariatric victim, Helen, was the subject of numerous calls over several years. Often in need of medical attention, we would be summoned to assist her to the hospital. These complex patients receive care at home through provincially administered programs, but they have limits. Mobility was her most significant barrier, often trapped in bed for days.

Helen would get enormous open sores on her legs and hips that we would find covered in dressings. Bandages were usually improvised using folded menstrual pads. It was a terrible sight; unable to care for herself, her dignity vanished. When she needed immediate care, we would respond to transport her to the local ER.

On one such occasion, I was called to the apartment, now working as a supervisor. Five paramedics stood deliberating on safely getting Helen out of bed, freeing her from the cramped room. The second phase was also difficult due to the smaller elevator. Our contemplation probably sounded like a gaggle of geese when there was a knock from behind us at the propped open door.

By the crest on his jacket, the fellow was delivering for a local pharmacy. Expecting medications, I stepped to the door to accept the package. Our patient was unable to get up. What I faced was a depressing sight. Startled by the unfamiliar greeter, the man held up six plastic shopping bags.

Three held two-2-litre bottles of a sugary soft drink. The other three bulged with 200-gram bags of potato chips. I accepted the roughly 11,000 calorie consignment with regret.

That was a turning point for me, realizing that a bariatric condition is truly an illness. This young lady was blessed with a good sense of humour and a pleasant personality. Over time, she received treatment for the condition. She lost several hundred pounds, having started at 700.

During her recovery period, she wrote the medics an open letter. The unsolicited note apologized for the undue burden she caused the crews. She announced her commitment to following through with her plan. This was one of those heartfelt letters that you knew took some strength to write.

Sadly, she fell off the recovery plan and succumbed to the illness. As much as you might think there would have been some remarks by responding medics, this young lady received all of our empathy. The experience mimicked an alcoholic falling victim to the disease once again.

Bacon, skip the eggs

Now one of my favourites, Walter, a middle-aged fellow, was plagued with problems. We had all seen him on the streets for years, most often carrying a plastic bag with pirated (shoplifted) mouth wash. It was a quick source of alcohol. He was a harmless soul who led a regular lifestyle before a string of bad luck. Drifting from place to place, he appeared in all corners of our city's core.

Working alone as a supervisor, a call came in for a collapsed patient. There were enough identifying details to raise suspicions that it was Walter. We were out of ambulances at the time; I was just down the street. It was a hot day, one that caused most of us to sweat just standing still.

Arriving at the scene, this was a busy thoroughfare for afternoon traffic escaping the downtown. Yes, Walter was lying on the boulevard. At his side was a large plastic bag. Marking my presence with emergency lights, traffic changed lanes as I exited my parked vehicle.

Walter had his medical issues, though most of the time, he was merely intoxicated. This latter condition tends to reduce a medic's initiative to do an assessment. That preconception should end with the realization that the state is indeed a disease worthy of care and support.

Rolling around on the ground, Walter announced he consumed one and a half family-sized bottles of a mouthwash breath freshener. It is a feat most of us could not perform.

To address his concerns about abdominal pain, I asked to examine Walter's belly. He was less than cooperative, a typical behaviour. Receiving permission, I began to systematically touch the area through his shirt. We were out in the open so exposing his abdomen was not practical.

At the same time, I also asked if he was hiding anything that could hurt me. Asking about needles and knives and receiving a negative response, the risk factor was resolved.

I ran into a bulge that you could quickly feel through the patient's shirt and my examination gloves. The thin blue vinyl gloves became the standard for personal protection in our industry a few years back.

It was a hot day; my hands were sweating in the gloves adding to my startled reaction. What I felt after working my way around the bump gave me a sick feeling. Finding a squishy, warm mass that felt flesh-like, I asked if it hurt when I pushed.

Again, an unremarkable finding. Pushing firmly but gently for a final time, I jumped to the conclusion that Walter earned himself a colostomy along the way. The exposed bowel tissue forced out of his belly was now protected by a sterile plastic bag.

The bowel, prolapsed or protruding from his belly inside the plastic barrier, posed a possible surgical emergency. Curiosity got the better of me as the responding crew radioed in my earpiece they were on route to the call.

If I could lift Walter's shirt, the yellow-stained one, hanging loosely over his waist, the view would confirm my interpretation of the warm mass. No blood or feces was staining his shirt. Hopefully, the bulging bowel and blood were trapped in the colostomy bag, a receptacle intended only for waste.

Lifting Walter's shirt, there was no containing my surprise if you were within viewing distance. Breaking into a belly laugh, it was likely interpreted as unprofessional to passing afternoon commuters. My pose went from squatting to collapsing onto one knee. Caught off guard, I was unable to stand while laughing at the moment.

It was a relief to see Walter wasn't ill. I mean, seriously. He didn't need the grief. He would die a couple of years later from other medical complications.

Tucked partway into Walter's waistband was a 454-gram plastic package of raw maple-flavoured bacon. Shoplifted, likely at the same time as the two-one litre containers of alcohol-based mouthwash in the well-worn plastic bag at his side.

The bacon had long since surrendered its cooler temperature from the store. It was reduced to a slimy, squishy mass in its clear plastic package. Eureka, the secreted breakfast meat relinquished its disguise, no bowel to see here!

Cathy and Gary, the arriving ambulance crew, would usually be disgusted to see Walter rolling around on the ground. We had all dealt with his shenanigans before. The only upside was his fresh minty breath. I was hoping my goofy smile was interpreted by them as; this is your call. Really, the smirk was, have I got a secret for you! Their laughing response returned on cue as; thanks a million, pal.

In my haste to throw the crew a light-hearted curve, I missed the approaching police car, now parked behind my SUV, blinking out a warning. The medics and the officer shared the lane along the curb, following my lead with their emergency lights.

The constable was not in a pleasant mood, seeing a frequent flyer, now denying any malady. The constable was unable to hand off to EMS; the shoplifter was his.

In what could best be described as a marginally medical report to my captive audience, I included the details of Walter's libation today. Before I lost their attention, the news also shared the discovery of the abdominal anomaly. The cop missed the humour and went on the offensive, asking about the mouthwash and bacon's origin.

Walters apoplexy was not a clinical condition. I believe this was his measured response having a litre and a half of the minty fresh alcohol solution onboard. If he had a conscience, it was a sad attempt to cover his inability to produce a receipt for his partially consumed possessions.

The last the three of us could see of Walter was the back of his head swaying from side to side in the police cruiser's rear seat. All while telling the officer he wanted the bacon back when he was dropped off at the detox centre to sober up. At least that's my educated guess.

Bottoms up!

Dad told very few stories of his service in WWII, though a favourite was being piped into battle in Sicily by the Black Watch. I witnessed dad's tears at my wedding when we hired a lone piper to surprise him; it was also his birthday. There are Irish and German roots in our family way back somewhere. I am unable to explain my soft spot for the pipes.

They say treating patients like family would take you down the right fork in the road. A persistent caller, Scotty, fought in the second war and paid the price. He suffered from "shell shock"; today, we call it PTSD or post-traumatic stress disorder. Dad suffered a similar version of the wound.

Both men shared several things in common. Dad and Scotty gave service to God and Country, had fragile sentiments and a relationship with alcohol to cope with the emotional pain. Our city continues to care for our veterans. It was Westminster Hospital in the day and now our Parkwood Hospital.

Introduced to Scotty for the first time, I didn't pick up on what my senses were trying to tell me. Our meetings began to follow a regular pattern. Calls were more frequent at the first of the month. Trips into Westminster Hospital were the routine.

Adding to his pain was the recent loss of his wife. Scotty returned to the same treatment for his sadness, rye whisky. Each month when the cheque would come in, he would pay the rent. His second assignment was a trip to the liquor store, making the journey by taxi.

One of my early calls to assist Scotty was after a slip and fall while carrying a case of his favourite brand from the cab to his door. The driver called for the ambulance via his dispatcher and stayed with him until we rolled up. The cabbie called him by name, a sure sign of a regular customer.

Not injured, we helped the veteran up the one flight of stairs to his apartment. I carried the case of booze up, so he could focus on the climb. It was an early assignment as an enabler. I carried similar things for dad.

When the supply was fresh, we would see Scotty daily. There were days when he would call, crying and lonely. Neighbours would add to our call load when Scotty would fall inside his apartment and attract attention through the locked door.

The building superintendent knew Scotty well. Also, a veteran, the superintendent was sympathetic, letting us into his apartment to assist him up into his chair or back to bed. Most calls we attended were for assistance and not to transport him to the hospital.

The calls for help went on for over a year when it dawned on me. If you interrupt the supply, our business might drop off. We went almost three weeks a month without a hail for assistance. I thought about it and waited for the opportunity to try out my theory. It was a different time then.

Responding one morning with my Supervisor, Harry, the day started out with a bang. A young kid was struck by a car crossing the street to join friends on the way to school. As luck would have it, the winter coat and brushing off the side of the vehicle limited his injuries to bruises and a scare. One that would leave him bragging about how tough he was to his friends tomorrow. Barely clear of the ER, we were reassigned.

Both recognizing Scotties address when Steve droned it out, we recounted how it was a new month. I missed the most recent call reports, so I suspected we were first in line for his inebriated antics. Harry gave him the benefit of the doubt. Also, a veteran and very religious, he did not drink and was involved in helping others with the problem.

Arriving at Scottie's apartment, we left the stretcher in the small front entrance. The stairs required our folding chair if we needed to carry the patient. The hall at the bottom of the stairwell was too narrow, another reason to check the situation out first.

Sitting on his sofa, Scotty called us through the door. Announcing the open door, you could hear him sobbing from the hall.

Sitting on the gold couch, the furniture showed its age and experience. Cigarette burns dotted the arms. In Scottie's one hand, a cigarette, the other, was reserved for a half glass of his whisky. It was only ten-thirty in the morning. My liver shivered silently in sympathy.

Harry stepped aside to let me address Scotty; I was attending. Despite being against drinking, Harry was empathetic and sincere as he patiently let me search out the reason for today's call. Scotty missed his wife, a common cause of his emotion. The tears were brought on and probably exaggerated by the alcohol.

Speaking vet to vet, Harry stepped up to ask what we could do for him today. I stood and stated I was going to find Scotty's medications. I was really on a "seek and find" mission for the booze. I was rewarded when I reached the kitchen just steps from the living room.

Sitting on the end of the counter in a heavy cardboard box were eleven bottles of rye. Next to the box was bottle one, over a third gone. It was the second of the month. Scotty was a day behind.

It was an experiment. Interrupt the supply, and maybe just maybe the call load would drop off and bring Scotty to his senses. It was worth a try. Calling Harry to keep him busy, I only worried about twisting the first cap off.

Turning each quart upside down in succession and leaning them against the side of the sink, the glug glug was deafening to me. It took a few minutes; each bottle was re-capped and set back in the box. Just as the last bottle began to drain, Harry stuck his head around the corner, curious about the delay.

Shaking his head, I replied to Harry's disapproval with "this is his only hope." It was also our only hope to pare back the calls. Job complete, I returned to our patient to confirm that he was "ok" and not in distress. Scotty was calm now. We wished him well and told him to call back if there was an emergency.

Clearing the apartment, I bet Harry we wouldn't be back. I left a bug in Steve's ear when we returned to the office to send me on any runs to see Scotty if he knew I was on shift. Checking daily, we went a whole week without a call.

I went on to meet Scotty a few more times. He smoked like a chimney, but I never found a case of booze in the apartment again. He couldn't be hiding it; you couldn't hide the calls. I never saw him cry again. That's not to say he never had a sad moment from time to time.

The last train

One sad, recurring predicament with the lion's share of life's regulars is their inability to break the pattern. Stuck in a loop, they are often helpless to escape the limitations that life's circumstance has held them, prisoner, to. My patient described here beat the odds. Bravo!

Dennis and I worked together regularly over the years. Coworkers first, then enjoying recreational SCUBA diving, we chummed around. Sporting some similarities in our sense of humour, we enjoyed the shifts.

On this tour, we would both meet a fellow for the first time. This gentleman was down on his luck. I would realize years later that there are always two sides to every story.

Dennis was a cop in a previous life. Some of his cynicism lingered in our industry. I forgive him; I worked hard to balance my doubts in people seeing them on their worst days. It is a real job as a responder to avoid falling into the trap of becoming a professional skeptic.

Receiving a hail for the report of someone lying on the railroad tracks would be incredible for some. Having seen several deaths due to a railroad misadventure, this incident was just another day at the office. Most of the calls were made after the fact. The damage was done. We were only there to confirm the caller's findings.

Oscar, our patient, chose an excellent time to seek help. It was daytime; bright sunlight blazed overhead. The air stood still and was as hot as hell. The engineer could see the trespasser way before he could stop the passenger train. Wheels screaming steel on steel, the locomotive and train went hundreds of feet beyond the point of impact.

Getting into the ambulance at the office, I thought the drama would be over in a heartbeat. Dennis echoed my synopsis. Both seasoned for a couple of decades in the business, it was all over but the paperwork. I was attending the call. Even as a shift supervisor, Dennis owned the ambulance service and was my boss and driver today.

The call details from dispatch were for a person lying on the tracks a few yards above a road running parallel. Intersecting close by was a major thoroughfare; the tracks over it were supported by an old steel bridge. Our hearts were in our mouths at the thought of having to climb a steep embankment for an obviously dead guy.

Arriving at the scene, railway staff walked back to see the damage left behind by the five-car passenger train. The feeling of complete helplessness cannot aptly describe the emotion when an engineer is involved in a collision. I have talked to a few. The pit of the engineer's stomach must turn over as the engine under his control strikes a trespasser on their tracks.

The man at the top of the hill waved us up as if by habit. Composed and not frantic, the methodical motion of his arm read, "come on up, I have something to show you," not "holy shit, I just ran over a guy, help." The nonchalant gesture would contradict the facts in less than a minute.

Climbing up the steep incline, rocks the size of apples covered the hill. Castoffs from the roadbed above, the moving stones induced trips and stumbles all the way to the top. Grabbing on to sumac stocks provided the only lifeline to avoid a Jack and Jill moment. Sorry, Dennis, for this story, you are Jill.

I was sweating like a pig, well before reaching the tracks. Dennis fell behind; it was a shame. He would have to make another trip down and back before the call was over. I looked after number one and left the first aid kit at the bottom of the hill. You needed both hands.

Reaching the rails, there were multiple sets of tracks. Off to my right, the train station sat nearly a half-mile off in the distance. Another railroad man a hundred feet away stood over the patient. A human figure lay between the tracks. Halfway to the two, the victim helplessly raised a hand. The conductor backed away with the motion.

Surprised that the patient was still moving, I figured there was no collision, just a close call. It had been an intentional close call. Within the last ten feet approaching the victim, I could see why the railroader moved back. The waving hand was dripping blood.

Lying between the tracks was a tall slim fellow. In his early twenties, he wore jeans and a plaid short-sleeved shirt and runners. You could tell he laid in the sun for a while, face and neck burnt to a crisp. He was either stoned or very stoic; he had not shed a tear. One leg and an arm straddled the now idle tracks.

The trainman confirmed that he talked to his dispatcher on his walkie-talkie, and the tracks were shut down for the time being. Passenger trains were just slowing down here in anticipation of the train station a minute away. Still nervous, I turned a couple of times to the sound of a passing truck below and behind me.

Standing beside me, Dennis was equally surprised at the live victim. I had just started to check him out. Touching a track, my knee was repelled by the hot steel. Talking as if intoxicated, I asked the young fellow what happened. The crying started.

A backpack lay next to the tracks. With the crying, it was time to have a look for clues. Sending Dennis back for some bulky trauma dressings, I called dispatch for an ETA on our police response. We could use the help, finally portable radios to save steps.

It was apparent the train ran over part of his hand. Crushed flat and turned black were his left pinky finger, the last half of the ring finger, and a small section of his hand where the smallest finger joined the palm. There was not much blood, a common sign of a severe crushing injury. The bleeding now came from waving and shaking the hand.

Years before this incident, I treated the victim of a lower leg amputation caused by a train. That wound was sealed from the pressure. There was about a tablespoon of blood that day. Train trauma often induces a version of shock beyond the physical part that leaves the surviving victim speechless. The absence of pain is a delusion for a brief period.

Listening to me, the young fellow let me hold his hand to examine the injury. The rest of his body did not have a scratch. The engineer beside us now described how he spotted the patient lying between the tracks feet first towards the train.

In the final moment, the victim purposely lay his left hand partly across the rail. It looked like the train wheel grazed the hand, pushing it down inside the rail away from the force. Dispatch replied with our unit number " two minutes," my hands were too sticky to acknowledge the update.

It was not good fortune that he survived the passing axles, air hoses and steel undercarriage hanging from the train. He must have laid very still. There was not a scratch on the rest of him after rolling the patient on his side to check. Broad marks crossed the victim's back and legs. Evidence of having lay on the oil-soaked wood ties beneath him smelling of the petroleum-based wood preservative creosote.

The sun was baking us all. There was no time to waste. I wanted to be back in the air-conditioned ambulance quicker than quick. I was convinced that this kid could walk after his near-miss. We just needed some help to get safely to the bottom.

Dennis followed the first cop up the hill. Dropping some large pressure dressings, stretchy Kling gauze, a foam board splint and a bottle of sterile water by my side on the railroad ties, he commented on the heat.

The constable, balding head never mentioned the heat. The sweat ran off his bright scalp, minus his forage cap. Good thing there was no sergeant around to catch that detail. You could tell looking into the cop's eyes, this was his first railroad slash crush injury, turning away as if there was another reason for being here. I had never seen him on a call before today.

I told Dennis I thought we could walk the kid down; he looked relieved at the notion of not having to do the whole spinal board thing. Our victim reacted to the decision by attempting to sit up. I wasn't ready for that. Placing a hand on his chest, I motioned to lay still until I finished dressing the hand.

Wetting the bulky gauze pads before covering the crushed digits, the pain of removing the dressings in a few minutes in the ER would be lessened. I used the foam splint in the pile of supplies to support his hand and wrist. Explaining that he had to stop moving, the command penetrated his intoxicated head.

He did not smell of booze rather a sour chemical smell. Diabetics have a similar "ketone" smell to their breath during an emergency. The smell today was one I was not familiar with. Not able to answer our questions, I asked the police officer to look in the backpack. I was expecting to see drug paraphernalia.

Not knowing what he was unpacking, the cop brought a plastic shopping bag out that held a can. Opening the bag, the odour wafting out in the heat resembled our victim's breath. Paint?

Turning the open can for my benefit, the officer did not recognize the contents. It held a few hundred millilitres of wood glue. The brown pasty product was partly a paint thinner or similar chemical that sped up the drying process, leaving behind a hardened wood-like filler for repairs.

Working near a couple of communities rife with vulnerable teens, I learned the effects of this stuff a few years back in northern Ontario. Wood glue, gasoline or model airplane glue; can induce a poor version of euphoria. The lasting effects are horrible. It was cheaper than booze or street drugs but left some permanent damage.

Our patient stood without a hitch when we gave him the go-ahead. Slightly unsteady on his feet, we would be there to help him down the hill. Dennis found a nearby path used by locals as a shortcut. Remaining on the slope, the trainmen and constable were a minute away from reinforcements arriving.

A sergeant exited his cruiser as we arrived at the roadside. With his forage cap tilted back and a swagger in his walk, I had seen his confidence on other calls. The cop on the top would be in for a "jab" for his missing headgear. Hopefully, the sunburn on his head would hurt worse than any discipline for being out of uniform.

The nurse on the radio patch asked for a confirmation on the injury being the result of a train. In the cool shady confines of the ER, I guess it didn't make sense to be up and around after that report.

We left our young fellow to the trauma hawks in the emergency room. A couple of young docs heard the nurse announce the incoming patient's injury after hanging up the ambulance patch phone. The plastic surgery team would have their hands full with this kid over the days to come. Or that's what I thought.

Sharing the story around with medics after the call, it didn't take too long to hear this guy hit the "regulars list." Behind the market building downtown and in alleyways, he cropped up intermittently for over a year. The healed hand injury was the earmark to inform the responding crew that this was the wood glue kid.

Wood glue was Oscar's choice of intoxicants. He was really on the shortlist with visits to the ER for intoxication. No one seemed to get the more significant issue. Substance abuse, although not from alcohol or street drugs, was pointing to an illness. Where was the cure?

Going on a year later, Brandon, my partner for the night tour, had me hopping. A lot younger than I, he was savvy with the nurses and had to be poked with a stick to get out of the ER's at times. Clearing the department following a routine transfer from a nursing home, the medical patient would not be returned tonight. He was too short of breath.

As a supervisor, I had the pleasure of working in the core for over two decades. The heart of London is the mecca for street people and regulars. Clearing a call from any of the three hospitals, you could be sent anywhere in the city.

The hospital was in our rearview mirror as we planed our midnight snack. There were several options up in the north end. Announcing your availability on the radio is mandatory. Expressing our disappointment in facing a reassignment was optional. We exercised the opportunity with a mutual grumble as I lit it up, heading for an unconscious patient in a stairwell in an apartment building.

On the way, we agreed that a returning resident to the building would have to wait to let us in. Other apartment dwellers would not answer the intercom with a request for help from a random choice of buttons in the lobby.

Luck was with us; the pathfinder led us to the patient as we left our stretcher by the door. Oxygen bag in hand, Brandon followed the fellow who discovered the victim after returning home from an evening shift. I begrudgingly carried our new semi-automatic defibrillator, hoping to leave it in the case for some younger, more ambitious medic in the morning.

Arriving in a back stairwell of the three-story walk-up apartment building, the nook under the concrete stairs was dark to begin with. Unlit from the failed bulb above, it was inky with only a sliver of light from the rear parking lot through an emergency door.

Rolling out from the cranny under the cement steps were a few unintelligible sounds. I could see how quickly passing by and seeing a running shoe poking out and receiving no response could lead the caller to the unconscious part.

Brandon received a responsive grunt when he slapped the victim's foot. A wake-up from the beam of my flashlight changed our game plan. Young Oscar raised his head from his backpack, doubling as a pillow. It had been a year since we had faced each other. Only his legend bridged the absence.

Wearing an ankle-length dark coat that was split up the back for riding horses, jeans and runners, our regular propped himself up on an elbow. Looking out from his cave as if cheated out of his nightly shut-eye, he came around quickly though never acknowledging he recognized either of us.

Hand well healed now, he grabbed his bag when we told him to come out of his resting place before the cops rolled up. Our greeter agreed he did not recognize Oscar as a resident. Suggesting we go to the hospital instead of getting a trespassing charge registered through his befuddled senses.

Leaning in for a closer smell, old faithful was back. Asking Oscar to open his knapsack to prove he did not have anything that could hurt us, he obliged. The plastic-covered can of his favourite wood glue lay across some books. Some soupy contents darkened the inside of the shopping bag.

Denying anything else was bothering him, he asked to go to the hospital. This was a change. He carried on a short conversation on the way past the waiting stretcher that we towed back to the ambulance. Returning the unused gear to the truck was a welcome alternative to working an unconscious or cardiac arrest call.

The ride into the hospital was a bore; Oscar sat slouched in the jump seat at the front of the patient compartment, looking at me through the divider. Strapped in to avoid rolling out of his seat on a corner, our victim missed most of the trip. Taking him to the ER in the core, he needed more help with substance abuse and mental health issues than the closest hospital could offer.

Dropping Oscar off with the emergency room staff, it was a busy night. The hustle and bustle must be from walk-in traffic; we were having a good night. A disappointed nurse stood listening to Brandon's report as a familiar doctor passed by with a suture tray in hand. He shook his head with an air of disgust.

Leaving the department in a couple of minutes after talking to Gail at dispatch, we cleared with our eye on the goal. Food awaited us downtown.

Pulling up in front of a favourite souvlaki stand, we both sealed the deal on a foam box of shish-ka-bob and some fries. The danger; the contents were an absolute artery clogger but the reward of choice for a night shift. Besides, we had the rest of the tour to work it off.

Eating in front of the television in the upstairs lounge seemed like the right thing to do. There was work to do later, but that could wait for now. That was until the carbs sunk in. Then neither of us could get out of our chairs.

The only phone on the second floor rang three times before Brandon could get to it. The other crew had not returned yet, so we were up for all calls by default. Things had picked up. Setting the red handset into its cradle, I could tell from Brandon's stare at the wall below the phone we were assigned a call neither of us would like.

"We know this guy" was not the introduction I was looking for. Hearing that someone had a train run over their hand in one of the rail yards didn't click at first. It couldn't be. It had only been two hours since we left Oscar in the ER.

Going for the upside, if there could be one, I suggested that an engineer or someone fell off a train segment shunting cars in the yard and suffered the injury. As terrible as that could be, it seemed more likely than Oscar since the scene was almost three miles away from the hospital.

Gail broadcast the update to look for our patient at a phone booth near the street. The patient walked out of the yard for help. Our caller still sounded like a frantic railroad employee trying to get to help on a night shift. Maybe his walkie-talkie was smashed, and that is how we got the hail instead of through the train dispatch centre.

Pulling into a commercial plaza in front of the train switching yard, I visited this phone booth before. Calling for a heart attack patient in a car in the day was not convenient; only a lucky few owned cell phones. Tonight, a dark figure stood at the door of the aluminum and glass enclosure.

Any suspense we harboured was dispelled in an instant with the long dark coat. Pulling up close, I rolled the window down. "Oscar, what have you done?" brought on the tears. Telling him to stand still, he obliged in a defeated stance.

Rolling the stretcher up to Oscar, a morose silence surrounded our patient. Coming from the same hand, as the legendary injury, blood dripped steadily on the pavement below. Brandon opened the kit and began preparing bulky dressings. Things changed slowly in our business; the powers that be in pre-hospital health care started to supply gloves.

Having covered our hands in latex on the way down the road, we were ready for the red stuff. Neither of us really thought we would be with Oscar again on the same shift. Hearing the call was for a victim near the tracks, a quarter of a mile from the downtown ER, the possibility of a repeat patient would have been a no-brainer.

Tonight marked the loss of Oscar's ring finger, second finger and his hand up to the wrist. Left from this pulverizing insult were his index finger and thumb. Hanging from the uninjured portion of the hand were shreds of fingers and shattered bones, exposed. On this occasion, Oscar remained outside the tracks laying his left palm onto the rail.

Flattened, blackened skin and tendons still moved involuntarily from the input of the remaining appendage. The sight was frightening. Now wrapped in a bulky dressing, Oscar's hand still fit up the riding coat sleeve. We obliged his request of "no blood on my coat," in turn, he complied, willingly climbing onto our stretcher.

In a repeat conversation from the first train call, I asked if he was injured anywhere else. His weak reply cleared our suspicions. Brandon asked before I could get the thought out, "What happened?" His thoughts clear now he knew what the problem was. "They let me out."

Rolling Oscar into the ambulance's rear, Brandon and I agreed it was time for a code four run into the same ER that we delivered him to earlier. Looking over the sheet and blanket covering our victim, he offered a surprise exclamation.

"They let me out too soon." When I asked what he meant, he replied, "If they keep me in, I clean out." Asking if that's why he put his hand under the train to get some time in the hospital, there were "puppy dog eyes" and a flood of tears that Brandon had to face for the ride in.

Our trip was fast and thoughtful. The radio patch did not elicit an inquiry to do with patient familiarity. I did not include the hint that might give someone a chance to arm themselves with an attitude. This kid was hurting in more ways than one.

Arriving at the hospital, there was little fanfare until we arrived in the room set aside for trauma patients. As luck would have it, the doc from the previous visit finished his shift between the two ambulance calls. I think I would have spoiled our relationship.

Sending the charge nurse the stink eye, I motioned to her that I wanted to talk outside the trauma room. I explained the first run to pick up Oscar on the shift in a nose-to-nose talk. She was aware of the history, so there were no wasted syllables.

Appealing to her sense of compassion, I shared the second incident and our patient's request for help. Taking the position that Oscar stuck his hand under a train twice to earn himself some extended time in the hospital to detoxify, she agreed.

The nurse promised to take the attending doctor aside and recommend a social worker and psychiatry referral. Making my thoughts known just made me feel better after our victim fell through the cracks earlier.

So, the doubts laid out in my introduction to frequent flyers painted a stock picture of some paramedics' impressions of the helpless. Everyone is entitled to a helping hand; Oscar was no exception. Our paths never crossed for years.

On a day off, I sat idly at an intersection, delayed by a traffic light; something caught my eye on this sunny afternoon. Standing at a bus stop waiting for a ride was a young fellow in a jacket bearing a college's markings. Slung across his back was a backpack chuck-full; it too took the same college insignia.

Seeing the fellow marking time for the next bus, his hand reached up to adjust the heavy pack. Missing the requisite fingers for a match, it was Oscar. He turned himself around, cleaned up and looked as sharp as a pin. He wore glasses now.

I have never seen him since, though second first impressions must carry some weight. He looked like he was on the road to success enrolled in some course. I never want to meet him again. I hope he carries the same wish.

The Author's Musings

Regulars can make you want to; laugh, cry and stomp your feet, all within the same call. Repeat clients will always be a part of our public service. It would be irresponsible to blame anyone for the resources and effort required to serve those who demonstrate the greatest need. Correcting the issue will not be a short-term task. It will involve our legislators, healthcare, education, our judicial system, and the list goes on.

A simple response would be to react negatively when faced with repetitive clients, no matter what discipline you work for. Taxpayers expect the public service delivery system to do just that, deliver. It is difficult for responders to avoid some cynicism, burnout or judgement after years of service. Most experience these reactions to one degree or another. Others come to work each day up to the challenge; they are professionals.

Personal experience will also affect job stressors, both positively and negatively. Organizations serving the public go to great lengths to maintain professional standards through training, supervision and consistent performance. I still believe the person shouldering the ultimate responsibility for helping is the individual putting the uniform on and hitting the street each day.

9

Vignettes from Richmond Street

(Emporiums or vomitoriums?)

Every town has a main drag. In my teen years, London's Dundas Street was the "drag." Running between Ridout Street and Adelaide, the stores and bars were magnetic. Our parents went downtown for a drink and to listen to Jazz or the Blues. Kids were dragged downtown to buy clothes and gifts, returning annually by the carload to see the storefront windows decorated for Christmas.

There were some excellent restaurants in the city's core. Bars that did not serve food were referred to as; "beverage rooms." Separate areas were defined for men and women to drink. Liquor laws were different then; draft beer sales were expressed in "gallonage." Dad would recite and brag about the statistics. Young drivers with muscle cars could be seen doing "burnouts." That was until the police pulled them over.

Sidewalks were dotted with teens and street folk in the afternoons and evenings, all looking for the action. It was a place to meet friends and hang out. You were legendary if you were seen cruising in a muscle car! Returning to school on Monday, kids at my high school would be huddled in groups. The topic was either a party or what went on out on the drag on Saturday night.

People lived in the core in apartments above the stores on Dundas. Still, others resided in hotels, often billed out by the week or month. Then there were the street people living in alleys, nooks and crannies or homemade shelters behind buildings.

Somewhere along the line, Dundas Street faltered and was all but silenced. Theatres went dark and re-located, a family-run seafood outlet dried up. Beverage rooms fell out of favour as the laws became more liberal. Others updated their approach to licensed liquor, food-serving establishments.

It was an early attempt to recover and adapt to the changing times. A real hit was felt in the heart of the city when our anchor stores: Simpson's, Eaton's and Hudson's, went the way of the new malls situated outside London's core. Some survived by moving. Others disappeared.

Facing the loss of stores, affordable living and even grocery outlets, downtown seemed to wither. Office buildings kept the area alive but in distress. The historic market building survived until time and circumstances permitted a welcome revitalization. The formation of a retailer's association continues to propel the core to new heights.

The most significant anchor in the core now is the arena and entertainment centre. It is home to our Ontario Hockey League team, the London Knights. They were one of the few attractions in our city that came from London's fringes to the core. A winning move for all, the venue hosts concerts and events between the team's matches.

A few retailers envisioned opportunities that others missed or continue to monitor cautiously when it comes to retail. Although not referred to as the main drag in past times, Richmond street was always there, plodding along. A preferred location for some, an experiment for others. Some smaller "one-off" shops were purveyors of designer clothes, accessories, and specialty items in the eighties.

The older brick and mortar infrastructure was starting to see a resurgence of retail and services. Boutiques, flower shops, chocolatiers, and carryout eateries appeared in a rather phoenix-like phenomenon through renovations and unique ideas. The Grand Theatre survived and looks grand, surrounded by a variety of shops and restaurants.

Richmond Street was being resuscitated financially and socially. I know that sounds somewhat Utopian. Guess where the new "drag" is now. Stretching from York Street north to Oxford, Richmond Street, branded as Richmond Row, the route is rarely idle.

Licensed specialty restaurants and bars are flourishing. Microbreweries are not seen as a fad anymore. Crowds of socialites from the university and college regularly fill the streets. Locals frequent the eateries and watering holes, many offering specialized drinks and foods for the discerning palate.

Adding to the reasons to visit Richmond Street are those special occasions. The days and nights when the younger crowd overwhelm the streets enjoying the experience, libations, sights and sounds. Homecoming, St Patrick's day, and Halloween, to name a few. Friday and Saturday nights continue to provide the steady infusion of business, keeping the drag prosperous.

During the daytime, retailers depend on the curious for an opportunity to offer their goods and services. As the day wears into evening time, the crowd morphs into the socialites, the early birds. Some do the dinner thing and a stroll, while others clear out before the night hawks descend.

Lights on, the stores, restaurants and bars compete for your attention and business. In the warm weather, the spots with patios overflow onto the street. Bars have security staff with taped-off lanes on the sidewalks to define their anxiously awaiting patrons. For the life of me, the process of lining up to drink escapes me.

In colder weather, including sub-zero nights, arriving patrons exit vehicles sans winter clothing to protect them. You might think that it would only be a short stroll to the front door of their favourite establishment. Leaving coats behind might even save coat check costs.

Nope, it comes down to looking chic. Ladies, sporting that little black dress, bare shoulders, tight jeans on the guys. Colourful tattoos adorn both men and women arriving to party the night away. It's cheaper than an online dating service.

It gets cold out there. Lineups, sometimes exceeding one hundred, routinely delay admittance for over an hour. Many late arrivers joining the end of the line never see the inside of the clubs. It's all about socializing while stuck in the queue.

You would think that spending time with others in an upbeat environment would bring out the best in folks. My sister and I were raised to be on our best behaviour. Mom spit-washed my cheek before sending me to that birthday party with a gift under my arm. I thought I was prepared for anything. Sometimes, the opposite behaviour befalls the Richmond Street crowd.

Inquiring minds might question the long introduction. Getting past childhood memories and history, the answer is simple. With these attractions come people in throngs. The very reason that EMS exists is to serve people.

The most innocent are simply curious. Shopping, dabbling in the eats and a drink. If they feel robust following their meal, there might even be a stroll up and down the drag to see the sights. The following memories did not seem so innocent.

Cool Cat

Halloween, for some, simply put, is about the treats. Wearing a costume in your younger years, you are empowered to be that character. Who wouldn't want to be Superman, a Princess or a Ninja Turtle for a night? Over the years, it was a fireman, soldier and hobo for me. For some older kids, the night is about tricks and treats with alcohol.

One such Hallows Eve found me working with Joanne. We were busy earlier with a nursing home run for a fall. The patient required sutures or stitches to the chin. Luckily for the patient, the mishap was benign. It dictated a return call for us to get her safely back to her bed. In the day, our service was responsible for all patient transports, both emergencies and routine. That changed in 2000. We are strictly an emergency service now.

Following the return transfer, I dragged Joanne up to the dispatch centre to collect the daily paperwork. The radio room was located above the train station on York Street. For every call, there was a dispatch form and a patient form. The documents had to be filed together daily. In my early days as an EMS shift supervisor, I was still enthused with the paperwork. Besides, we could chat with the dispatchers and get a look at the big picture.

Standing in the radio room overlooking York Street, we were treated to some mini chocolate bars. Our uniforms were costumes, sort of. One dispatcher wore a headband, a tiara. That's when the princess waved her imaginary wand and sent us to a bar on Richmond Street just around the corner.

Exiting the second-floor communications centre, we were going for an intoxicated female. It was a weeknight. We hadn't paid the dues to get to Friday or Saturday yet. Before we went mobile, another crew was dispatched further up Richmond for a fight.

Our portable radio crackled to life with updates for both crews. Our patient was out in front of a bar. The other unit was directed to hold back pending police arrival. What did the police know that the crew needed to know?

Pulling up in front of the bar, it took a quick U-turn to get the loading doors next to the sidewalk. We were protected from passing traffic. Stepping out onto the street, you could see a trend here. People in costumes lined the sidewalk. The bars were holding competitions for the best outfit. Music spilled out onto the street from dance floors.

Joanne and I were met by singing patrons, poorly conceived outfits on some. There were no prize winners here. Walking past us in costumes were a police officer and princess wearing a wedding dress from years ago. Our approaching patient was being supported by a witch carrying a black plastic cauldron. In it were her winnings, a "T" shirt bearing the name of a favourite beer.

The cat. Our patient had seen better Halloweens. Dressed in a skin-tight black bodysuit was a generously proportioned young lady. I would bet she could not arch her back tonight like the traditional silhouetted cat in the cartoons. Not passing judgement; I am an overweight guy, but a bodysuit. Ummmm, not this guy.

The preparation and makeup before the escapade started were outstanding. Frisky black ears were attached to a deely bopper style headband, replacing the original bouncing antennas. The eyes were done well; the tip of the kitty's nose blackened.

The whiskers were comical. Pussy cats fuzzy black pipe cleaners, now bent, were still stuck to her cheeks. Was there crazy glue involved? That would hurt coming off later.

Slung around our cat's neck was a brass-coloured plastic saxophone. Hanging limply from her back, she was dragging a three-foot-long tail. It was attached at the waist, coming from the bottom of a black belt, a good plan. Adding a liberal amount of alcohol was a doomed variation from a successful costuming scheme.

Our patient was in trouble. She was incapable of standing unassisted. Kitty experienced some nausea before the hail for her EMS trick or treating characters. Fresh cat food, AKA mushy potato chips, ran down her chest. There looked to be some debris in the mouthpiece of the sax, sidelining an ill-conceived musical.

Then it struck me. There was a musical currently on Broadway that featured cats as the main characters. Our casualty was an actress that got off the bus too early. Wrong, she was a Halloween reveller gone astray.

You would think kitty would just return home to curl up in front of the fireplace. It was not to be. Friends left her with a witch and bid her goodbye. A criticism offered by her crutch sporting the pointed hat. I could hear our counterparts further up Richmond. The dispatcher updated their call details with a cancellation. The police arrested their patient before the crew arrived at the scene. No paperwork, bonus!

Loading the wobbly feline into the side doors, she denied any other ailments. The cat's discomfort was relieved by propelling the treats onto the street and her faux fur earlier. I was driving on this run. Joanne was compassionate but short when Kitty started to wretch slowly, then more violently, gaining speed. It was a wonder she didn't pull up her claws. I am referring to the patient.

The brief ride to the ER gave our patient time to consider her plight. A crying cat with runny makeup is so sad. She was doing better now and declared she would make it into the hospital under her own steam. With the witch in tow to register the cat, we delivered our vomiting feline to awaiting nurses. There were no costumes here.

The last we saw of the cat lady, she was behaving very well. Cats can have a conscience too. The witch had gone mad, screaming through the porthole in the plexiglass that separated the waiting room from staff. The sorceress was insistent that she be allowed to sit with the cat at her side, what a scene.

Observers

Very early in my career, I was mildly intimidated when under the scrutiny of a manager or supervisor. There was nothing to see here. It must have started during adolescence. My sister dumped me in the soup once when she told Dad I hit her.

The victim of some corporal punishment, the sentence was a spanking. It would be my last. I was taller than Dad shortly after. The truth came out later that there was no assault when sis had a massive guilt trip. My mood was somewhat reticent after snickering when she got a spanking for telling a fib.

Our call rolled in at lunch hour. Jimmy was working on a sandwich in between rings on the phone and "10-4's. In a whining voice, he announced, "a motorcycle just wiped out at the Canadian Pacific tracks on Richmond just south of Oxford." Rob and I already responded to a collision earlier on the 401.

It was a no-show; the drivers sideswiped each other in a failed passing move. Both cars were in the ditch, interiors covered in dust from open windows. The rubber was still on the road; there were no injuries. It had been almost two hours since we moved.

Hugh and Art were into their lunch, Rob volunteered us up for the call. Standing within arms reach was our assistant manager. Oliver, in his late fifties, was an ex-military fellow. The word in the lounge was, he served as a demolition expert.

There was so much doubt. This fellow was a bundle of nerves; his hands were constantly shaking. Oliver would stand around talking, chewing on the ends of the arms on his glasses. The ones with huge lenses, they were in fashion.

He tried to talk the talk like he had seen it all in his service to the country. Maybe he was a cook? I guess he could have experienced something exploding in front of him, perhaps a soufflé. That would make me shake.

Oliver spoke up in his "take-charge" tone, "Let's go, boys, I'm going on this call." Responding in a three-piece suit with a huge tie, he was the best-dressed medic. What had we done to deserve this? Working in 150 today, it was a 1972 SUV equipped with off-road suspension and four-wheel drive. An oldie, it was still in the blue and white colour scheme. The truck cab had a bench seat, so the three of us scrunched in together.

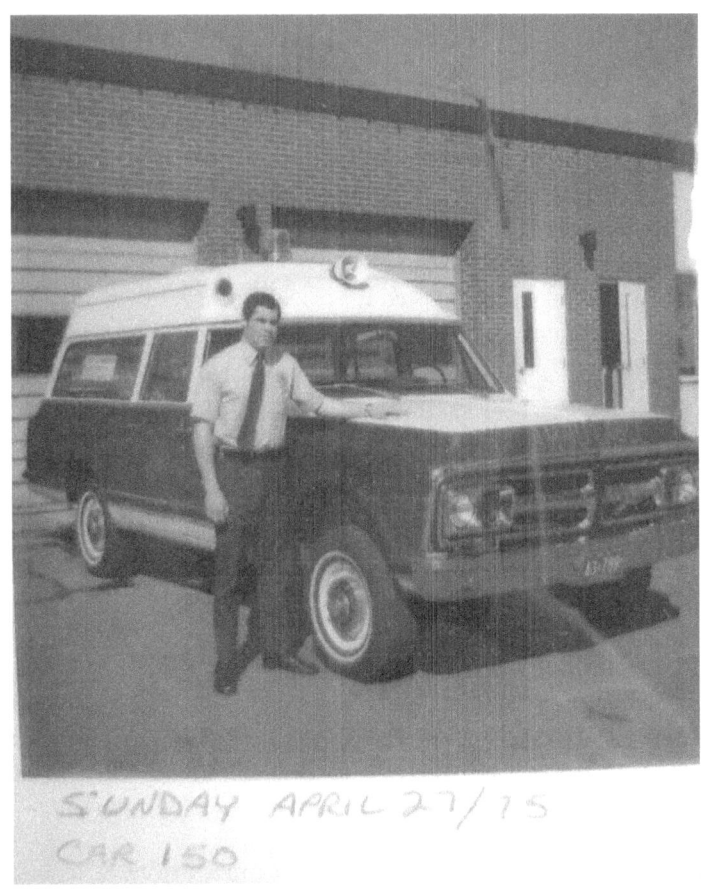

Rob could hardly reach the siren control mounted under the dash, now hidden behind Oliver's swaying left knee. His feet were next to mine; the 4X4 floor-mounted gear shift precluded great posture. This was worse than being on an overbooked school trip on a bus. Giving the ride of a dump truck, the ambulance bounced over the CN tracks around the corner from the office.

I was doing the radio work; Oliver was blocking Rob. He had enough on his plate. Jimmy piped up, "the call is right on the tracks; I had the cops call CP to stop the trains." As I acknowledged the call, Rob looked over at me, leaning around Oliver. We exchanged the; is this going to be a nasty or what look? Our manager resembled one of those dogs with the head bobbing from the back deck of cars in the day.

It was midday on Richmond before it became the drag. There was still lots of traffic around. Drivers were dodging the crash to get to their all-important lunch meetings. As we climbed out, a citizen approached us, offering his name as a witness; he was pale. Both of us replied in unison, "Wait for the police."

Following us around, Oliver looked more like a guard dog than an observer or our manager. We loaded a backboard, first aid kit and oxygen on the stretcher. Leaving the rear of the vehicle, we walked around the ambulance and up to the tracks.

A group of onlookers stood taking stock of the situation. None offered first aid to the patient. The witness was nowhere to be seen now. We were starting from scratch, with no first aid or story. The patient was on all fours, like a wounded dog unable to limp.

The biker appeared to be a seasoned enthusiast, clad in leathers and a poorly modified helmet with a sticker to indicate the make of his motorcycle. On the rear of his headgear was the official declaration of his blood type "B positive." It was a typical American soldier's move during the recent war in Vietnam.

Kind of a rugged-looking guy; he was not to be messed with. He was whining like a child. I was thinking, what would other bikers say? Is all this over your smashed bike?

Kneeling to greet him, his injuries took me by surprise. The wailing stopped; his greeting was more of a grunt; "I lost it." There was no car around, so what could have caused this? I had been to several minor motorcycle crashes where the rider laid the bike down to avoid an impact. Bikers spent more time inspecting their ride in sorrow than on their injuries. It should have been a walk-away incident.

Doing a quick turn, I surveyed the scene. The black bike, leather saddlebags and lots of chrome from front to back lay on its side. There, just south of us in front of the ambulance, was a nasty pothole. Popped out of the cavity was a crumbling asphalt divot the size of a melon.

It looked like our biker hit the pothole, or did he hit the solid divot? Turning the front wheel abruptly, the rider was thrown from his ride. So, it should have ended with a western roll and recovery. That was what our gym teacher taught us, learning the high jump. Remember, I was the chubby kid; I never got it right. Unfortunately, neither did our patient today.

Forward motion and gravity came into play after leaving the motorcycle; you can't fool with science. The leathers prevented a single scratch on the victim's torso. That's great, I thought. The well-worn, gauntlet-style leather gloves protected his palms.

The problem, physics, did take its toll. The traction provided by the gloves stopped the rider's hands on a dime. Well, actually, their forward motion was ultimately quashed by the first rail. The palms of his hands went down into the space running alongside the railroad track, locking them around the steel ribbon crossing Richmond.

The arriving police officer climbed off a beast, similar to our patient's. Still wearing his helmet, I looked up to see the expression on his face. "That could have been me." His second expression threw me off. His eyes were riveted to the crowd behind us. I turned to see Oliver, pacing at a feverish pitch.

Oliver was not cut out for this stuff. He attended the intro course to EMS when he was hired. That was a formality. I've got five, 1975 dollars says he would faint if he got blood on his hands. No shame in that, though he invited himself; he was no help.

Continuing to grunt now, our patient rolled over onto his buttocks. He was holding his hands, palms up, writhing in pain. All I could think at the moment was, *this must hurt.* He's probably embarrassed that he is crying.

Crap, I know why he is crying now! There pointing out from beneath both wrinkled cuffs on his leather gloves were his shiny blood-stained radius and ulnar bones. Once upon a time, the forearms were connected to his wrists. Shattered at impact, the force drove the sharpened bones out through the skin. Looking more like a Spiderman pose now; the injury pushed the hands back.

Call it a compound fracture for the experts. The once-over assessment, luckily, did not net another single complaint. There is no discount for multiple injuries.

Our patient's extended hand position was frozen in place by the protruding bones. This was an injury that I had only seen in a black and white photo in a textbook. A pilot came to a grinding halt striking the ground on an ill-fated flight.

Both ankles were fractured off at right angles. The leg bones were visible as they stuck out the ends of his shattered legs. Splintered bones stuck out past the plane's rudder pedals. It was a similar terminal velocity with today's abrupt stop.

What to do now? This would not be a typical splinting job. The guy escaped the incident without another bump or grind. He was "self" splinting in the seated position, wrists balancing on his knees.

Loose, bulky bandages would cover the injuries once we removed the gloves. I wet the dressings down with sterile water, a move to keep the wounds from drying. That accomplished, the whining started again when I got my shiny shears out of their holster.

Designed to cut through anything, including zippers and leather, the buck stopped at the jacket. The rider's weathered coat was a badge of honour, demonstrating experience, passion and association with the elite. Memories to be cherished. There would be a real war story in the future explaining the repairs to both arms. The verbal pushback halted their field alteration temporarily.

Initially refusing the offer to disentangle our patient from his heavy coat, the first attempt to move him to the stretcher changed his tune. The slightest move aggravated the bony injury; his arms maintained the perfect angle for the exiting bones. We made it clear there was absolutely no way to remove the coat with those wrists bent back.

It was going to happen here on Richmond or in the ER lying on his back. The second option was a sure path to the destruction of the hide. I painted the picture, the upside of the bragging rites to the leather repair for the rider. Receiving our victim's permission to cut both sleeves up to his armpits, the shears were drawn.

Mimicking a maneuver fit for a tailor, I cut up the coat's seam inside of each arm from the cuff. It was a slow process but necessary. There was no need to rush; it was all about the preparation.

Rob and I worked together to pull the coat slowly over the patient's back. The plan was to miss the bandaged wrists as the jacket cleared his injured extremities. We were on the same page. Looking to my side, Oliver was stooped over like a "rubbernecker," hands-on his knees, glasses in one hand as he looked on.

Placing our hands under his arms, Rob and I stood the fellow up and turned him to face away from the stretcher. The police officer pushed the cot behind him as he sat on the stretcher, hands in the air. Using the pillow on his bent knees, the patient could lay his wrists on the pad to continue to keep them comfortable. He would be the only one that could ensure his comfort, splinting the fractured extremities.

Oliver was in the way now. In a weak attempt to look like he was part of the solution, he beat us to the truck's rear and started to open the first door. Hesitating, he stood looking puzzled when he could not find the latch to open the driver's side of the rear door. Rob pushed him out of the way, releasing the inside latch to the door.

Without hesitation, Rob ordered Oliver to get in. Thinking our observer would follow, I jumped in beside the stretcher. He was there for the ride only; Oliver ran to the cab's passenger's door and hopped in, already maxed out with the sights and sounds.

The transport was uneventful; the rider only asked once about his bike. Police would send it to the dealership supporting that brand on Wharncliffe. Our drive was taken slowly to avoid bouncing the victim's wrists on his knees. The splinting job was a variation from the norm. No one I talked to could suggest a better method to treat the injury.

Arriving at the hospital, Oliver remained in the cab. Not a single word was exchanged between our manager and Rob during the drive. In the ER, the unusual injury attracted an attending orthopedic doc's attention as we transferred the victim onto the gurney. The day hit an all-time high when the suffering rider was immediately given something for his pain.

Returning to the truck, we found Oliver leaning against a fender, nervously puffing on a cigarette. The ride back to the office was short but informative. Our quality assurance inspector offered high praise for our efforts; he never rode with me on a call again.

A brief spin on a small dirt bike in a parking lot before starting an EMS career, and I can honestly say I never got bit by the bug. This job reinforced the prejudicial notion that I would never ride a motorcycle.

Cashed out

"Apathy: the lack of emotion, indifference or lack of interest." That technically describes the environment on my first emergency call to an ATM, the future of banking. The financial vestibules were initially located adjacent to bank branches and were a popular cash source before the advent of wireless terminals brought to your tableside. Today the electronic currency substitute is the standard.

Now, locate one of these gold mines in the entertainment district, and it was a recipe for success. Close to a bar, it was a hit. The downside, there was no reason for some merrymakers to quit drinking; more money was steps away.

Combine the convenience with heat and shelter, your banking experience was a pleasure. To our less fortunate citizens, it was a close second to bed and breakfast accommodations. Partiers on a mission to restock their pockets with cash provided a steady flow of traffic. You would think that someone would question why a person was lying silently in the well-lit space.

Though I find the practice unacceptable, it is common to see people panhandling. Standing on the island between two lanes of traffic, others sit on the sidewalk bearing a small sign and a paper cup, begging. The plight of the homeless and destitute should touch everyone.

Our victim at the bank tonight was not making a withdrawal or begging. Unless it was for help.

The call was for an unresponsive male on Richmond at the ATM. Gord and I hit the road from our base just down the street at York and Waterloo. A block closer to the core, the former central fire station was a minute closer to the action. You could see your breath in the evening air, jacket weather.

People were getting their second wind with the infusion of cash at the terminal. Arriving, we could see a commotion from the sidewalk through the glass. It was like looking at kids watching fish in an aquarium. Onlookers were pointing, exchanging opinions.

This was one of the first calls I responded to, where the good Samaritan summoned us with his cell phone. Still in hand, as we arrived, it was the size of a brick. Our caller realizing that the 911 call was free, was all too eager to help.

We were sporting a new EMS feature, another tool in the paramedics kit. The AED, an automated external defibrillator, was designed to correct life-threatening heart rhythms. That, along with CPR and oxygen to assist the patients breathing, was a turning point for pre-hospital cardiac arrest. When the patient's ducks were in a row, it worked.

Pushing the pile of gear on the stretcher up to the door was like a short game of dodgeball. Strolling night hawks stopped to see what the commotion was all about. Getting through the door was difficult, with several people waiting for their turn to conduct a transaction. The caller was quick to point out that his good deed was done. With that, the Samaritan left us at the door and was off into the night.

The smell as we entered the irregularly shaped room was noticeably foul. The victim losing all control, our workspace now smelled of feces. Money was obviously a greater priority than a pleasant environment for some. Looking out through the window behind the spectators, two new red, white and blue police cruisers arrived in unison. It was a real sideshow!

Lying on his side, this fellow was dressed in hand-me-downs. Two layers of pants visible were not enough to shield him from the pending midnight temperatures. His back was up against the low stainless-steel enclosed heater. The same source of warmth kept the floor-to-ceiling windows from fogging up. Moreover, it was the catalyst working in tandem with the excrement to foul the air. He must have been warm now, though. Several layers of sweatshirts covered his torso.

A quick check yielded the expected result; he was pulseless. People were continuing to talk and laugh in line, oblivious to the emergency in progress. Police, entering the door into the glass room, looked for an answer. Reporting that we were starting CPR, their mood took a turn. The constable's only question: "Has he been robbed or assaulted"?

I could not answer, honestly. Telling the officers that the victim was "dead" shut the room up, like when I dropped a rose at dinner. As a matter of fact, the foul smell was evidence that our victim had lost control of his bodily functions when he became unresponsive. Add that to the heat, and no amount of money would drag me in to finance a night's drinking. People's expressions turned now to an escape plan.

With that came the very loud announcement; "You are all under arrest, move over and give these guys some room." There were six citizens, four responders and the motionless patient trapped in the enclosed space. All of us, wanting to escape the overwhelming smell, enhanced following the patient's roll onto his back.

Slashing the man's sweatshirts up the middle drew a gasp from one female viewer. Peeling the backs off of the defib pads, Gord connected the AED to the victim's bared chest. Care began with an airway and the bag-valve-mask ventilator. I joined in the process with the first series of cardiac compressions after the pads were connected.

The machine was activated. Following commands, I sat back on my shins as the small electronic "doc in the box" declared, "STAND CLEAR, analyzing." Contained in the shiny new computerized gadget were over four thousand heart arrhythmias. The software sampled the patient's rhythm, then compared the findings to the life-threatening examples on file. The decision proclaimed, "no shock indicated."

For all the training and declaration from our electronic master, the plan; continue CPR and drive fast to the ER. The doc in the box determined the patient's heart rhythm would not benefit from the new approach. I secretly hoped to shock the crowd with the patient's response to 200 joules of current bolting through this poor fella's chest.

The evolving party crowd full of self-importance was now agitated at their temporary capture. They would soon be released. The rank smell providing the only lasting effect of their imprisonment.

The trip to the ER was fruitless. The patient had long since expired. The heat in the room probably accelerated the fatal process. I suppose our homeless fellow could just as quickly have died unwitnessed in his sleep on the banks of the Thames. In this case, passers-by opted out of his chain of survival.

This call begged the question; how could people walk around, step over, or be in the presence of our victim and not wonder? He hadn't moved in some time, though most witnesses were here and gone in a couple of minutes.

For some, the story would end after a coffee break on Monday.

Ralph, NOT the person

So, I promised you a story about vomit. What, like you, haven't heard that one before? Probably the busiest weekend on Richmond Street is centred around the annual Homecoming celebration. The call to higher education brings thousands of students to our city. Their mission? To study, achieve and land that career that will launch them for a lifetime.

The alternate assignment for a lot of scholars is to have a great time and social experience. Some alumna or alumnus from past graduating years, a.k.a. mom or dad, believe that the social experience ranks as important as the educational component. They would have you believe that it is the "rounding out" process. There is a need for balance.

So, there I was, driving fat, dumb and happy up Richmond on the critical night of the celebration. Our home team cleaned up. Two separate radios were crackling with calls for both EMS and our counterparts at the fire department. The computer showed ambulance icons broadcasting their GPS signal as they travelled around the city.

A crew requested the supervisor at the ER for a fresh set of stretcher straps. Theirs were hopelessly soaked in recycled beer by a student leaving a local establishment. Reversing course, I dropped down to Commissioners Road to the cities busiest emergency room.

Issuing the straps to the crew on the ramp at Victoria, both medics mentioned the heavy traffic on Richmond now that the parade and game were behind us. Seasoned paramedics can read the street like a book. A simple drive-by suggested the crowds were ramped up for this particular Saturday night. I returned to the core.

On a regular weekend evening of "clubbing," crowds arrived later. Tonight, the experimental and sentimental groups hit the street early. Sidewalks on Richmond were filled with student's current and past, ranging from their late teens into their seventies. Most were sporting school colours on their clothing, some with painted faces. For this occasion, it was all about getting a seat for the duration.

Several establishments toward the north end of Richmond displayed school colours with ribbons and balloons to attract customers. Line ups were overflowing and very noisy. Making the first pass up the crowded street spelled work. Thankfully, not everyone that is under the weather needs or requests an ambulance.

Getting just north of Oxford, a few frat house partiers could be heard from the road. Students covered the front steps of a century home, all bearing their favourite drink. For some, it was their first bust out at a university party. Others took it in stride, pacing their refreshments.

With a quick loop around the block, it was time to head back to the core. Crews often ask for support on a call with a difficult patient for safety issues. Other teams request a supervisor to act as a witness to sign off the victim who is refusing care. Staying mobile in the core saves the time it would take to pack up and leave the office. There was always time for paperwork when the streets calm down.

The sights on Richmond Street can change in the time it takes to turn around. This tour was the worst for witnessing vomiting in my career. People watching is part of the job. Driving slowly is a small benefit of the marked supervisor's vehicle.

If you read closely, the theme here is food, specifically pizza. Don't let this turn you away from the cheesy treat. Most people keep theirs where it belongs. For some partiers, the end of a long night brings on a voracious hunger.

There are lots of hot spots on Richmond Row for a late-night snack. A slice and a drink is a cheap closer after a great time out. With no dining rooms, the purveyors of pizza turn their patrons out to the street. Some sit out front; others walk, talk and eat. Multi-tasking is a youthful talent.

Driving south, the first pizza guy had a fresh slice in hand, but there was no seating at the location, so he improvised. Perched on the top, I mean the very top of a fire hydrant, was an intoxicated fellow. With a slice in one hand and the paper take-out triangle in the other, he was having a good evening. Swaying, eyes closed, he could have passed for a bull rider at Gilles Bar in Texas.

Now, intoxicated and eating pizza simultaneously, and my personal dance card would have been full. I slowed right down, fearing our rodeo rider was about to fall off his cast-iron beast and hit the sidewalk. Swaying uniformly from side to side, I could tell he had the whirlies.

Addressing the other urgent matter, the hydrant valve that he was sitting on. He must not have felt that operating nut pushing squarely up his, you know! Ah, the pain reflex, alcohol, dizziness, nausea; one or all finally caught up with our reveller. It started as he was going for the next bite of his oven-baked delight.

Taking him by surprise, his expression told the tale. With the pizza at his lips, the man's last few bites suddenly passed the current portion. They were travelling in the opposite direction. The ABC pizza (already been chewed) flew out onto and over the remainder of the midnight snack.

Retching, he finally tipped sideways off the hydrant. Shocked that "rodeo boy" didn't wince as he disconnected; I think his long legs in a wide stance kept him from falling. He was a trooper, though. The remainder of the slice was still grasped firmly in his fist, though I would not want it anymore. Gillies would have given him a Stetson for his performance! A honk of the horn from an impatient motorist behind, and I was off down the street.

Looking out at the pedestrian traffic on a busy night is distracting, to say the least. Thousands of people wandered up the street, talking and laughing or hailing a ride home. Standing out from the crowd was a tall, athletic man wearing school colours.

Looking more like a basketball enthusiast than a football player, the fellow leaned against a hydro pole at an intersection. It looked like he stopped, taking a moment to ponder life and have a cigarette.

Others around him took to the crosswalk when the light changed. I could see his pizza snack now. A smoke and a slice, it looked so simple. As he stood up and away from the wooden pole, his unsteady stance tipped him back against the oversized crutch. He raised the slice up, eyeing it as if to say or think; I have pizza.

With the smoke still in the corner of his mouth, he was saving that hand to steady himself. Using the other hand to aim the snack, he took a bite. On occasion, I remember my Mom sipping pop through a straw with a cigarette in the other corner of her mouth. That was different; it was a long time ago. I don't get it. I'm a non-smoker.

It was a balancing act to get the pizza in without losing the smouldering stick. Success with the first nibble, and it was off to the races for our sportsman. I was stopped in the curb lane a few meters back. Morbid curiosity kept me focused on our smoker. I put the vehicle in park to avoid an incident.

We have all seen a dedicated smoker miss a beat and cough from the inhaled cloud. That's what I thought I was witnessing, but only for a second. The tall guy's chest heaved. In an instant, cheese, dough and condiments came spewing out through pursed lips. Luckily the approaching pedestrians cueing up for the next opportunity to cross were outside his effective range.

Splashing on the sidewalk was a foamy, chunky concoction. The late-night grub was under pressure, airborne over a meter. The closest couple disconnected hands to step back and avoid the splatter. I re-focused now on the expressions of the hurlers surrounding revellers. The friend took on a grimace turning her head, then her body to escape the upchucking volley.

Two more regurgitative moves, and our fellow turned to head south. The last I saw of his head, reaching well above the shorter pedestrians, that cigarette was still smouldering. I will never understand the value proposition of saving the cigarette.

Pulling away from the curb, I got a wave from a young lady. She was sporting colourful deely boppers painted in Homecoming colours. It's only polite to wave back. For those that are wondering, I was old enough to be her father.

Easing back into the southbound stream of traffic between taxis and "J walkers," the pace was slow. Both lanes were alternating stop and go to avoid pausing cars and pedestrians. There was a buzz of white noise as I drove along, windows down in the warm September air. People were hugging in groups, likely classmates from graduating years past. Other gatherings suggested a family tie of mature graduates and their children preparing for next year's class exodus.

Seeking a safe haven, I pulled into a lane alongside a downtown church; it is home to police and EMS on busy evenings. The location exiting onto Richmond Street offers a panoramic view of three clubs, a couple of take-out eateries and strolling partiers.

A lone walker shuffled northbound on the sidewalk in front of me. His footwork resembled a television zombie, suggesting a current condition and not a pre-existing disability. The man was not dressed for the weekend festivities.

Held down by a thumb on a paper plate was the remainder of two slices of pizza. I knew the shop they came from. The owner, a retired military medic, was always kind to EMS. Our corpse would take a couple of steps. When his unsteady forward motion required realignment, he would stop. It took a moment to eat a few mouthfuls of pizza, then carry on.

After several stops, he was at the bumper of my parked SUV. Setting the crust from the first slice down, I assumed he would take a few more steps. Good thing I didn't buy a lottery ticket using the same instinct. Leaning forward, the staggering singleton erupted in a pizzanomi. Showing good form, he clearly missed his still active plate of food.

Only two steps this time, the sleeve on his sweatshirt served as a napkin to remove partially expelled debris. With a memory like a goldfish, the pizza-eating corpse went right at the second slice remaining on the now collapsing plate. Two bites and the taste tester retched into the next eruption of pizza. Oh, the humanity. I couldn't take it anymore and pulled out around him to attend a call further south.

The experience did not dash my love of the marginally Italian dish. Chicago natives would have you believe they were the authors of the recipe. That tidbit I learned on an outing to Chicago eateries featuring their deep-dish version. I finished the tour without another hint of second-hand pizza.

Dogpile

Paramedics compare their neutrality to the Swiss in the Second World War. We provide care, do no harm and get you to the hospital. Generally, we don't care how or what has happened. That is unless it pertains to understanding the injury or illness as it relates to patient care. The exception would be in the case of our safety. For years, medics would routinely walk into calls, not completely informed of the reason for our response.

The theme of violence is inescapable. We would not knowingly walk into a call involving weapons where the bad guy was reported to be lingering. The same would apply to a fight call that has not been resolved. It is bad enough when medics attend to the loser from the altercation. To walk into the line of fire with the pending winner is foolhardy.

The problem with the decision-making process; call details are not always precise. A recent example was the elderly lady reported to have collapsed. It turned out that she had been assaulted (elder abuse) by her grandson; that was a jackpot. The call takers at the Ambulance Communication Centre and the dispatchers at the 911 centre at police headquarters do their best. Our safety is in their hands.

Cruising back to our station, Bernie and I were having a few laughs over his most recent posting. We just left the old Victoria ER. Taped to the wall was a cartoon of the registration area at the front of the department. The sketch portrayed the staff on one side of the plexiglass and some hilarious caricatures exaggerating the client's peculiarity regularly appearing at the window to register.

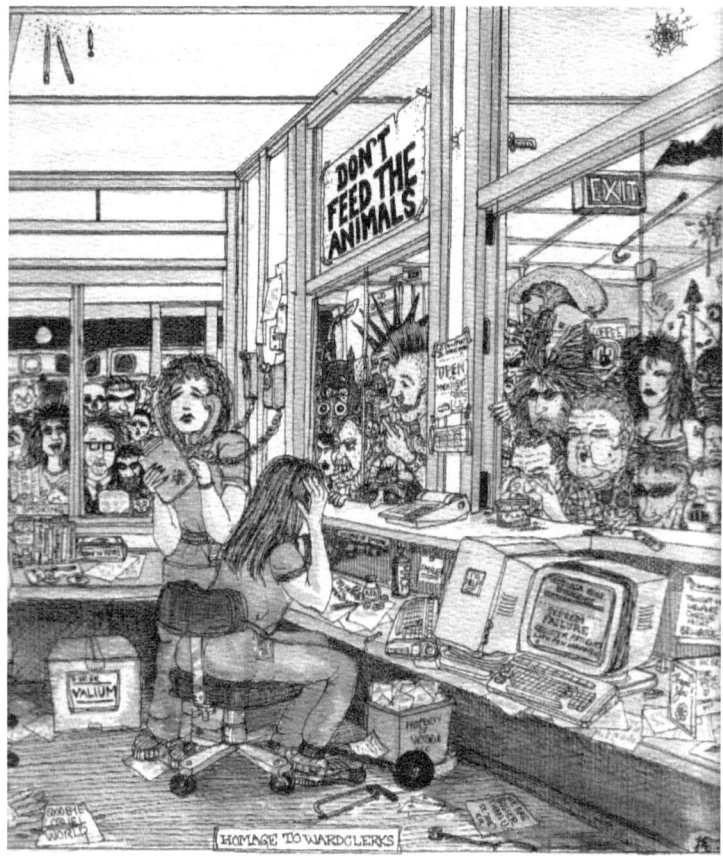

Bernie is a world-class published cartoonist, in addition to being a compassionate paramedic. A common subject of his humour, our craft and associated professionals. Delivering the cartoon to the unsuspecting clerks and nurses, the image was assigned a prominent location instantly.

Joe's voice came up on the radio; "Code four to Dundas and Richmond for a laceration over the eye. It's right in front of the sub shop". There was no mention made of any evil component to this response.

More cuts over the eye are the result of a simple misadventure than violence. With one brutal call under your belt, you could take the stance that everything and everyone will present a danger to you. The experience is an excellent reminder to keep your situational awareness up, not a reason to enter with fists drawn.

We were only a minute away and rolled up, figuring an inebriated person missed a step on the way in or out for a sandwich. Standing in the street were a group of four locals. From experience, they appeared to be street dwellers. Two men and two young ladies standing, talking, one female pointed east on Dundas.

I was driving on this call and positioned the ambulance crossways in the westbound lane. I was closer to the crowd as we exited the vehicle. Bernie was a couple of steps behind, getting the first aid kit. Walking up to the group, the straightforward inquiry "who is injured" caused the withdrawal of three of the four.

Within arms reach now, the female pointing east as we arrived remained stationary. Bringing up the hand that was not raised initially, she produced a long knife. Her three comrades standing behind me blocked any exit. I was too far from the truck to retreat. Bernie was nowhere to be seen yet.

It was a quiet moment. Too close to turn around and escape, I backed up a step; my shadow followed me, knife still raised. The young lady was not waving the utensil, but that didn't reduce the lump in my throat. Responding with "Put the knife down. Put it down now". I raised my right hand, intending to push the knife away if it came to that. The other hand went for the radio microphone clipped to my left shoulder.

Squeezing the transmit button several times harder than it took to activate, the monotone message likely didn't raise Joe's eyebrows to start. "London 159, 10-2000 in a fight with a woman with a knife" Dundas and Richmond." Releasing the mic, there was an opportunity to distract now. She knew help would soon arrive with the radio hail.

Waving the hand that sent the signal caused her to look in that direction for a second. Grabbing the woman's left wrist with my left hand, the knife hand with my right, I yelled in her ear to drop the weapon again. I'm not much of a strategist when it comes to fighting; my crisscrossed arms were defenceless.

The tone escalated for the moment as she refused. Releasing my left hand, I reached up and wrapped her shoulder-length hair around my hand, pulling her head towards the ground.

She was a small lady; the plan was to force her downwards to the sidewalk, causing her to drop the knife. Things can change in an instant. The male standing right behind me was the tallest member of the group. He was wearing a long Australian oilskin drover coat designed to break over a horse's back. I could feel the man's coat sleeve encircle my neck as I struggled with the female.

This was not the time to let go of her knife hand. We were stuck together like a couple of peas in a pod. Adding to the mix, I had this loser trying to choke me and pull me over backwards to free the friend. Bernie's voice broke the silence.

For the life of me, Bernie's words were a blur. I can only guess they were not pleasant. It was a standing dog pile now, the three of us weaving and staggering. My partner was doing his best to pull the tall guy off my back. At one point, we struck the front window of the sandwich shop.

Faces from within were looking at the melee. I hoped we would not crash through the plate glass. There were not enough bulky pressure dressings in the ambulance to take this scene on. I couldn't shake this guy. My grip on the knife hand tightened out of fear.

Salvation: the night air was broken with the wail of multiple sirens. London police recently installed the updated warning systems. For years our police responded silently to emergency calls, victims of a past chief bent on his older English policing model. Thankfully he had not recalled their guns.

A few blocks away when the sound started, their approach was brief and the catalyst to quell the confrontation. As patrol cars pulled up, the death grip on my neck released, followed by the sound of the long, black-handled knife hitting the sidewalk, a welcome relief. Several familiar faces bounded up and took control.

The story came quickly, with police taking over. Our knife-wielding lady ducked into the sandwich shop and reached over the counter to take the knife. She intended; to use the weapon on the fellow that had punched her boyfriend, leading to the ambulance call. The cut to her friend's face drew the 911 call from an employee in the shop behind her.

When she came out, her friend was already walking east following his assailant, hence the pointing. The situation calmed down now with the uniformed response. A sergeant approached to ask if we were all right. I was scared for a moment. Police constables separated the two to get their stories.

Returning moments later, a constable informed Bernie and me that there was not enough to charge her with assault. It seems that grabbing her before she waved the knife at me zeroed out the intent. Ok, so no harm, no foul.

Now the tall guy was another thing. A police officer had this fellow up against his cruiser several yards away. While radioing the police background check, the dispatcher returned with the information on their system. The long coat in past criminal incidents had been the perfect cover for a Bowie knife.

Although he never used it, police confiscated a knife on previous occasions. Yep, that's right, more than once. He replaced the weapon after more than one seizure. Tonight's search was negative, much to my relief. It didn't matter to me that he had never used it before.

With the original patient nowhere to be found and the scrum safely over, we drove away. I considered myself lucky, with no injuries and a partner that stepped in. We needed a coffee; it was my treat.

Top twenty

What is more relaxing than a Sunday drive? Actually, it was Saturday night, and I was in a new SUV assigned to the supervisors. Equipped with a new laptop computer and all of the latest bells and whistles to glisten and pierce the night. The supervisors each had a portfolio in addition to minding the store on the shift. Mine was fleet before vehicle management was a job unto its own.

Planning the vehicle design features with the brass was a bit of a sales pitch. In my favour was the history that my superior liked bells and whistles as much as I did. The boss would never get to drive the unit. A real shame; it's a blast.

It was not the inaugural shift in 1344; the first few finished quietly. Leaving headquarters, I was intent on visiting the stations, part of the routine. The audio system was simple, but tunes are tunes. There were years of no AM/FM radios in the trucks. With the change from Provincial to local vehicle design and purchase, radios were now standard. The local FM station used Saturday night to stick to the top twenty popular hits.

The communications centre dispatched a truck to Richmond Street north of Oxford Street as I cleared the base. The call involved the report of a fight with a couple of injuries. One of my favourite songs just started. It didn't take much to let dispatch know I would be responding. Multi-tasking is one thing. Most of us turn the radio down or off when responding. It just seemed like the thing NOT to do this time.

Turning onto Richmond at York, the song was hitting the second verse. North, I went, volume turned up, and the window down several inches to listen for converging emergency vehicles. The last thing a responder wants it to hit is another responder. It happens.

Probably not what some superior wants to hear, but it was a hoot with the radio on, screaming up the street, lights flashing, siren wailing, then yelping as I crossed every intersection. A current top twenties artist entertaining me verse by verse. Don't mistake the thrill ride for an utterly irresponsible act. The call seemed worthy of a supervisor. The time was right, the speed was under control, and the roads were dry. That's not to say they weren't busy.

Approaching the busiest crosswalk on the drag, the orange overhead lights were activated, authorizing pedestrians to cross; they weren't yielding. Coming to a stop was not an issue, just a delay. Cutting the siren for a moment, the noise just seemed useless during the pause in the action.

That's when it struck me, a young lady crossing in front of me stopped halfway across the marked path directing the pedestrians to the other side. The look, confusing at first. Was she waiting for me to continue north, my lights were still on? The song hit its peak, and the stroller began to wave her hand in unison to the music. Crap, my secret exposed to the taxpayers.

I laughed out loud through the open window when I realized we were both on the same tune. As quickly as my progress was halted, I was back on the road again. The drive was uneventful for the last few blocks. The evidence quieted before arriving. EMS crews or a cop might not see things the way I did for a couple of minutes. The song still brings on a laugh when I hear it while driving, not code four.

Pankegger

During the Homecoming celebration weekend, there are several ways to entertain the masses. Drinking and eating are two that immediately come to mind. Combining the two works well when done in moderation. The same stipulation goes for early rising students bent on seeing a parade followed by a football game in a couple of hours. Well, not so much.

Vomiting students on the festive weekend are the norm. The drinking and antics early in the day are limited to silly acts of overindulgence. The nasty stuff comes in the evening after the game.

Responding to the report of multiple intoxicated patients would not usually attract a supervisor; this weekend was different. Two crews were dispatched to a frat house gathering right on Richmond.

Arriving with the first crew, the party was in full swing. As if we were invisible, the participants did not break from the tasks at hand. Students worked at tables; extension cords lead to griddles cooking flapjacks to order. Others were mixing and preparing in assembly-line fashion. Now I like pancakes with real maple syrup, a favourite. But with beer, the mere thought verging on sacrilege.

Perched high atop the shallow shingled roof over the traditional-looking veranda, a group of students huddled at one end. This behaviour could very easily add a fall to the call details. It would be fifteen feet to the dirt with a missed step. Someone famous once said; teamwork makes the dream work. This was an exhibition of that philosophy.

A student sitting on the shingles straddled a glistening aluminum keg. The type I knew to hold fifty-eight litres of beer. Don't ask me how I know; I never attended university. Another student protected the second keg from rolling off the slanted roof. I could see these were engineering students, redundancy in their plan.

The student assisting looked like a budding plumber. Do plumbers need university certification? Guarded with one hand, the pupil held a spigot at the keg's outlet. The other grasped a clear plastic tube. It was a good fit; there was no leakage from my vantage point. The remaining student, a military future for sure. A bombardier. He was leaning over the end of the roof, directing the tube to hit the target.

The target, student's mouths, lined up, waiting to get bombed. They looked like robins being fed by a parent in a frat nest. If you have not heard, the term is sometimes referred to as "shotgunning." The act of drinking beer without swallowing.

Beer, coming from a pressurized source or assisted by gravity in quantities too large to swallow, passes the gullet into the stomach with a slight tilt of the head. Believe it or not, there is a knack to the technique.

A small-scale method is to turn a beer can upside down and punch a hole in the bottom. With your spare hand, you position your thumb at the ring tab. Then, draw a vacuum, sealing your mouth over the bottom of the inverted vessel. Quickly right the can, at the same time releasing the ring tab, the contents shoot down your throat. Again, don't ask. I just know.

Choosing the bulk method for supplying the beer was likely the work of business students. The term "economy of scale" would be an MBA thing. A keg is cheaper than canned beer, keeping the unit cost in check. It was obviously a widespread practice, given the lineup of participants.

The second crew rolled up behind us now. I would have responded even if there was a door charge to see this event. The pace equalled the service at any fast-food outlet.

Sitting on the grass off to the side were a couple of breakfast aficionados. Looking worse for the wear, their expressions painted a grim picture. The hosts became concerned when the seated participants suddenly became silent. Rolling off her bum onto her hands and knees, one young lady looked to the side. It was more of a "help me" look than "look at me." Drool fell from the corner of her mouth. It was a countdown.

Standing her up, the first medic crew could also see we were heading for a touchdown or a splashdown. The girl's look changed to horror; the warning was over. Through pursed lips came a solid stream of pankeggers. In her favour, she had taken a deep breath just before she hurled the breakfast. The emergency over, a friend stepped up to take her somewhere to recover.

That's one trait you see in students often lacking in your garden variety partier. Many kids are from other places, causing a bond that does not end with some nausea. It also saved a crew the transport.

The other crew was not so fortunate. A vomiting copycat hung over the side of their stretcher, the attending medic having given up on the small plastic kidney basin to catch the pancakes and beer. The failure of the blue pan was a combination of volume over-pressure, physics. That's higher education for you.

The event was back in full swing now. Light-coloured debris in the grass was far enough away; it was ignored. Young people, strong stomachs. The second crew disappeared down the road, bound for the closest hospital to deposit their victim. Our work here was done.

Patient, orderly and loyal to their colours, the remaining participants were painted and clothed in anticipation of the activities happening later today. They continued to eat pancakes; the syrup had run out. I only hoped that the feast did not preclude their attendance at the parade and game. The entertaining events were about to begin.

Red rover

There is a mountain of human suffering and grief thrust at paramedics. There comes a chance now and again to serve in other ways. We study anatomy, physiology and emergency patient care to provide support, do no harm and transport our patients to the hospital. Sometimes it is only possible to achieve the first two steps. There are times when that is good enough.

Ask any medic with road time, and they will admit that one of the worst calls to respond to is a "kid call." That goes doubly for responders who are parents. Underlying speculation is often; that could be my kid.

Art and I were clearing from a call ending at the ER at St Joseph's. I was chatting with an old friend, Sister Suzanne. She was the administrator of the department. Quiet, determined and blessed with a heart of gold, she understood people. She even liked a joke now and again, a clean one.

The red phone rang at the counter as Art was stepping away. With a quick, dramatic reach, he leaned back, popping the red receiver out of its cradle into the air then recovering it. His greeting "153 here". Silence ensued during the brief message, followed by an, mmhmm and a hang-up. "Darbs, a kid, hit by a car; Richmond and Vanier." Sister Suzanne, hand over mouth at the call type, offered her "good luck" as we passed her, our stretcher in tow.

It was just around the corner. Windows down, the run got lots of siren use. Sidewalks were busy, school kids were out and about. If the plan worked, the noise would keep the students off the road and on the sidewalk where it was safe. Arriving, there was a small crowd on the walk. Several drivers left their vehicles abandoned in the street to help the victim.

Police were not there yet; we approached the group around the patient. The stretcher was loaded with gear in anticipation of finding an injured child thrown from the impact on the roadway. "Plan for the worst and hope for the best." It doesn't always turn out that way.

Expecting, no hoping for crying. A sobbing child illustrates it is not as bad as it could have been. Silent, sick or injured children raise the index of suspicion in any medic. Crying inconsolably infers a conscious patient with an adequate airway. A stethoscope confirms it.

The gathering did not part with our announced arrival, a bad sign. Bystanders were not deferring to the patient caregivers; that's wrong. An audible bark came from behind the guy looking down over a kneeling woman.

Stepping back, several onlookers retreated to expose a first. Sitting next to the kneeling Samaritan was a full-sized Irish red setter. The lady must be a dog owner. Her patient was sitting calmly as she held a blood-soaked "T" shirt draped in layers over the canine's head.

Two police cruisers screeched to a halt at each end of the abandoned vehicles. Coming from opposite directions, they angled their cars to block the northbound lanes. No one was going to disturb the accident scene. There were measurements to take and statements to record.

The woman looked at Art, eyes glistening, offering the story. She approached, driving her car as the dog ran off the boulevard in front of her, narrowly missing the animal. A passing car going the opposite direction also missed the pet but blocked the driver in the far curb lane from seeing the dog. Having avoided two vehicles sprinting across the four lanes, the hidden car's front corner clipped the patient. Our victim retreated back across the road, likely heading for home.

A couple of anxious cops popped up behind the concerned gaggle inciting their departure, save and except the first aider. As surprised as we were to see the dog, the officer behind Art called on his walkie-talkie to advise their radio room that it was an animal struck. He also cancelled the responding sergeant.

Luckily, Art and our helper were dog owners. She qualified herself as a dog owner, as my partner spoke up. Exchanging the breed of their own pets, they affirmed their intent on helping the victim. Stepping back now, the officer assigned to document the call returned to his patrol car. Following him was the driver of the third car for his statement.

I was driving for the call, so I opened the kit to assist Art with his plan. "Sterile water" from the truck was the first request. Retreating to the ambulance for a moment, I retrieved the small plastic bottle. Announcing to Art that I was going to update dispatch, the delay gave him a minute to start caring for the dog. Our patient was remarkably calm, considering he narrowly missed several cars and was still around to bark about it.

 I waited for some barking or a yelp as I opened the driver's door and called Steve. "London 153. 153 go ahead. It wasn't a child struck here; it was a dog". "Thanks, mate, that's good news."

Explaining our delay, I offered the closing information. "London 153, Artie is doing first aid on the dog; we will be clear in a couple of minutes". There were too many witnesses to spin the truth or a tail.

Looking back at the patient, Art was uncovering the head wound. The bloody "T" shirt concealed a severe scalping. A nasty flap of his scalp lifted at one end was still attached at the back of his head. He likely got under the corner of the car for a moment. Gently, Art peeled the loose skin back and poured the water into the wound to cleanse it.

It was a move that surprised me. I would have bit Art's arm off receiving the water on the exposed tissue if it were my scalp. The dog was silent. The woman held the dog's collar; you could see the ID tag attached. Our victim sat motionless, receiving the care.

Returning to the sidewalk, Art was applying a bonnet to the dog using a triangular bandage. The first officer advised he notified animal control to respond and take the dog to a veterinarian for care.

Our canine victim stood a good chance of having his scalp stitched back in place with the early cleaning and dressing applied to the injury. The downside, if it didn't heal, I don't know of any dog toupee stores in the city. Here's hoping for option one.

Leaving the dog with the woman and police, we did not have the time to wait to see the outcome. Things have a way of working out; the odds were in the dog's favour. We were always up for an adventure. Kudos to Art for the doggie first aid. The triangular bandage was an excellent fix for the injury. With any luck, we would stay off the supervisor's hit list for treating an animal. There is probably a rule in Toronto for that.

Opening night…or day shift

Did you ever aspire to be on stage? Some of us have dreamt of bright lights, a stage or a microphone in our future. Paramedics are routinely on stage. Every time we provide care in a public place, people stop and watch our every move.

Today, most crews can attest to turning around to see a citizen capturing the action on a camera phone at an accident scene. It can be innocent or lead to some difficulty, depending on the circumstances. One such occasion had our Deputy Chief receiving a Tweet from a local radio station.

As a crew and I stood on a sidewalk at a reported accident scene, we were captured in a picture. It turned out the incident was resolved before we arrived. None of us were wearing helmets or yellow vests. A policy is in place for our safety. An innocent mistake, but I got some paper on it, no time for an excuse, GUILTY as charged.

Hugh and I worked a shift one bright summer weekday; the morning had been quiet. There were lots of chores to do around the office.

Harry, our shift supervisor, was all over us to clean the garage floor. Wetting it down, then squeegeeing the surface dry was a regimen instilled by our fleet guy Preston.

Both were ex-military officers. Great to work for, but in proper military fashion, they hated seeing their staff idle. On a dead day, you were given rags and varsol. Cleaning the grease out from under the hood was just busy work. The same sentiment was expressed when given pliers to remove stones from the tire treads. We escaped this morning with a quick floor cleaning.

Before lunch, Kelly punched up the overhead speaker in the garage with "gotta code three for you guys." A code three is a medical emergency of sorts but not immediately life-threatening; no lights and sirens are required. Hugh returned our squeegees to the closet while I went to the radio room for the details. With the great escape from the garage, a late lunch was a small price to pay.

We were sent to an upscale shop on Richmond Street. The call was for a dislocated knee. I knew it was upscale when I looked at the tag on a dress; $200.00. My jeans that summer cost thirteen bucks, give or take a few cents. We pulled up in front of the store to see a couple of women standing in the front window, naked mannequins. Thankfully, it would be another twenty years before cell phones with cameras hit the street.

It looked like the business was getting ready for a sale. One mannequin was partially dressed, another disrobed model was pushed to the side to make room for the changeover. To this point, the action in the window had not drawn much attention. It was showtime.

Getting the stretcher out, Hugh admitted his wife shopped there before. As we turned, the call unfolded before us. Lying across the floor in the front window was a young woman. Some clothes gathered in a bunch were under her left leg at the knee. She was crying before we arrived. Staff were offering a tissue to clean up.

Our patient grimaced with the pain. Lying on the stage, she clutched the post coming out of the mannequin's rear end attached to a plate on the floor below the model's feet. Dislocated knees are painful. I was finding it difficult not to smile at our predicament. We were all on display. Passers-by stopped to see what the ambulance crew was up to.

The patient's co-worker explained that a missed step up onto the raised floor in the window caused the accident. Our patient spoke up now after blowing her nose and wiping the tears away. In her twisting recovery from falling, she lodged her foot against the edge of the platform.

The move caused the lady's knee to give out, repeating an earlier injury. A history of figure skating falls brought this incident to number three for the "trick knee." Previous tumbles ended her skating career; dressing mannequins was supposed to be a safe sport.

Our priority to start was preserving the patient's modesty. Hugh was the most compassionate medic I will ever have the pleasure of working with. In a simple move, the sheet destined to cover the patient on the stretcher was deployed early. It now spanned from the lady's waist to her ankles. The task of immobilizing our victim, then moving her, would be complicated by the growing crowd behind.

We needed room. Taking the models out of the window to make space to lift the patient took a surprising turn. When I raised the first figure by the torso, it no longer had a base. Lesson one; there is a post on some that go into the butt. The others were steadied with a bar into one foot. When you lift a mannequin up improperly, freeing it, you are left looking like you are dancing. The problem: she is very stiff, and you are forced to lead.

Friends that worked with the patient laughed out loud at the expression of a passing businessman. He must have thought we were helping change the window over until he spotted the partially covered woman on the floor. Like I need to be on stage. The inanimate dancers were graciously handed over to the ladies.

Hugh took my lead and transferred the second form to another shopkeeper. With room to work, we slid the bases aside. I directed our patient to move the good leg next to the injured one. Using triangular bandages, the two legs were cinched together.

Following my direction, the woman stiffened the sound leg, which splinted the bad one. The trick was to avoid flexing the sore knee.

Chronically dislocated joints develop a common characteristic. The more times they become displaced, the more able they are to repeat the painful move. To that point, we took care to place the lady on our stretcher and used our pillow to support the bent knee. A smooth ride would lessen the pain on the way to the ER, where she would receive some pain medications.

It was a short ride up the road to St. Joseph's ER. The other half of the dislocating story needs to be finished. A chronically injured joint will sometimes reduce itself or go back into proper alignment when the pain subsides, and the supporting tissue relaxes. As careful as we were, the twisted knee realigned itself when we lifted the stretcher on the ramp at the ER.

Arriving in the department with the freshly resolved dislocation is tantamount to going to the doctor with a sore throat unable to cough. With the bandages still in place, I was confident the nurses believed my report. At least the patient was happy; most of her pain was gone.

Not every tale on Richmond Street is a sad one or ends up badly. The broad range of calls that medics respond to on the "main drag" keeps it interesting. A crew returning to headquarters on a Friday or Saturday night announcing Richmond is busy gets the stink eye from others within earshot. It's like saying, "what a quiet night" you have released the curse. Under their breath, most medics are waiting for the next nasty one. It keeps the adrenaline pure.

It shot the proverb: Luke 4:23 *Physician heal thyself*, right in the proverbial foot. Thankfully I am surrounded by great colleagues offering genuine support and expert advice.

Approaching the end of a warm, quiet night shift, the lounge door was propped open. The silence outside the base was palpable, no traffic passing by, just a few bugs and a single bird offering a morning hail to its pals. We were on the home stretch.

It was a slow shift, only a couple of calls behind us tonight. Cal and I started with a midnight fall, causing that inevitably fractured hip. In the wee hours, there was the call for a guy wandering down the street. Apparently ailing, he had a tottery-looking gait from a distance.

The senior favouring a painful hip got our best TLC. Triangular bandages were applied in three convenient locations. Tied around her hips, knees and ankles, the cloth band secured the unstable and audibly uncomfortable injury. The patient sheepishly admitted her misadventure was attributed to floppy slippers and a dark, sleepy walk to the bathroom.

Night shift nurses in Saint Josephs ER were quick to drop their knitting. It was no time to be making wool booties. They quickly attended to our patient, a kind elderly woman. She was entering the next phase of her life. It would be a fair wager that this fall marked the loss of her independence. She would now require assistance with some of life's daily activities following surgery to fix that shattered hip.

Our wobbling buddy strolling downtown along York Street was in no great hurry. The passing motorist was a dozen years too early. He was unable to do something immediately satisfying and cost free. The "drive-by 911 call". An option we now take for granted, the non-invasive act of helping, was not technically possible then.

A citizen calling on behalf of a patient out in public used to be reserved for epileptic seizure victims flailing around on the street, a very upsetting vision. Another common sight, coming upon a vehicle accident seeing patients suffering a traumatic injury. In most cases, callers drove to find a cop or a location offering a telephone. In the day, there was no easy way to notify the emergency services.

Tonight, a vigilant citizen arriving home minutes after seeing the wandering creature called to describe the would-be patient's dilemma. The call initiated a very vague request for help. When we finally located the fellow in the caller's defence, he looked a little sketchy. It seems everyone hands off their problems to EMS and police.

You gotta love the calls for help; "there's a guy at the corner of." One of my favourites; "I'm calling from Victoria British Columbia; my brother is not answering the phone. He had a heart attack last year, you know". Police check on a lot of these calls before an ambulance responds. In most cases, the person is not at home!

Faithfully this morning, we strike out on a not-so-earnest mission to drum up a not-so-obvious patient. Locating this fellow, a man with no place to call home, was easy enough. We found him before the police. Our wanderer was heading up an alley several blocks east of our helpful citizen's original call details.

He hadn't a care in the world when we approached. I explained how we came to meet. Our target, the recent consumer of an untold quantity of mouthwash, was miffed with the uninvited attention.

Now, I'm all for fresh breath, but the associated maladies from such a wine list have reduced many a medic, some police officers and nurses to tears. That is after retching from the smell. The adage of "what goes up must come down" is easily converted in medical circles to; "What goes in must come out." It's never pretty, so leave it at that!

We were there already, cancelling the police. Our act of kindness already in motion earned the homeless man a ride to the ER. It also netted him a day-old turkey sandwich while sitting in the back hall of the hospital downtown. And here I thought you always uncorked chardonnay with turkey? Alas, I digress…

Our last run was a few hours ago; I enjoyed a snooze on a rock-hard couch in the dimly lit lounge. You could hardly miss a single snap of the two punch clocks.

 One clock sat on the desk in the radio room to stamp dispatch forms, the other in the lounge to record comings and goings for payroll timecards.

They methodically broadcast their minute-by-minute update. I learned to sleep or rest, still hearing the phone, most radio calls and those noisy clocks.

A crew went out to return an old gal to her east-end nursing home bed. The victim of a fall earlier, John and Art, begrudgingly peeled themselves off their uncomfortable chairs, passing by the rest of us. Positioned precariously on a couch, I switched to a chair. A change is as good as a rest.

After another half hour of miserable rest, the hotline rang twice in rapid succession. Harry answered as if on cue, hanging up and quickly responding again to the second request. Usually, our shift supervisor, Harry, was stuck in the radio room tonight when the regular dispatcher called in sick.

There was a short creak of the worn wheels on the office chair rolling out of the radio room. Harry's sometimes authoritative ex-military voice kicked in. "253 Haynes Street boys, the cops will wave you in from the end of the street. There's a guy on the front lawn waving a hatchet. The police dispatcher said there's a lot of yelling going on in the background".

Hello, that made my heart flutter. Never slide down in a chair allowing your neck to kink up and your butt to hang off the seat. The first few seconds of pain when you stand up will get your attention.

The other crew was up first. Donnie was a seasoned responder; his partner Ben a quiet fellow, was almost too innocent for this job. He had the thinnest skin in the place; the patients often played him sensing it.

Before the crew pulled out of the bay, another two lines rang in unison. Harry, not used to the pace, loved the action in the radio room. He quickly became empowered when the situation heated up. His military swagger full-on now; he was responding to the police line again. Fingers quickly diverting to the direct line into fire headquarters at Waterloo and York.

Harry's head popped out through the door into the still dimly lit staff lounge. He addressed Cal and me with more urgency than earlier. What's more urgent than a guy with a hatchet? "Get over to Haynes; sounds like the guy lit the place up after calling 911. The cops don't know if there is anyone in there. Watch out for the fire trucks!" He was like my father, overprotective.

The other crew was just pulling away from the bays. We were only a minute behind. As we entered the garage, the sun was preparing to pull up smartly into the eastern sky. There was not enough light to make things easy yet.

The silence vanished; with no air conditioning, our windows were wide open. We could hear Donnie and Ben ahead of us, their siren "bee bopping" away. The scene was just a few blocks from our station.

My family never lets it go when I can pick a siren's owner out of the air. It reminds them of the MASH character Radar O'Reilly when he could boast the same notice of approaching helicopters. A fire crew sounded off in the distance, taking the early morning air and thrashing it with their old "grinder" siren. Engine 3 approached from the west, coming from the Bruce Street station.

Pulling in behind the pumper, we parked near several other fire trucks at the scene from the central station on York. Their engines revving, the pump operators were anticipating the request for water. You could hear the siren winding down, growling coming from the already stationary truck as we arrived on their heels.

Some fire trucks competed with the traditional "fire engine red" units positioned ahead in a freshly painted bright yellow. They stuck out with the approaching morning sunlight through the tree branches overhead. We pulled up to see smoke arching out of a second-story window and wide-open front door.

The house was set up on a slight hill, a grass terrace guarding the wide front porch. The wood stoop looked intimidating for paperboys with weak throwing arms and Halloween goers looking for easier picks for treats. The place just looked spooky. That was before the smoke began pouring from the structure.

Donny and Ben were approaching the rear of their truck, stretcher in tow. Facing each other, having overcome a minefield of obstacles, they returned from the front lawn. There were discarded white dressing wrappers several yards from the sidewalk by a century-old tree.

Their unit was wedged between two city police cruisers, front and behind. The ambulance was in a static convoy of black Chevy's lining the street in front of the residence. Police were stationed across the yard, one officer giving light to the gravity of the situation. He was returning his revolver to its covered leather holster; the sight was a first for me.

Ben's patient talked and motioned with a partially free arm; it was handcuffed to the stretcher side rail. There were signs of a forearm injury to the opposite side; blood seeped through the white cotton gauze-wrapped extremity. The arm aligned in a yellow canvas splint was held down by a strap to the stretcher. Police constables looked on as Ben quietly attended to the patient.

Donnie yelled now into the abyss of emergency vehicles surrounding us. "Someone get those cars out of the way." His demand was heard, though the response was delayed briefly while the officers spread around the lawn figured out who had the keys to the patrol cars in the way. It was a "who's on first" base moment as cops scrambled to clear a path for the exiting ambulance. Ben never uttered a word before jumping into the rear of their ambulance, followed closely by one constable.

As Donnie closed the rear doors, he leaned over, offering the tidbit, "he chopped his forearm off with a hatchet, it's hanging by a tendon. Shit". We were blocks from the old Victoria emergency room, good thing! Donnie had to take the long route going around the block. The ambulance quickly escaped the convergence of blinking black, white, red and yellow vehicles.

Drowning out any conversation or subtle sounds now were the arriving sirens from two more pumps. Geez, they are loud. Pulling up within ten feet of our back doors was Engine 5 from the Adelaide Street station. An old-fashioned open cab LaFrance pump that was built in the USA. It boasted a large chrome bell and siren on the front bumper, a benchmark for fire fighting.

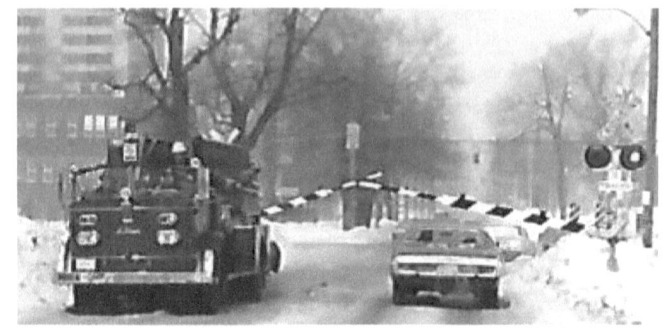

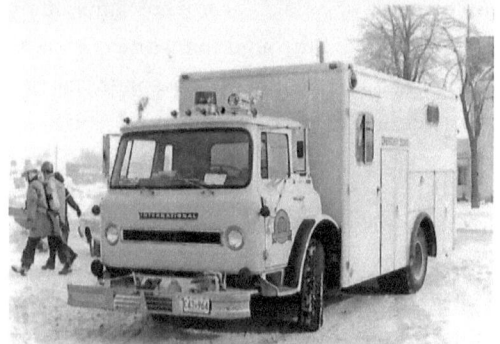

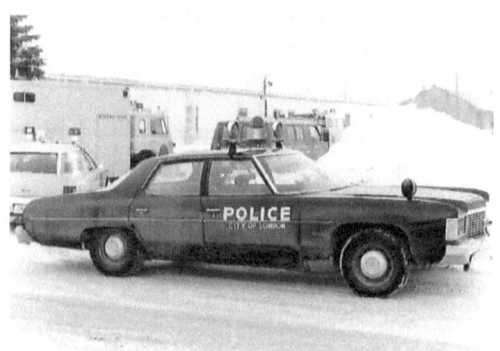

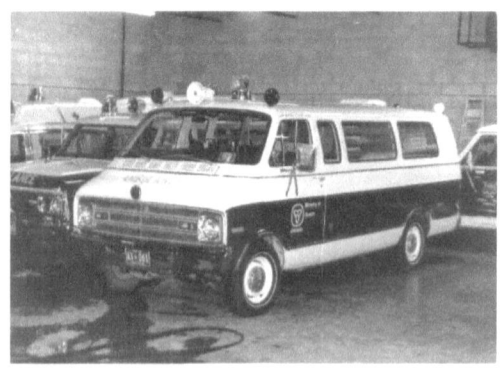

On the heels of Engine 5 in stark contrast, the new yellow Engine 9 from Wellington Road came to a gruelling halt. Discharging hissing gasps from air brakes on their shiny new King Seagrave pumper, it came to a halt. Between them, another police car made its entrance, driven by a sergeant inserting himself into the mix.

We were hopelessly blocked in for the time being. The only consolation, the latest fire units, were there to bolster the manpower compliment. They did not need to haul hose off their rigs to join the spaghetti already lying across the street. There were yards of hose line strewn around, leading to the smoking home.

As Donnie disappeared, a police officer running towards us yelled the update; "there might be a kid in the house." Disappearing into a cruiser, he was talking on his car radio. This was surprising since the police were issued walkie-talkies a few years earlier.

I glanced back as we opened our van to remove the stretcher, oxygen kit, backboard and first aid supplies. We were blocked in by a gasoline-powered pumper. The armada of running vehicles was creating a haze from the volume of exhaust in the still air at street level. Good old leaded gasoline fumes, yuk.

Cal and I pulled and pushed the stretcher over the curb, catching two wheels in our haste. The slippery wooden backboard nearly sent the loose equipment bags on it to the ground. Approaching the tree on the boulevard, we left the rolling aluminum cot there. We preferred to abandon it now rather than risk tripping over the bumpy surface ahead.

Bulging hose lines wiggled their way past us. They were charged with water, leading up onto the terrace to a ladder erected by firefighters on the front lawn. Aluminum rails spanned the gap over the porch to an upper window.

Another turgid canvas line stretched through the front door. Smoke belched from the top half of the shadowy opening, dispersing along the ceiling of the porch. We could hear a commotion coming from inside the house; two upper windows were open. Dark smoke exited the windows rising straight up into the still air, little evidence of fire suppression having started.

With police further back on the lawn and no one barring us, Cal and I carried our gear to the porch. We were eager to be close by if there were going to be any patients. Looking back, we were probably too close to the action.

Firefighters were all assigned a task. Several were off somewhere inside the acrid structure. Police standing too far away were preoccupied with their assignments to inform Cal and me of the danger.

You could hear muffled yelling through firefighter's air masks from within the home. Unable to see each other, they were actively chattering back and forth. As we climbed the front steps, a lone firefighter positioned on the ladder above us readied a hose nozzle at the front window. There was still no water spewing through the opening. It was probably just smoke there; the fire was further into the house.

As Cal and I stood on the porch, onlookers slowly appeared on the street. Some gawkers clad in housecoats; others looked dishevelled in quickly donned clothes. The noise startled residents into action, curiosity driving the rest.

A next-door neighbour with a great vantage point called down to Cal standing with his back to that end of the porch. It took a couple of seconds to realize the call was from a bedroom window behind and above him.

After getting Cal's attention, I could hear the voice say, "he has three kids," an unwelcome communique. I was on the opposite side of the front door under cover of the porch roof when I heard the approaching rescuer.

Turning to look in through the front door, the top half of the entrance was obscured with heavy grey smoke. That acrid-smelling shit that would have been much more tolerable from the curb. Beyond the door against the left wall, a staircase ascended into the smoke-filled home like a tall building into low clouds.

Coughing slightly now, I stuck my head into the doorway to see the results of the first fire suppression efforts coming down the wooden stair treads. It was a pink-tinged water runoff from fire fighting efforts. The mixture was a sure sign of terrible things to come.

Closely following the pink warning were sounds of footsteps from hip-high rubber boots and an earnest voice coming through a protective mask.

Appearing at the bottom of the steps was a single firefighter. He was carrying a victim slung over his shoulder in the traditional "fireman's carry." What Cal and I saw next was the most unwelcome first glimpse of a lifeless teenager.

Causing a temporary distraction, the lone rescuer stood on the threshold of the door removing his life-preserving air mask. The victim still on his shoulder. A light-coloured soupy vomit spilled out of the mask's lower cupped area, designed to hold the user's chin. For the moment, this guy was my hero. Anyone who could rescue this kid and exit the building still wearing the partially obstructed mask deserved a medal.

In a second, our attention turned to helping lower a young female victim from the firefighter's shoulders. The lifeless teen rested partially on the yellow cylinder carrying the rescuer's air supply. The patient's waist crossed the fireman's chest and shoulder. As if the smoke wasn't enough, the air was foul, tainted with the smell of last night's supper. It was running out of our rescuer's protective mask and down the front of his long black coat.

We rolled the victim onto her back as Cal and I lowered her to the wooden porch to start a quick assessment. Taking aim, we set her onto a now wet backboard. Our first look was at the patient's head.

The wet was a gruesome trifecta of water, mixed with blood and clear fluid running from within her skull. Lying lifeless on our board was a teenager sporting the worst head trauma ever in my career, except for a few decapitations. I felt the flopping, dripping appendage against my chest on the way down. Our young lady lay on her back, clothed in a damp and badly soiled nightgown.

The victim's head was missing what could best be described as a wedge of its contents. Starting dead centre from the bridge of her nose, arcing over the top to the back of the skull. Something akin to a wedge of melon. So much for a fruit entrée for breakfast.

Please accept my apology in a most sincere Canadian way. The description aptly captured the moment.

Blood, at first glance, continued to ooze generously from deep within the crevice. It was poorly illustrated in the early morning light. The greasy, brightly coloured brain tissue was trying to glisten in the still smoky air. It had an odour that would linger for decades, embedding itself in my memory bank only to be recalled from time to time in my occupation.

Early on in the industry, we were unofficially taught CPR. No Provincial body existed yet for training or certification. There was always the caveat that there might be some liability if something went wrong. Fortunately, when this emergency rolled around, we were trained to American standards in the basic technique. Three of us at the ambulance service were qualified as instructors.

With the shock value behind us in seconds, we stepped up to the challenge. Starting with the A, B, C's, Cal opened the oxygen kit and quickly retrieved an oral airway for our patient.

She lay motionless as we started CPR, coming up empty-handed with a pulse check. There was no doubt she was pulseless. I checked twice with bare hands. To date, only physicians enjoyed the personal protection afforded by gloves. This would change just a hand full of years later with the world's introduction to AIDS.

In an embarrassing moment during a lapse of situational awareness, it suddenly occurred to me we needed help. Our ambulance was temporarily wedged between a host of other responders. Our victim needed what we couldn't immediately offer, rapid transport.

At the time, we only staffed three crews on the night shift adding to the traumatic conundrum. In a fortunate twist, I had a helper close by, forgotten at the moment with all the excitement. Strapped to my belt was a resource not regularly afforded to the EMS industry in those days.

Sitting in its leather holster was an ancient walkie-talkie, nearly three times the size of its modern-day counterpart. The grey rectangular squawk box not yet turned on, a minor oversight, laughable at best. There was only one in the service. I attached it to my belt earlier, discouraged at the time when it was catching against the arm of the lounge chair.

Hearing the "peep" when the radio came to life, I called Harry. "London, this is 158", a brisk "58" the reply. "Where is 155? I think we have three kids here, all code 4's". "55 London" was his reply and address to John and Art returning from the east. "London 155, we are at Dundas and English".

That's all I needed to blurt out the retort; "Johnny, get your ass in gear to Hayes Street. I have kids here all code 4's". Luckily it was the night shift. The media hopefully turned off their police scanner and went home earlier.

Setting the blood-stained portable back in its holster, the device saved dozens of steps. I was never quoted, just laughed at later during an informal debriefing.

CPR was done for a couple of minutes or less, preparing for the move to the street. Firefighters suddenly appeared on the porch, evidence of the reinforcements for the general fire alarm. There were lots of hands to help escape the veranda and terrace. A firefighter's wet and filthy coat came from nowhere, covering the girl from chest to shins. Lifting the backboard went off without a hitch.

I was still not sure what to do if there actually were more kids to treat and transport. From the end of the short street came 155, silently doing a three-point turn to ready themselves for a quick return to the Vic. We moved slowly to allow Cal to ventilate the patient.

It was a steady pace with the slippery, blood-soaked backboard as we made our way over hoses and the curb. We wove our way through a fleet of blinking lights standing between us and 155. I quickly turned to a captain and appealed to him and his followers to move enough vehicles to eke out a path between our unit 158 and the open street.

By now, Cal and I were bloodied from chest to waist, visible on the light blue shirts. Who knows what hit our dark blue polyester uniform pants below? Gravity could be cruel. Winding around a revving pumper, we met John and Art with their stretcher lowered to a working height.

After loading the kid, we left them to take over, guessing out loud our suspicions that the patient's father had chopped the girl's head open with the hatchet, then lighting the house on fire. There was not much of a medical report; it just seemed obvious at the moment.

With the rear doors of 155 still open, Cal and I shared the same thought, take their backboard. Picking up our blood-covered ventilator, mask, oxygen bag, and their board, we jogged back towards the porch.

In my haste, I stepped on a fire hose, twisting my ankle, a rookie mistake for a volunteer firefighter. Knowing what I stepped on instantly brought about an awkward recovery.

Approaching the porch, the scene was different this time. Several firefighters disappeared through the front door; the grey smoke whitened and was subsiding now. There was more activity from within the house. A red helmeted captain leaned out of an upstairs window pulling aside his air mask.

Pushing the twisted screen aside, he stretched to see his coworkers on the lawn. Calling for help, he announced there was "another one!" On this round, the action on the stairs was obvious.

Two firefighters descended the wooden staircase on the run. It is still a mystery to me how no one fell in their haste to exit the building. This patient was only wearing underwear. To avoid a delay, I tossed the spineboard onto the porch.

He had similar injuries to his sister, missing a smaller portion of his head. There was blood on his chest and back over one shoulder. More blood was bubbling, frothing from his nostrils. There were shallow injuries to the side of the gaping hole in this fellow's skull. It seemed that the gashes were likely missed attempts to inflict deeper blows.

Firefighters rescuing this patient would set him on the backboard for us. One firefighter stepped on the edge of the board, positioned on the shallow porch. His hip-high boot slid on the varnished surface. He, too, made a good save, only dropping the kid the last few inches bum first.

Where did this kid get the drive to breathe? Was he on autopilot? Asking around after the fact, the theory posed by an ER doc: the victim's brain stem containing the medulla oblongata must have escaped the direct impact and penetration required to immediately interrupt the breathing process. This kid had a strong pulse! Cal and I looked at each other, an incredulous sight.

Offering no warning, our patient snorted one agonal inhalation. It was followed by a brief snoring sort of flutter going in the opposite direction. Surely it was a function inconsistent with the cerebral chasm before us.

Surprisingly there were no burns visible. Beyond the blood, some dark soot covered the victim's front, not his back. It explained the position he was lying in when he was attacked and his posture during the fire. The collaboration of smells from his injuries was striking. Firefighters looked at us as if waiting for a reaction.

Cal brought the oxygen ventilator out and gave this struggling kid several breaths. Where did he get a pulse from, with a head like this? The breathing never improved. His intermittent gasps were still out of sync with the measured intervals between Cal's ventilation efforts.

In rapid succession were a couple of slobbering breaths. The attempt to breathe was followed by silence. Sounds of water being discharged above and around us broke the brief quiet. Cal ventilated several times and spoke up, requesting help carrying our second victim to the street.

Squawking now from my hip was the antique portable radio performing like a champ. Booking on the air, Donnie and Ben in 157 were clearing from Victoria. I wondered if they took the time to complete their first call report, such as it was.

Imagine filling in a legal document with a pencil today; see you in court. There were only three lines for the written description of patient care rendered. Detailed vital signs not included, literally! I guess their paperwork could wait. We were happy to have the help.

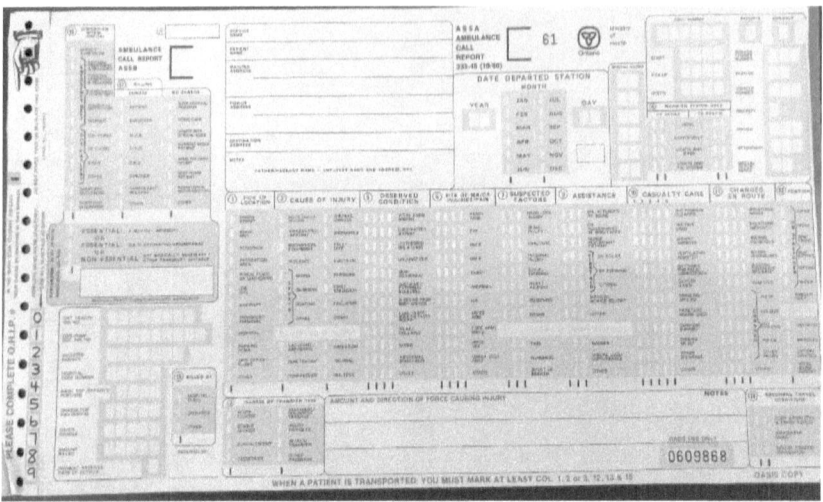

AS5A - patient care form

Donnie was wound up. He later explained that he had been stationed at the ER entrance, cleaning his stretcher when 155 rolled in. He must have been startled, being upstaged from his patient with the mostly amputated forearm. His old race car driver mindset and firefighting background kicked in. Hearing from John sailing through the door, bearing the news of more victims.

Always a team player, Donnie loved the excitement. Grabbing up Ben, they had made a beeline back to our now bustling scene. Grateful, I used the portable radio again to tell them to be prepared. We would meet them at their truck.

Most of us referred to the ambulances as trucks. Historically the original ambulances were cars adapted for ambulance and funeral work (sometimes the same vehicle did both!). My first boss used to ride us when we used the term truck instead of the accepted "car" on the radio. Traditionalists?

We passed our cot with all the help, abandoned on the front yard in lieu of the gang of stretcher-bearers. With a generous supply of hands, the stretcher levitated to the paved roadway towards Donnie without interruption. It was a welcome favour; our gratitude was expressed to our fire friends with a smile.

Donnie was not nearly as gentle in repositioning the van as John had been for his earlier departure. Don's turn included mounting a curb, increasing the likelihood of a damaged tire or a premature front-end alignment. Our fleet guy Monty, a retired military leader, would never understand it next week taken out of context.

Over the hoses and around the remaining vehicles, we arrived at the rear doors of 157. Ben offered a disturbing look at the sight on our arrival. With an uneventful transfer, they took over. Once again, we grabbed their backboard.

Still, on the street, a voice from the terrace drew our attention. We caught sight of a platoon chief from the Waterloo fire station, standing back from the steps. Not used to hearing a chief yell, it attracted the undivided attention of all. Another patient was waiting on the porch.

Equipment in hand, we travelled in a pack now. There were more firefighters than medics crossing the grass to the steps then up to the porch. Our final casualty, a young male, lay lifeless. He arrived before we could offer the backboard to avoid the transfer.

Setting the board down beside him, Cal grabbed another plastic airway and the soiled mask and began breathing for the boy. I checked; there, on a sticky, blood-covered neck, was a pulse. Moving to the spine board was easy with the extra hands

As we lifted the backboard off the porch, hands found the holes around the board's perimeter to steady the platform. I was at the head with one of my hands at each corner, giving signals by twisting the plywood back to level when it became uneven. The command was given to lift the feet higher for a safe transition down the stairs.

The firefighters lifting the feet were a little overzealous. The board, patient and the associated blood and water on the board slid my way, landing just above my belt onto my uniform. It was a small price to pay and soon forgotten. Cal kept up the patient's assisted breathing walking alongside.

The onlooking neighbours watched as the group moved to our stretcher. For a third time, faces reflected their disbelief with glances of sadness and empathy. The morning sunlight left no detail veiled in the shadows. We made our way back to our stretcher abandoned earlier on the lawn.

The street was bright now. The morning sun came piercing through the trees in our "Forest City." Extra firefighters not tasked with a suppression assignment were very apparent on the front lawn and curb. Several wet and tired smokies were watching the EMS side of things carry the scene. Thankfully our friends don't just attend fires. They often respond to more complex calls. Having to move patients over the terrain single-handed would have painted a different picture to onlookers.

Our cot was no trouble to lift over the grass on this leg of the journey. Leaving the street, the retreat required a short trip backwards to a laneway to turn around assisted by several spotters.

In about a minute, I had Cal on the ramp at the old ER. The driveway was spotted with nurses, orderlies and doctors arriving for their day shift. Oblivious to the incident and the arriving victims, their imminent shift report would change that.

 We were directed into OR 1. A room reserved for critical or pulseless victims of illness or trauma. Familiar faces were showing signs of frustration and overload as they greeted us with a clean stretcher. They got a warning from Harry of the incoming patients. The first two kids were pushed off to the side to make way for the final assessment. The room's layout and equipment were designed for a single stretcher patient.

From under the now taut white hospital linen sheet to my left came a sputtering. We heard the same sounds earlier in a much more dimly lit circumstance. We almost missed the transfer to the hospital gurney with all the staffs' help.

They say, "many hands make light work," which is true in the ER. Without the opportunity to offer our patient report, we were promptly ushered out of the OR into the hall.

A nurse closed the door behind us. Appearing briefly from an indirect path to the same room, a middle-aged charge nurse returned to the area behind the front desk. She retrieved something from the meds cabinet and disappeared with the same haste. No one offered an explanation, though thoughts wandered around a theory.

Three ambulances lined the ramp at 7am with no place to go, thankfully. It's times like this that are often disrupted by an early morning abdominal pain or a VSA. We were fortunate. The EMS Gods left us to our own devices to recover from the most violent and tragic experience some of us would face in our careers. We were on until eight am, only having a few minutes to clear our heads.

The incident would ruin one EMS professional and his career. It affected the others assigned to the call for the immediate future, some for more extended periods. Who knows what toll the scene took on firefighters and police?

Looking around at the other five medics, we were a nasty bunch. Our light blue shirts bloodied; the skin hidden beneath likely stained as well. There were a dozen hands and arms marked with more of the same.

The patient compartments of our ambulances were adorned with blood. Looking closely, a couple of small pieces of brain tissue and hair stuck to the floor and the wall to the patient's right in one unit. Layered onto this already confusing sensory challenge was the concentrated odour of smoke. We all stunk from the ordeal.

When you visit a loved one in the ER following an incident, they have been cleaned up. Vomit and blood-stained clothes, wounds and most odours have been addressed. Seeing the dressings, medical appliances, and monitoring equipment on the patient is upsetting but reassuring. There is no diminishing your emotional response to seeing a person suffer.

Nurses, doctors and paramedics routinely take in intensely disturbing images and experiences. Without hesitation, they assess, treat and sanitize the sick and injured. All in a day's work, some would boast. That statement scares me. We have all said it in the hopes of appearing brave. The affects and effects run deep.

Paramedics at the scene work within an arm's length processing these sights. Victims are often found in the position that the predicament caused.

To describe a scene as messy is an understatement. Low light, noises related and unrelated to the incident and the smell leave their mark on your memory.

You might think that you could filter out the undesired. Sometimes you can and do. Despite everything you do, your brain is like a multi-track recorder. It captures everything, storing it forever.

Paramedics transporting the patients from the scene sanitizes the next caregiver from the raw sights. ER staff continue exhaustive efforts to stabilize each victim. They still get the picture attached to tissue and clothes through injuries and the patient's actions and statements. It is not unusual to have something a paramedic, patient or police officer says in the ER leave a stressful mark.

The medical community resorts to triaging patients when they appear in multiples. A French word, the technique is used for distinguishing the more seriously injured and ill from the less acutely affected. The skill ensures that the patients in the worst condition arrive in the emergency department first.

Medics and nurses often repeat the triage if a patient remains in their care long enough. Patient volume causes delays and compounds the stress. Multiple screams of pain or seeing the life drain from a patient's face is unforgettable.

First responders are regarded by some as lifesavers. Conversely, others view emergency responders as nothing but civil servants. I am not looking for a handout here, but medics routinely provide the first round of skilled professional care. Far more than simple transport (substitute transport for ambulance drivers).

This professional pride is not intended to overshadow the efforts of the police. When they assist us, it is often under stressful circumstances. The public they protect is their worst critic. In some cases, they are at risk while protecting the public and other responders; they deserve kudos.

Firefighters often share the same sights as medics. They enter the scene before any intervention, sharing some raw visions. In this case, they found the kids lying in their respective beds, having sustained the most traumatic and disturbing injuries imaginable. Their task was complicated by having to work in a fire and smoke-filled home.

Anyone with children can relate to a midnight check, a simple look in on their sleeping child. Finding their child in their bed is usually a safe zone. In this case, it was the scene of the teens undoing, unimaginable for most. Now, add trauma, fire and hold the light, all adding to the surprise factor. Responders will tell you that after caring for children, most are prone to more vigilant midnight checks. That's stress.

In addition to seeing the "worst" cases, paramedics align themselves daily with the pressures and stressors of human suffering. In the same fashion, paramedics begin to think everyone is unwell for one reason or another. It doesn't have to be an injury. Dealing with medical and mental health crises is both tiring and sometimes dangerous.

Spending a lot of their time with criminals, it is not a stretch for the police to think that many people are criminals until proven otherwise. Both professions usually stick to themselves socially. Coworkers understand the talk and accept the walk.

The interaction with patients experiencing their worst day inevitably includes absorbing a modicum of their stress. Anyone believing otherwise is in denial. It has been my experience to witness the toughest paramedics crumble at different points in their careers. It is a common by-product of the demands and hazards inherent when offering patient care during a crisis.

Stress surfaces and presents differently with each personality; the hurt is there. Everyone is an emotion-gathering vessel, waiting to overflow. Much effort is directed to support and cure those who accept the responsibility to care for others. Keeping stressors at a manageable level is a task assigned to every responder. By association, the same obligation goes for coworkers, supervisors, their employer and family members. (Please insert a sigh here.)

Meanwhile, back at the ER:

Everyone was running on the dregs of an adrenalin hit. We cleaned up our stretchers and equipment with disinfectant and hospital rags. Some stains, primarily blood, just smeared, spreading with the cleanser.

Coming clean now, the trucks looked good. It would take a couple of shifts for the odour of smoke to disappear. Or was that us and our uniforms? The cleaners definitely needed attention.

A man exiting the department passed us with his wife in tow, looking sidelong in our direction. He steered her away, avoiding eye contact. He likely had a good view of the action as we passed through the waiting room with our patients earlier. In those days, there was no back way into the treatment areas.

To the innocent, we probably looked more like the purveyors of violence than caregivers. In pairs, we ducked into the clean utility room. The small closet in the back hall of the ER was reserved for cleaning supplies and dumping bedpans and urinals. The shelves were well-stocked.

Several past experiences led me directly to the hydrogen peroxide shelf. Like a weaker form of bleach, it breaks down blood proteins while also acting as a disinfectant. Off with our shirts, wet them down, then add the peroxide. Blood foamed in its presence, evidence of its action. A quick rinse, then wring out the fabric in a towel. We were off to the office, pretending that there was nothing to look at.

Back at base, the day shift was wanting their trucks back. The medics were fresh and eager to take on the day. We faced a few questions to follow up on what Harry shared from his vantage point. Art and I would soon be heading south from the office en route to our respective destinations. We were still too amped up to fall into bed.

As a fast-food lover, it occurred to me that a quick stop for breakfast and a cup of coffee would hit the spot. Caffeine offered a meagre effect, rarely keeping me up. Overhearing us, the others, even one medic who never went for breakfast after a shift, jumped on the bandwagon. I sensed it might bring our teams some closure.

Arriving at the counter beneath a couple of golden arches, we received quizzical stares from staff. Likely it was the presence of the six of us bearing the same crest with a tiny red cross on a gold disc that restrained them from asking. There was really no doubt looking at us what the dissipated stains on our shirts were. Lord knows what the peroxide, body fluids and smoke smelled like.

In a humorous effort to break the ice, I ordered six "Happy Breakfasts." Receiving a round of laughter from all left others within earshot to wonder what we had been drinking. Can you drink adrenalin?

11

Strictly Crashes Act II

Bashfulness was never a trait that rooted itself in my makeup. Ask me the question and sit back; the answer won't be brief. I am known for not filtering the details at times. Even in an attempt at self preservation.

Saved by a double-double

Never let it be said that paramedics, including the author, are specifically immune to having the odd collision. Andy and I just returned to the office with hot coffees and a baked treat. The dispatcher surely knew if she kept track that we had just enough time to make the pick-up. We were due for a break; this was sabotage

Still perched on the ramp in front of the bay doors, Gail at dispatch down the road droned out the call for 1171. Answering the radio for my partner, I never liked doing all the radio work. As a supervisor, it was not about jumping on all the jobs or exercising the newfound authority or avoiding either.

Chest pain calls for the ambulance service are our bread and butter, those and abdominal pain runs. It would be no surprise to another medic reading this that we routinely drink and eat on the way to calls. Not saying that it is the right thing to do, but after hundreds of interrupted breaks and meals, stuff happens.

I was busy driving, so the paper cup on the driver's side remained in its holder. The bagged doughnut slid back and forth on the engines cowling.

Peeling back the tab on his double-double, Andy would not miss the opportunity to wash down his freshly baked chocolate brownie with the cup of Joe.

We came to a stop for a red light at the intersection before making the left turn as our lights blinked and sirens crooned out their emergency signal. The warning systems are intended to declare a clear message. It's their job to remind you of your responsibility under the highway traffic act. PULL TO THE RIGHT AND STOP.

A driver sped through his green light coming from our right to beat us. He hoped we would continue straight through the intersection after stopping. Taking a hard left into the underpass beneath the downtown railroad tracks netted a grunt from Andy. The ride was a little jerky for a chest pain call.

Heading down under the tracks, the siren echoed off the concrete walls, lights reflecting faintly off the same grey surface. We were in the left lane, another routine held by emergency vehicles unless turning right. Our jackrabbit driver was hugging the right side now, doing the speed limit. Still greedily trying to keep his pace up, what was his hurry?

Replying to dispatch following their patient information update, there was only one hand on the wheel. The other was now smacking the engine cowling with the radio's microphone, looking for the clip beside my cooling coffee. Andy was riveted to the task of completing his break en route to the medical call.

Confirming with Andy that we would be turning right ahead when we came out of the tunnel, I glanced to my right for a second or two. As we approached the speeding motorist, he caught up to the car in front of him. With a quick yank to the left on his wheel, he popped up right in front of me.

The smack was solid but brief. The minivan was overlapping the front right side of the ambulance. Rear-ending any vehicle generally means it is your fault. For the moment, I let fly with a one-word curse. Both vehicles were not stopped yet. There was a gurgling to my right.

After turning off the siren, I parked the now stationary ambulance. Siren silenced, the red and white lights still glistened as they broadcast our position. My wounded ego wanted to pull into an alley out of sight. Moving the vehicles before the police could investigate would interfere with the facts.

There was that gurgling again. Andy was choking. He turned to me with a minor look of panic but could not get any words out. Expecting an outburst judging my driving, I was ready for the worst. We had our belts on, so there could not be any injuries. Is choking an injury?

Swallowing hard, Andy went for his coffee. The emergency was over in a single gulp. The brownie, a.k.a. airway obstruction, was cleared by the creamy coffee. With a short burst of "this ought to be good," I hopped out to check on the other driver.

Andy grabbed for the microphone to announce our misfortune to dispatch. The sarcastic tone in his message earned a slam of the driver's door. It was my fault; I had hit the left rear corner of the vehicle. The rusted van looked like it was heading for the junk pile. A dented tailgate, the result of a previous mishap, eased my conscience.

The driver was still in his van. With the vehicle's ownership already in hand, he knew the drill, refusing to look out his window. Growing impatient, regardless of fault, our vehicles blocked both lanes.

Finally, tapping on the glass, the fellow turned and would not open his door or window. In a booming voice, I opened the path for assuming responsibility. "Are you ok?" Still no movement, just a simple nod in the affirmative. Finally, the door opened, allowing the three-word remark to fall out the crack; "the windows fucked".

The rude comment was followed by a dismissive turn back to his insurance and ownership. I announced the police were called as I walked away. He acted as though he couldn't care less. There was no corresponding inquiry into our condition.

Returning to Andy, I was happy to see that the damage to our van was cosmetic. The shattered plastic grille, dented bumper, and a cracked red lens on the intersection light would all be a quick fix. "Five minutes for the cops" was the salutation. Telling him about the other driver and his indifference, my partner thought we would be in the clear.

Pulling up behind us was a familiar face. Parking the shiny blue and white police cruiser, the emergency lights were activated to make it official. With a shake of his head, Don strode past our vehicle without a word. On the job for several years, he read the signs.

The story from the other driver would be the clincher. That's probably why he went to the other guy first. Hearing in his words what he was doing at the time of the accident would spell it out. The driver jumped out of his vehicle to address the officer. He was quickly ushered to the concrete wall in safety.

Approaching my window several minutes later with the driver's documents in hand, Don asked: "Did this guy pull out in front of you as you went to pass him?" "Yup," was my final answer. Directed by Don to pull the ambulance around and ahead of the minivan, it cleared the left lane. Relieved drivers trapped in the underpass pulled slowly past our group.

The minivan driver walked back to the cruiser and waited to climb into the rear seat. After a short conversation, his statement concluded, he returned to his van and waited.

Minutes later, Don climbed out of his patrol car, walking up to the other driver with his papers. He attempted to pass the first two through the window. Through the same crack at the rear of the door, words were exchanged. When Don leaned in to address the fellow, the door opened slightly.

When the brief exchange ended, he handed the driver what looked to be some yellow papers. With that, the door was slammed closed. Don sent him away with a parting comment, then stepped out into the lane to stop frustrated drivers from working their way around the blinking obstructions. Our collision buddy pulled past us, not turning to wave or glance our way.

Don was at the passenger's window before Andy could roll it down. The opener was almost laughable. Don asked the driver what made him pull out in front of an emergency vehicle. The guilty driver fell short of an honest answer.

When Don quizzed him about the previous damage on the same corner, the deal was sealed. His last ticket was for an unsafe lane change. Today the citation was not yielding to an emergency vehicle.

Was the drive-by with no acknowledgement of the incident an act of submission and his shame for the doubleheader. It was my turn to give a statement. Papers in hand, I got the front seat, likely a cleaner perch.

Minutes later, Don sent me off with the completed accident form in hand. Cleared from the call, there were no pending assignments from Gail. After announcing we needed a vehicle change, we skulked back to the office. It was a short drive to exchange our bruised ride for a new unit.

There was still lots of paperwork ahead; trust the government for that. Besides, there was a mug waiting to rejuvenate the cold coffee. The chocolate donut disappeared in four patient bites: no choking here!

Look before you Jeep

We have all seen vehicle stunts on television. You know the ones with crashes, flips and explosions. If they were taped, you could slow them down, look closely and, in some cases, see spectacular explosive flashes coming from under the vehicles. Designed by brilliant professionals to dramatize the incident, experts rarely get injured in the process.

Rank amateurs out for a thrill often don't think things through. The consequences can be just as sensational. Though not often caught on film, they can end with injuries. That's reality!

Sent to a property just inside the city boundary, a stream meandered through the fields along the bottom of a sharp sandy cliff. Hikers and dog walkers frequented the area. In this case, a witness became a good Samaritan. Walking out to the road for help, it was years before we routinely carried phones in our pockets.

Having owned several Jeeps in my day, it was challenging to find new obstacles to traverse and trails to follow. Make no mistake, it is easy enough to get a four by four stuck. The problem is; when they get hung up, they get really stuck. Too bad the dilemma wasn't so simple today.

Responding to reports of a Jeep in a creek, there were exchanges between Artie and me on the way, repeating the rhyming words in the dispatch details. Dispatched with another unit behind us as a backup, the story was that several people were in the vehicle when it crashed into the creek. Cathy and Ben were miles away.

We expected to find the off-road unit tipped into the water and someone ejected onto the ground. Although never having been on the farm, the lure was visible from the roadway. The chance to drive through water in my four-by-four would have to wait. Offroading on this farm was dismissed in the past since it is private land, a no-no for four-wheelers.

A rubber-booted lady met us at the roadside, pointing to a gravel access path for the farmer just a few yards down the road. Our van would be no match for mud, and there was no clearance for rough terrain. It would be slow going.

The landowner had the right idea; take the high ground. The track was well-packed from the weight of equipment and harvested crops over the seasons. Lucky for us, it was summer; the mud was history.

Our pathfinder explained that the vehicle was in the creek. She was a regular on the walking route and thought that our ambulance could not drive down to the flats along the waterway.

Asking where the rutted route would lead us, the woman with her retriever on its leash explained we could get up on the hill above the stranded unit. We would then have to walk down to our patients.

It seemed simple enough as we followed slowly behind our guide. Calling our dispatcher Kelly, he passed the directions back to the second unit, still a long way off. The dust behind the ambulance as we drove up the inclined path quickly settled. A reassurance that traction was not an issue.

At the top of the trail, we passed the Samaritan now pointing off to her right. I knew we were on an elevated piece of land, but the surprise in seconds was startling. Hitting the brakes, the ground dropped off abruptly in front of us.

The more calls a medic has in their repertoire, the more you assume your situational awareness is as sharp as a razor. This call will be a cinch, I thought; not so fast. In my mind's eye, I had the creek sitting around twenty feet below us. Although it would be a pain, the four of us could easily navigate the obstacle when the second crew arrived.

Standing on the precipice of a sandy field, the ground dropped away from years if not centuries of erosion. Over fifty feet below sat a roofless jeep, upright in the middle of a shallow stream. Rocks and other debris were visible on the creek bed from our vantage point.

Sitting in the driver's seat, a lone male. Motionless and not responding to Art's attention-getting yell, we looked at each other; now what? Next to the stream sat his passenger, bleeding from lacerations and other injuries too distant to assess from the surly bonds of our vantage point.

We were in over our heads, really. Returning to the van, Kelly was waiting for information on our patient's condition. The exchange included a request for the rescue squad and an update to Cathy and Ben, still several minutes away.

Telling the crew over the air to watch for the dog walking lady, I turned to her beside the ambulance and asked her to repeat her trip to assist the other crew and the fire department. She disappeared behind the ambulance as I met Artie at the side doors for the game plan.

A couple of years earlier, I purchased a body harness for rescue work. Equipped with rope and a lack of nerves, I convinced Art to head out to meet an old school friend at his farm to try some rappelling down the outside of his silo.

Sliding down the rope on stainless steel fittings following the directions, we escaped injury. Brazen and dismissing the risks, we descended a second time. Sliding yards at a time and using the fittings and gloved hands to control our fall, it was a thrill before winding up the nylon line and calling it a day.

A weekend course in high-angle rescue at the Elora Gorge later that year filled in some blanks but made me shudder in retrospect. My luck would run out someday.

Each ambulance was equipped with one hundred feet of rope. Unsure of the line's actual intent, it was there for the "whatever" moments bestowed upon ambulance attendants. Give a medic enough rope, and he will hang himself out to dry.

We imagined a simple scheme. Tie off to the ambulance and rappel down to rescue our victims. The others would soon be here to help us get out of the gully. We had watched too much television.

The dangers associated with the absence of a harness and carabiners to descend fifty feet on a rope eluded us at the moment. With the cheap rope provided by the ambulance service, we stood at the edge of the steep hill looking down. The silo was ninety feet straight down to the ground; there was dirt to walk down here. Where's the problem?

Inside the crew bench near the rope were two sets of plastic garden gloves. I planned to go down first, then have Artie pass me some gear. A first aid kit and backboard for a start. Running the rope around my generously proportioned behind, I held onto the two strands in front of me using the gloves.

The plan was to squeeze and release my hands with the two ropes passing in opposite directions, slowly walking backwards down the hill. There were a couple of missed steps; the creek came up quickly without a fall.

I turned to the first victim still in the driver's seat and called to him with no response. His friend sitting a few feet away on the gravel next to the water admitted the driver had not spoken since the Jeep landed in the creek. The end of the rope slithered up the hill and quickly returned with the blue tin box and backboard tied to the end.

Walking into a foot of water and mushy sand wasn't as bad as I imagined. We could work standing next to the vehicle. The price paid, a pair of soaking feet and work boots. Our patient moaned; he was breathing in a snoring fashion. I forgot to ask Art to send the oxygen kit down with the board.

Hearing a voice from the hill, I looked up to see Artie sailing down to meet me. Did I make it look that easy? Was he trying to outdo my descent? The cursing started when he was just a few feet from the bottom.

Hosting a flurry of un-Christian-like one-word bursts, Artie began to shake his hands at lightning speed. When he opened his bare hands, the shredded palms told a story. Too fast, no gloves, self-inflicted wounds.

With Art out of commission for a few minutes, I had a good look at our driver. There were no seatbelts in the ancient off-road icon. It was in poor shape before its flight. Landing on all four wheels, the impact inflicted a compression motion when it stopped.

From the hilltop, Cathy stood near Ben, calling down with her offer of assistance. I was just underway with my assessment and asked for the oxygen kit. The driver still had a partial airway but likely suffered a fractured neck and internal injuries. He sputtered blood from his mouth and nose with each breath.

Jaw clenched, there was a chunk of his tongue sticking out between blood-covered teeth. Still partially attached, the tongue would have to wait. The driver's jaw was snapped shut like a vault door preventing good suctioning and a more detailed look. It took a minute; the oxygen bag rolled down the hill, caught up in the last few feet of rope intended to lower it.

There was no opening for inserting an oral airway. Our victim got the nasal airway treatment. Assisted by jelly to lubricate the nasal passage, the slippery stuff squirted out of a small foil pouch that looked more like a ketchup packet. I could smell the drying blood as I worked in front of the victim to protect his airway. The jagged, dripping, flopping piece of tongue looked nasty.

Running down the creek, fanning out on the surface of the water behind us, gasoline or oil spread a multi-coloured tint onto the once clean brook. There was not much of a chance of fire here; water splashed under the vehicle on impact wetting everything down.

The jeep must have bounced, rebounding from the force of the impact. A few feet away, sitting even with the water's surface, was the vehicle's battery, torn free from its mount and thrown clear. Another voice from above, a familiar fire captain, leaned out over the edge and sized up the scene. Announcing we needed a basket and some help, the faces of the pumper crew disappeared.

A second delivery from the hilltop arrived. Attached to a backboard for the trip down was a cervical collar. Designed to support an injured neck preventing further injury, it was time.

There was not enough help to keep in line traction and protect the injury at this point. The unconscious patient was relaxed and motionless; the collar went on without a problem. Art sat the ventilation kit on the jeep's hood, feeding oxygen to the driver, leaving to assess the conscious passenger sitting off to the side.

Ben disappeared from the hilltop, abandoning Cathy. He headed off to find a less challenging route to the creek bed. It would be an excursion.

Gathered on the hill now were a group of firefighters from the pump and rescue crews. Heavy coats abandoned, yellow waist harnesses cinched tight, the first two firefighters started down. It was an anti-climax to our earlier descent without an audience.

Our driver awoke now, a great sign. With any luck, he would not be combative for the extrication and ascent to the ambulance. Still drowsy and slobbering as he tried to speak, moving his extremities was a surprise. He stopped moving around when I grabbed his blood-covered hands, suggesting he likely had a neck injury.

Artie's hands looked like they were painful. He didn't make a peep as the well-equipped fire rescue crew arrived at our side. Working beside the Jeep in shin-deep water, I was glad for the help.

Usually, at accident scenes, we roll the stretcher up next to the vehicle. Sliding the spinal board partly off the cot and under the patient's butt in the car bridges the gap. Moving a seated patient out and then flat onto the level board with lots of hands to support the upper back and neck was usually simple.

Today, the eighty-pound aluminum stretcher was fifty-odd feet above on the hill. We had a limited number of hands available; it was time to improvise. The firefighters, lucky fellows, had rubber boots on and dry feet. Each held an end of the rescue basket as we slid the spinal board from inside the basket to the edge of the driver's seat of the drowned vehicle.

Looking for Ben, he was nowhere in sight. Other firefighters reached out as Artie, and I described how we would support the victim. We lifted him from his less than aerodynamic vehicle, now resting silently in the stream, transferring him to the board suspended slightly lower than the seat.

The patient sat on the backboard to start. I held his neck as Art's and several firefighter's hands came in from the sides behind his back and laid him flat on the board. The basket was set on the shore while he was strapped down for his trip back up the hillside. It was the minimalist approach to accomplish the rescue and avoid more delays.

Shouting up to Cathy that our patient was likely a head, neck and back injury, she replied she was ready. Still no Ben? Asking for a second, collar and straps, our attention was focused on the driver. Artie sent a board down earlier; neither thought of the accessories as we worked alone.

Artie announced he would go up with the immobilized driver. Having to lay supine or flat on his back, the patient spat and sputtered blood from the partially amputated tongue. The tissue around the mouth is very vascular, presenting a challenge to control bleeding.

Offered a harness sent down with the basket, Art strapped in like a pro; his secret was safe with me. One firefighter clipped his waist belt to the foot end, while the second rescuer took the opposite side to Artie. Fellow rescuers used the winch on the rescue to tow the patient and crew to the top.

The second pair of firefighters and I had the easy job of sliding the passenger onto the spinal board after applying a collar. He was strapped down while we waited for the basket to return for the second trip. I felt a hand on my arm.

Slipping in silently behind us, Ben appeared from nowhere. He was a quiet fellow, but a little warning would have been appreciated. For a split second, my mind raced to thoughts of a previously undiscovered victim climbing from the weeds further along the creek. Nope, just Ben.

Covered in burdock burrs to his waist, Ben took the long road. He quietly admitted to finding a path to the bottom but was forced to go several hundred feet downstream and zig zag his way to our level. He hated heights and turned down the job of rigging up and ascending with the passenger.

As much as it begged a snicker, I thanked him for the help and suggested he return to help Cathy. She would need help with this patient when he arrived at the top of the hill. He turned without a grumble and headed out. That's Ben.

The worn and now dirty Stokes basket bounced off the face of the hill as it hit bottom. The spare safety harness intended for me was strapped to a hand hole along the one edge. Strapping into the belt, firefighters set the patient in the basket and fastened the cross straps.

The cable leading to the rescue unit above tightened up on the firefighter's command. I clipped onto the basket and began the assisted walk up the hill. Missing a few steps when loose gravel gave way, my difficulty was shared by the rescuer at the foot of the basket.

Secured to the edge of the wire "Stokes" basket, we were not about to fall and roll to the bottom. We could walk up the hill with some assistance from the half-inch steel cable from the rescue truck above.

Arriving at the top, I thanked our rescuers. The prospect of hand-bombing the patients on spinal boards up the hill via Ben's route gave me the shivers. Where was Ben anyway?

Cathy and Artie loaded the driver in the back of our ambulance, now suctioning blood from his mouth. Conscious and aware, he slobbered out the experience of his ride to the creek.

He and his friend were offroading for the afternoon. As they sped across the field, the passenger spotted the dropoff first and bailed before the driver could swerve. The Jeep sailed over the edge with enough speed, fortunately or not, landing on its wheels. The stop must have been terrible.

Rolling over the edge, the passenger took his own ride as he tumbled down the hill to the weeds. Covered in cuts, scrapes and sporting a fractured wrist, he was the least injured.

Ben showed up at his ambulance's back door as a firefighter, and I loaded the stretcher. We did ok, considering my assistant never lifted a cot before by his own admission. I handed off the passenger to Ben. Returning to my ambulance to get the low down from Art, I announced to Cathy her patient was loaded. There was a beehive of activity in the back.

Art finished the assessment and determined the fellow likely had a fractured neck and pelvis. We transported our patient to the closest hospital, which was not the best choice. The best place for trauma was miles further. Our orders in the day did not allow for heading directly to the best place for accident victims. It would be years before a trauma by-pass directive hit the streets.

I was the proud owner of several four-wheel-drive vehicles in my day. Hills, creeks and mud are the mainstays of any true blue "off-roader." To this day, the advice of *"look before you leap"* reminds me of that call.

Skidmark or question mark

Everyone has a different threshold for excitement, danger and acceptable risk. Friends and family thought I was crazy when I built, then flew, a small ultralight airplane. Less than four hundred pounds of aluminum, steel and Dacron and I was off to the wild blue yonder. Cautiously climbing to ten thousand feet well clear of the established commercial airway routes one afternoon, I acknowledged the feat included a tolerable risk. Really.

A quick ride around the lumber yard on a small motorcycle a year before joining emergency medical services was admittedly fun. A co-worker offered his Yamaha bike to try. I concede I was curious.

Before the next riding season could start, I bought my first new car, then started a career in ambulance work. It didn't take too many shifts to see my first motorcycle collision. I lost the bug to ride before I got out of the gate.

A couple of years into the occupation of picking up the unfortunate victims of accidents, I met a fellow I could not stop feeling poorly for. He was an innocent passenger on a motorcycle. There is a theme here after reading the last story. Passengers are left out of the decision-making process when it comes to risk assessment. It always comes down to judgement.

Anytime you take a passenger for a ride, you should never assume they know all the risks. That is especially true for unconventional rides. Whenever I give the "doom and gloom" briefing about some upcoming activity, I take a hit from the family. It keeps them laughing at me.

So, there I was, once again, riding along fat dumb and happy on a sunny day with my mentor Hugh. Cruising south on Richmond Street, we passed bike after bike, enjoying the "large" day. Hugh pointed out the safer drivers from the crowd, noting their helmets, leathers and gloves. It was warm out; fashion did not prompt the riders to wear the hot coats and chaps.

It wasn't more than a couple of minutes when Jimmy piped up with "151 London, your 20 (location)?" In an instant, we were off to a "motorcycle down" call. It was no coincidence with the day. With several bike accidents under my belt, including a fatality, I was beginning to feel seasoned. There is a first for everything, a variation on a theme.

A few minutes later, we pulled up to the scene in front of a school at a crosswalk. Who was injured, the rider or a kid hit by a speeding biker? Parked along the curb down the road was a low-slung bike with a helmet dangling from a set of "ape hanger" handlebars. The crowd blocked our view, so I assumed it was a kid hit by the bike.

Surprise…lying flat on his back was a fellow that had me by a hundred pounds. Helmet off, his friend, the real biker, crouched over the victim. This fellow had leathers on with heavy boots, the whole get-up. Concerned for his friend, he waved wildly for the crowd to back up with our arrival.

The patient was a passenger on the bike. Helmet still on; he was screaming as if mad at someone. Wearing a thin buttoned nylon shirt, shorts and leather sandals held on by a loop around the big toe, he hardly looked the rider part.

Kneeling beside the patient, I started with the basics; "where are you hurt?" Expecting to hear his back or neck was the complaint; the response "My fucking back" came as no surprise. When paramedics hear "back," we think of the spine. Taking in the scene now, the injury was lining itself up with clues trailing out behind the fellow.

Have you ever seen a skid mark from a driver's violent braking to avoid an accident? How about the wiggling black line left behind on asphalt when someone does a "burnout"? Down the road was a short dark streak on the hot pavement, signalling the beginning of the end.

A few yards closer, a pair of shattered sunglasses lay abandoned. Closer yet were intermittent shreds of cloth that matched the patient's shirt. The front of his clothing was intact. Behind the victim, small pieces of pale pink and then yellow, shiny dots lined the remainder of the path.

Screaming now for his rescuers to "do something," our victim began to cry like a baby. The writing was on the wall. The initial skid mark was rubber. The closest skids were shirt, skin, then fat. Jeez, no wonder he's screaming.

Writhing on the ground, the shrill outbursts were a helpless cry. Unsure what to do, our rear-seat passenger squirmed as if itching himself like an animal on a convenient tree. There was a smell, not gasoline, not exhaust.

Insulted skin and fatty tissue offered up the fragrance, wafting off the hot pavement. I knelt beside the victim, assessing. Sounding more like a dying animal, he reminded me of a fellow that I treated a year ago with deep burns. This incident was before medics carried pain medication. We could offer no relief.

There were no chances to be taken. This guy was going for the "full ride," collar, board and straps. Using the traffic cop to hold the backboard for us seems now like cruel and unusual punishment. The view from behind the victim was gruesome. The constable arrived moments earlier on his own Harley. A skilled professional rider, he was dressed for the job.

School kids and their teacher watched the action through a chain-link fence. Having a hunch, I sent Hugh back to the Suburban to grab up a cotton pillowcase and the two bottles of sterile water. There was one bottle in our tin first aid box; it might fall short of the mark.

The biker was beside himself, now hearing the screaming and crying coming from his passenger. Later, I would learn that the intense emotional response stemmed from guilt, marking ownership of his friend's predicament. You can't take this one back, buddy.

Rolling the fellow towards the schoolyard was an excellent move blocking the ghastly sight from the kids. Nearby witnesses and gawkers gasped as the patient's back arrived at a perpendicular angle to the road. I could hear the teacher shouting to turn the kids back to their school.

Stuck to a large field of exposed fatty material, shredded skin and tatters of a once cool shirt: a small truckload of gravel. This was the poster child for dirty wounds. Over one foot in diameter, the irregularly shaped cavity oozed a clear serous fluid, along with a generous measure of blood along the border of the injury.

There was a lot of skin missing. Well, not really; it was easy to spot. It was underneath and nearby our victim, leaving a greasy streak behind him on the roadway. Smeared on the hot asphalt, the detached tissue created the most dramatic superficial injury I faced so far in my two years. You would think the fresh air would be a relief. It was way too early for healing to start.

Soaking the soft pillowcase in sterile water, there were no bandages large enough to span this massive abrasion and now avulsion. The remaining two plastic bottles of cool, clear water were poured over the patient's back, a vain attempt to clean the hollow where tissue and fat once resided, intact. The smell at close range was unmistakable.

Stretching the dampened cloth over the wound, we rolled the patient onto the waiting board held by the cop. The look on the professional rider's face made me regret my decision to enlist his help. Unfortunately, we needed the extra hands for the moment.

The screaming resumed when the fellow was lying flat on the board. With most of the gravel gone, the moist cloth would be a temporary fix. The mix of sticky pale yellow body fluid escaping from the massive divot in the patient's back would dry quickly.

This fellow escaped severe, life-threatening injuries. Head, neck, femurs and belly intact, he won the life lottery. Small consolation for the pain he was experiencing coming from the edges around the insult to his back.

Now missing most of the tissue and gouging deep into the fat on his back, sensory nerves were long gone from the middle of the wound. With that loss would be no feeling, a permanent condition. Where the victim's skin survived around the outline of the crater, nerves went into overdrive. The pain would be relentless until brought under control by our friends in the ER.

With the patient hoisted onto the stretcher positioned next to us, Hugh started some oxygen, attaching the green plastic mask to the wailing fellow's face. It wouldn't do much, if anything, but psychological first aid and appearances are everything.

It was a real grunt lifting this fellow into the ambulance. Three hundred pounds plus was my guess. That, in addition to the eighty pounds for the older model stretcher. Working under the bright sun, we lost as much sweat as this fellow lost in blood and body fluids, minus the pain.

The patient received the lights and sirens treatment for the ride to the ER. His vital signs were stable, but the pain increased the further we got past the incident. More intact nerves were coming back online and hurting like a burn. A brownish fluid now ran out from under the patient's back, over the board's edge onto the linen below.

Leaving the patient in the hospital to go onto the next call would typically be the end of the story.

This story deserves a brief epilogue. Sitting in the waiting room at the same ER that we delivered our unfortunate victim to only two fortnights ago, something made me look up from my paperwork. It was the voice that drew my attention. The bike passenger was responding to another guy walking behind him, something about parking.

The unlucky passenger walked past me on a course leading from the outpatient area. It was the plastic surgery clinic's turn today. Stooped over, he was still in pain. Wearing another summer-weight shirt, this one was unbuttoned, exposing an oversized bare belly. The loose shirt offered no restriction to the dressing on his back, probably changed following a check-up in the nearby clinic.

Did you ever look at someone you were familiar with and wonder what was different? New glasses, a new haircut or colour. There was no prize for missing the obvious. Still wearing cutoff jeans, this fellow had fresh dressings covering both thighs. The legs are one site used to harvest skin for grafting.

I looked at the man and received no audible response. The connection struck a nerve though, he lifted his head up and back, acknowledging my presence. Following behind at a safe distance, his chauffeur. He was minus the leathers and helmet today.

As the patient walked out of the department, his shirt had the beginnings of marks or blotches. The grafted and healing injury was still weeping some brownish fluid. What a sentence. Pain, dressings sticking to the wound, and the impossible task of changing the bandage to keep it clean. The care would prevent infection and reduce the odour from the drying body fluid.

A level crossing

Every kid worth his salt has owned or played with a miniature train set. Picking up those tiny engines and making up trains with tank cars and boxcars, kids are intrigued. Heck, I have some great memories of riding behind the small engine in Springbank Park in Byron. Years later, its successor pulled my daughter and me around the quarter-mile oval to her delight.

Real trains are not cute. They are not toys, and you certainly can't pick them up and arrange them with your bare hands. They can and do rearrange most things they encounter at nearly any speed.

Over the years, responding to train incidents has never brought any sense of "this will be a cool call" after my first. The initial experience was a fatality and provided no medical challenge beyond confirming the "bloody obvious." Minimal bleeding and gross dismemberment were the highlights. That story is in chapter ABC.

Ok, enough idle chatter, back to work in the big smoke. In the lounge just before two am, Kelly set the Provincial Police line down, announcing, a train hit a car outside the city. Two am, you ask. It was just after "last call." We were the closest unit working out of our office downtown.

John, a laid-back fellow, never got excited on any call. Known for a snicker when the chips were down, it was his nervous tell. He could fall asleep in an instant. There was no surprise to have to shake his shoulder to get on the road. Waking him was like the old "shake and shout" during CPR training.

It was nearly fifteen minutes to get to the scene. The level crossing was on the edge of a small community out in the County. Trains routinely doing over fifty miles an hour blasted their horns before passing the white sawbuck warning signs and flashing lights.

This night was no exception. Tiny red lights glittered from the rear corners of the caboose in the distance. Railroads still had them then and for several years after this crash. The back end of the steel behemoth came to a stop almost a quarter of a mile east of us. A single black and white patrol car sat stationary at the crossing. Its red gumball machine-like emergency light rotated slowly, exhaust puffing out in a narrow white plume.

Sitting at the east side of the crossing was the front end of a heavy older car. The kind we referred to as a "tank" compared to today's lightweights. John and I looked at each other; this was a child's play. A fatality for sure.

Exiting the ambulance, I was ready to approach the vehicle to wave my hands over it, an act of presuming the death of the corpse mangled inside. The rear half of the automobile was missing, gone, not even a shadow down the tracks; the car was a four-door, as it turns out. One rear door on the driver's side hung off broken hinges on an angle, giving away the original body style.

Something made me grab the two kits that were expected at the patient's side on every call. Slinging the oxygen and first aid bags over to the car, I set them down. Standing where the floor would have been behind the driver before the impact, jagged, torn steel rested on the ground. A voice clearly called out.

"I'm ok, buddy; I never heard the train." I crouched down to peer into the interior of the car. Headlights from the patrol car aimed in the direction of the annihilated vehicle revealed an incredible sight. There were no headrests in this tank; the outline of a driver's shoulders and head appeared above the bench seatback. Looking out at the silent officer nearby, he had not uttered a word as we approached.

John piped up from behind me, announcing his assistance. He was returning to the ambulance for the stretcher, a backboard, collar and straps. It was eerily silent, the train's diesel drone well out of range. The car's headlights were still on, the engine stopped or stalled.

Asking this lucky fellow where he hurt seemed like the right thing to do. I expected his answer to be "all over." The impact, then twisting forces dispensed by the speeding train, could not have missed their mark. Coming around to the door, the middle-aged driver looked out of his window at me and denied any injury.

Leaning down to address him and have a look for myself, part of his salvation hit me square in the face. Alcohol. Breath tainted with the odour of a past alcoholic beverage belched out front and centre. Looking over at the pensive officer nearby, a quick point of my finger to my nose, then pointing back at our victim, drew an endorsing nod.

Warning the driver to stay still seemed a waste of time since he survived the crash and sat for who knows how long, awaiting his escape. He got the party line of "stay still and don't move your neck" for the sake of the mechanism of injury.

Returning to my side, John and I were equally surprised when the driver's door opened without hesitation on the first attempt. It begged the question; why had our victim remained in the car for so long. It would be fair to say that it would probably take some time to gather your thoughts if you were hit by a speeding train.

Pulling up to the scene, a pickup truck familiar to our patient stopped. The lone occupant confidently walked up, addressing the patient by his first name. Catching the waiting officer's attention, he motioned for the acquaintance to accompany him back to the patrol car.

Checking our victim from head to toe revealed no apparent injuries and no pain response to gentle squeezes of his neck, legs, arms, and chest. Indeed, a lottery winner. John and I turned the fellow out of his seat to stand up following the collar treatment. He transferred quickly to our hard plywood bed for the trip to the ER.

It was as if the attention paid to the patient was a total waste of time. The driver looked at both of us, then back at his car. Had his tank been drivable, likely, he would have driven off, fading into the night.

Loaded into our bright, warm ambulance, the conversation turned to the train. With the man safely strapped to our backboard looking at the ceiling of his new ride, the collision begged the question. "What happened?" A local, our patient, had been returning home from the legion. This smelled like court time.

The driver narrated how he regularly crosses the tracks and should have known better. His repeated claims that he'd never heard the train seemed like a distorted defence at the moment. Thinking that this fellow's children would be relieved he had survived, I expected their second reaction would include a generous browbeating.

Opening the rear door to our patient compartment, the constable appeared hat in hand. We had the fellow ready for the ride to the hospital when the officer asked how much he had to drink this evening. Not sensing the consequences of his answer, the response was a fait accompli.

A second officer stepped into view from behind the rear door. Hand around his Sam Brown leather cross strap, he leaned in, announcing he would be riding with us to the hospital. This would ensure the driver could not rely on a modification to his story. "Really, your honour, I drank in the ambulance." A great move to seal his fate and help us avoid court.

The absence of the train crew at the crossing was explained away by the first constable. Both the engineer and conductor returned to their caboose to write down their story when the cop arrived. The engineer had to be rattled witnessing the impact, though surprised and relieved seeing the driver survive the crash.

Yup, it was beer. Lying on your back after a few brews and a train wreck, now jiggling your way down the road, was a recipe for nausea followed by vomiting. It was a good thing our patient was strapped to the board. Tilting the immobilizing platform on its side and providing some suction prevented our guest from choking on his libations. Our Provincial escort did not look impressed as his evidence sailed up the suction tube to swish around in the reservoir.

For beer lovers, it always tastes and smells better on the way down. For everyone else, it just stinks.

Not my house

Cars belong in garages. If your home is of a more modest design, then the family ride belongs in the driveway or on the road, not in the house. The call for a car that has accidentally intruded into a dwelling is always unsettling.

There are lots of issues that come into play. Has it started a fire by striking the gas meter? Is fuel leaking into the structure, also risking a fire? Is the car inside the building far enough that it requires rescue to release the victim? Any single complication poses a host of hazards and challenges.

Responding to the call for a car vs. house, Brad and I raced to the scene to see if we could beat fire crews. The unofficial contest was not about speed, rather about control. Having a handle on the patient and the scene first is a much better starting point.

Arriving at the scene last always places paramedics in "catch up" mode. Taking a report from the rescue squad and trying to size up the job after everyone else was there first sucks. We lost; a pumper crew arrived before us. Fortunately, they were still setting up a hose line in preparation for the rescue.

Sticking out of the corner of the one-story brick ranch home was an older car. Headlights still on, we approached the car as if the patient was the only issue. Mistake one was on the books. The patient, a loner in the vehicle, spoke to a witness or neighbour standing at the driver's door. The door ended up just inside the remaining brick wall.

Strewn across the front lawn were shattered bricks and a small shrub. Lying close by, a chrome trim ring that once held a headlight. The front corner of the car hit the house first. Looking like a low-speed event, most of the car was still outside the building.

An eerie light glowed under the driver's door. Looking at the destruction around and under the car, a small hole in the wall revealed a couch below. The family room was empty with any luck, abandoned for an early evening to bed.

Replying to a captain that appeared at my side, I looked at Brad after hearing the firefighter ask what they could do to help. It was one of my earlier experiences where competition for control never got off the starting block. We all agreed the car would not tip into the home. We would still need help with the door.

A fire would have been a real problem; who knows what could happen? I let the captain know we would need extra hands removing this fellow from his vehicle. We were still assessing.

The fire officer asked Brad standing closest to the car if the ignition was off. Looking through the window, the key was safely turned off. Turning to share the news with his crew, the firefighter disappeared into the darkness between the houses.

Brad was headfirst into the car through the opposite window. Asking over his shoulder if he smelled alcohol, a quiet shake of his head from side to side was a relief. Both Brad's hands were visible; their motion followed his calm narration to the patient that he was protecting his neck with a collar. I passed Brad the oxygen mask, leaving the bag on the roof above.

So how do you hit a house if you are not drunk or being chased by the law? Tracks leading from the road across an adjoining front lawn to the impact pointed to a gentle wander off the road to the victim's destination. Was he a sleeper? That was more like a highway thing from fatigue and the monotony of the hashed line between lanes mile after mile.

Brad backed out of the car, announcing, "Let's go." Asking what the rush was, I could see our driver, head drooped down to the wheel and not moving. Our stretcher was set up, ready with the backboard.

The patient looked tired. Head tilted to the side, he looked like he had run a race. Impossible, this fellow was in his seventies and grandfatherly looking.

Turning to attract the captain's attention, I waved at a closer firefighter asking for some hands. In seconds, four eager fellows appeared, ready to help. The front edge of the driver's door was an issue; it was inside the wall.

The surrounding brick shattered, giving way to the force, leaving a small gap. As two firefighters grabbed the door by its rear edge, I could hear voices from under the car. Other fire crews were assessing the damage and risks from the basement.

It was time for some brute force. The captain stepping up behind his crew urged them to force the door open "gently," preventing the car itself from moving. Several extra hands appeared, grabbing the frame while a flashlight lit their way.

Opening without a hitch, a few creaks and groans of fatiguing metal cleared the path to our patient's release. We were free to transfer our victim to the backboard.

Brad whispered that the patient had a very thready pulse, and his colour was pale. The push to get him to the ER was on. Internal bleeding was Brad's guess, though I doubted it since the impact was not that great. The fellow was not wearing a seat belt but did not complain of any pain when Brad asked.

Sliding the board partway off our stretcher under the victims behind bridged the gap. Lots of hands supported his neck and back as we turned the man out of the car. Sliding him to a flat position on the board, then returning the board to the stretcher, the fire guys were on the mark. The oxygen wound up strapped between the victim's immobilized legs.

The lawn was still soft, not frozen for the season; stretcher wheels caught the soft earth. With relatively little effort, our helpers grabbed the stretcher. It literally hovered off the lawn for the trip back to our ambulance. The fellow was not talking but did respond to Brad's questions as we were loading him into the back of the ambulance.

He was losing ground. Climbing into the bright patient compartment, I helped Brad to prepare the victim for transport. Starting oxygen from the larger tank in the ambulance, I turned to cut the fellow's coat off one arm. Brad took a blood pressure from the other bared arm.

For some reason, I took our victim's arm that I just released from the suede coat and checked his pulse. No pulse. Shouting to Brad, I remember announcing, "he's arrested." With that, the patient started talking, and Brad blurted out that his pressure was under one hundred, though there was still a pulse on the other wrist.

Stepping backwards out of the ambulance's side door, I tripped when I didn't plant my foot firmly on the ground. There are no points for swearing in front of a patient, though I suspect he missed the curse. We were off to the hospital without a single thank you to our friends for their help.

Waving at a cop standing by the house earlier, I passed the news, we did not smell alcohol from the driver. He responded with a puzzled look and walked away, almost disappointed.

The brief radio patch to the ER nurse did not net much information. There were no obvious injuries to report. The driver's account of the accident was more like a dream. We could only pass on the mechanism of injury and the low blood pressure. The fact that he was boarded and collared was a given.

The trip was short. Opening the rear doors on the ramp at the hospital, Brad was bagging the patient now though he still had a pulse. You couldn't see a drop of blood. I assumed a puzzled look standing at the side of the stretcher lowering it with my partner. Not a mark on his chest or belly, Brad shared my bewildering stance.

In the resuscitation room, Brad described the "mechanism of injury." Followed by a guess at the car's unremarkable impact speed then narrating the patient's waning level of awareness to unconsciousness. Several surgical staff appeared for the event with the pre-arrival details shared by the charge nurse.

With his clothes now removed, our patient concealed no trauma secrets. Not a single mark or cut to be seen. Index and second fingers appeared from the four corners of the lowered gurney to feel for pulses. The blood pressure was almost zip. A doctor suggested looking for blood in the belly once the large IVs were in each arm. In moments, a catheter was inserted into the nearly clinically dead driver. Staff had their suspicions.

An intern I recognized intubated the fellow to ventilate him; he was losing ground. The invasive check of his belly was positive. A young medical student got the nod from the lead emergency physician when he suggested a ruptured "triple-A." "AAA" is an abdominal aortic aneurysm.

The aorta, a large vessel carrying blood from the heart, divides to supply both the body's upper and lower halves. In the doc's words, it "sprung a leak." Sometimes leaks start slowly for a variety of medical reasons.

The condition can also be caused by blunt trauma; I had my doubts in this case. But hell, I'm just a casualty care attendant. The one clinical sign or clue that swept clear over my head had been the absence of a pulse in one arm.

In a more aggressive move, the call was made for a surgical tray for the visiting surgery resident initially consulting on a patient in room eleven across the hall. Within minutes we were cleared back to a safe distance like wallflowers. The patient's abdomen received a quick prep of iodine. Orange belly pointing to the ceiling, a fist-sized incision was followed by a red tsunami that gushed from patient to gurney to floor in seconds.

Surgical snaps clicked from gloved hands attached to a tall fellow with a cloth mask dangling loosely on his chest. He barely entered the impromptu portal into the patient before declaring he had it. The dam had been plugged. It was a last-ditch effort to stop the flooding loss.

It looked like litres of blood. Red footprints tracked on the floor by staff circled the bed. Evidence of scurrying to connect unmatched blood to the victim. An out-of-breath orderly returned moments earlier with O positive blood. It is the universal donor type when there is not enough time to do lab tests to dial in the exact cross match for the patient's blood type.

"Intravenous fluid is great, but it doesn't carry oxygen," decried another doctor to a young observing medical student. The whole sight of the surgical procedure in the ER was an exception. Never having spent time in the operating room, it was a dramatic sight in addition to the makeshift "sterile field" technique.

It turned out to be an unsuccessful result; our patient succumbed to his aneurysm. It was likely a "pre-existing condition," as told to the medical student by our improvised mentor. We cleaned up our ambulance and returned to the office to share our experience with a couple of lazing crews at the station. Three medics never opened their eyes, instead choosing to search the insides of their eyelids for the genuine meaning of life.

Caught

Very little in this world is private. Just ask a politician caught on camera or quoted. A half newsworthy item can carry over several news cycles in a heartbeat. Unfortunately, your secret is at risk when caught engaging in an activity that should remain private. As unusual as this experience was, fortunately, it was not newsworthy.

Once you have seen or shared something, it is too late to take it back. Luckily this one didn't wind up in court. A Crown Attorney would have had a hay day asking me to recount the night. Again, this incident was never deserving of attention until now.

Joanne and I just cleared our dispatch centre. The short drive back to the office to do the shift paperwork was usually routine. The stop at the radio room to pick up dispatch forms was more social than work.

Chatting with dispatchers and looking at swaying patrons, leaving the bar across the street was entertaining. Work is work, and it was sitting on the engine cowling between Joanne and me, driving away from the radio room. The pink dispatch forms had to be matched with the call reports.

Approaching the intersection, the traffic signal turned green for us long before we reached the cross-traffic now stopped. A car halted for the red light to our left sat patiently. Hands-on the wheel, I just finished recounting the staggering patrons lined up for a drink at the bar.

It was hardly a two-word exclamation. "Look out" melted into a succinct warning, too late to divert our orange and white van from its eastbound path. Joanne tried her best when she saw the silver bullet approaching from our right. She leaned in towards me, having seen what was coming.

Rocketing out from the railroad underpass, the small pickup struck our ambulance on the passenger's side doors, usually reserved for loading the walking wounded. The impact shunted the van sideways. With our forward motion, we cleared the intersection before I recovered.

Parked just clear of the underpass, I threw the lights on to mark our vehicle, now uselessly blocking the curb lane. The dispatchers must have fallen off their chairs with the radio report of the collision. It should have been the mundane announcement that we arrived at the base.

Requesting police, Gail sounded relieved with the news that we were "ok." Joanne, unsettled from the collision, was still restrained by her seat belt. We both climbed out to check the other vehicle.

Looking down into the underpass, the damaged truck rolled aimlessly back down the incline. It rested; tailgate pinned against the concrete column dividing the opposing underground lanes. Approaching the driver's door, the female driver laid her head against the glass, eyes closed. Joanne walked around to the passenger's door, looking for a second victim.

First impressions are lasting. Leaning in against the partly open window, the question is always: "are you injured?". The obligatory introduction results in a "no" more often than you would think. The woman's eyes opened with a corresponding negative response and a curse. The air was not blue, though the odour of alcohol jumped out of the sedentary driver.

Paramedics are never to take the words of a would-be patient at face value. Victims are sometimes unaware of their injuries or their extent. Call it shock or simple confusion, the primary survey continued.

My small metal flashlight aimed in the cab of the disabled vehicle was quickly extinguished. Hearing me call out, Joanne looked back in the cab. Waving the temporary beam again, Joanne looked to me, then down to the driver's lap, where I motioned the light for her confirmation.

The driver, now sitting silently, had been busy before the impact. The fly on her jeans was down to the bottom. Pants wide open, her underwear bulged with her right hand resting inside. Still unaware that she had been caught "red-handed," our driver seemed oblivious to the observers perched outside her doors.

I stepped back. Making no attempt to exit the disabled truck, the driver sent us away for some reason. It was time to stand and take in the moment. There was an accident form for each of us to complete. One of my assignments as a supervisor was the fleet. Would the boss relieve me of the follow-up required since I was the medic driving the ambulance tonight?

Arriving in darkness, a police officer sizing up the scene positioned his car facing the wrong direction. Nose to nose with the pick-up truck, he lit up his cruiser, intending to warn approaching drivers to avoid the obvious.

The crash involving an ambulance was an official call. The officer donning his forage cap likely expected a sargent to stop by. It was an emergency vehicle involved that was worth a drive-by. As the constable walked up, I shook my head from side to side and opened with, "ya gotta see this." Joanne turned away, returning to the damaged ambulance.

The real issue here was the suspicion of an impaired driver. The pre-impact activity was just icing on the cake, something you would never expect to see at the scene of a collision. The official salutation from the officer awoke the resting woman, still no hands on the wheel.

Calling on his walkie-talkie for another officer to attend, his request was prematurely answered by a curious officer passing by. The two cops spoke through the open window. The second parked his ride, exiting to take the time to look at the driver for himself.

Returning to the basic story, the first constable got the picture. Advising that the driver declined medical attention or a ride to the hospital, he motioned to his co-worker it was time. He returned to the window and quietly announced to the driver, she would be going with them.

The official warning recited by the officer that she was under arrest as she exited the truck brought the driver back to life. Rearranging her dishevelled clothing was a priority now. Walked away to the second patrol car, the officer sat up front, writing notes as his passenger returned to a slouched position in the cage.

Approaching the investigating officer's car window, I handed him several documents needed for his report. I was irritated at having to delay my own paperwork back at the office. Relieved I would not have to sit in the rear of his cruiser to give my statement, I stood patiently. The paper report took fifteen minutes to get my portion on record. Documents in hand, I returned to the ambulance.

Joanne had been busy. Her statement was done and sitting on the engine cowling, on the envelope that held the blank reporting documents. Looking at me, I think she expected a comment about the drinking driver. I wasn't going near that land mine.

Several weeks later, I ran into (figuratively speaking) the investigating officer on another call. Smiling as I asked if I would have to appear in court, he relayed the crown attorney's response. Apparently, the woman withdrew her intent to fight the issue in court.

Surely the judge would take no mercy after hearing the story. The cop suggested that her defence counsel probably explained what the scientific evidence revealed in addition to the witness statement regarding her appearance when found still behind the wheel. Case closed.

Frozen

The city's newest east end station was generous for a two-crew base; there was space in the garage for four trucks. Repurposed from a mechanical repair shop, large overhead doors lined the front and back of both bays. The lounge was comfortable, though not very appealing, verging on dingy. The microwave and colour TV was its most attractive features.

The plus here was the station manager. He was old school and a clean fanatic. The title freak referring to clean should go to a younger candidate exercising a less measured approach. Sam, nearing retirement, took on a station with a slower pace than his previous routine downtown.

Crews respected Sam's experience and direction, though, at times, you could detect a veiled threat buried in his instruction. Sam was always carrying a cleaning rag draping from a back pocket to catch a spill or mark. He walked with a confident swagger disguising his small stature. The station was pristine despite the shortcomings in the furnishings and finishes.

Arriving at the back door for a station check and some administrative duties, the fresh snow crunched under my boots, stepping out of the SUV. It was the coldest night of the winter, and nearly 2 am. The crew tonight was experienced. Debbie was an Advanced Care Paramedic, working with Paul, a younger fellow, a part-timer taking hours at two services until a full-time opportunity presented itself.

Opening the station manager's office, paperwork lined the floor. Shoved through a mail slot, shift logs flew haphazardly, waiting for their daily retrieval. Sam called in sick for the tour; Paul jumped at the chance for a call-in. Any other night, the mail would be sorted and piled uniformly, another one of Sam's earmarks.

Sensing the dimmed lighting ahead, I offered a muted salutation. A hushed drama on the large screen at the other end of the room provided the only light. Awake but not needing the noise from the crowd scene to interpret the story, both medics issued a relaxed "Hi." The crew had not moved for hours, or at least since the snow started, a real treat. Tonight was not the night to disturb a team enjoying their break.

A piercing beep from the base pager over my shoulder broke the silence, sounding its alert to an assignment. The brief pause between the tone and message gave away the urgency of the hail. Announcing the crew's unit number, the call's priority, then a rural address, the communication ended with the report of SOB.

Shortness of breath fit the bill. Lying down for the night, some folks with a CHF history, congestive heart failure or COPD chronic obstructive pulmonary disease can only lay flat for so long. Puffing away, anxiety and fear flood in, followed by the call for help. Partly relieved by sitting upright, the condition is often only reversed with a trip to the ER.

Not excited at the prospect of heading out to fresh snow and cold air, the absence of grumbling was a surprise. The call would mean an hour's work before the crew could clear the hospital, pick up a coffee and return to their station. The bay door hit the concrete with a clunk. Out of context as a late arriver, the crowd scene on the television held no intrigue. There was another station to check, paperwork in hand; I turned and left.

Hearing the crew receive some additional information over the portable radio, there was little chance of a treat and release tonight. The long history from the spouse's description to the dispatcher spelled a visit to the ER for the patient. They were heading north of the city limits.

Climbing into the Suburban SUV, the vinyl seat was cold. The windows were dotted with freshly melted snow, a sign the cab would be warm again in a minute. The supervisor's vehicle was a four-wheel drive, another bonus tonight. Lights flickered with the startup, though the radios and laptop computer never lost their place during the brief stop.

Taking the back routes around the city broke up the routine of station runs. What should take an hour without interruptions could drag on during a busy night chasing crews on calls or stopping at the emergency departments to clear units and negotiate with nurses to offload patients.

Five minutes into the trip between stations, dispatch was polling for an available unit. Calling several vehicle's Louise was on a mission. Our service was just entering the age of GPS vehicle tracking. Small ambulance icons advanced a fraction of an inch refreshing the mapping screen to my right. I could see them; Louise must be looking for one of the crews at an ER.

Finally, a crew she could assign, the call went out for a single-vehicle accident. Advising she would get more units when they came available spelled trouble. The call location slid right past me the first time. When the medic asked for a repeat, I took my eyes off the road for an instant. A half-mile ahead on the map screen was the intersection for the crash.

Reaching into a box of examination gloves on the passenger's seat, the blue vinyl would provide no barrier from the cold. One glove on and the other on the computer keyboard; it was time to let dispatch know I was it. Supervisors provide first response support when they are close by a call, or no units are available; it was a twofer tonight.

Louise sounded relieved having another unit to assign to the crash. The caller was a patient in the vehicle and was trapped. The car struck a "hydro pole." This was not the ideal night for a rescue scenario; it was minus something, windy and slippery. Pulling up to the wreck took less than a minute.

Driving around town in a vehicle that needed to be kept warm for the medications and equipment in the rear compartment, I was that guy that was always in short sleeves. I hated being too hot. The winter gear and rescue helmet in the back was reserved for situations like tonight.

Smiles and laughs from medics and cops at the scene and citizens outside the ER seeing me in summer wear did not weaken my resolve in the cold weather. I would not go back to the truck for a coat until I was "good" and cooled off.

Reaching in the rear door behind my seat, tonight, it was time for the coat and hardhat. Exhaled breath rose in a faint white cloud as I stood pulling on the jacket. The breeze carried it sideways in the shadow of the SUV.

At the end of broad tracks scraped sideways in the snow, a compact car sat behind the far side of a utility pole. The wooden post looked more than a foot and a half in diameter, not giving an inch from the hit.

Reading the marks in the fresh snow, the car spun around, crossing the road. Striking the passenger's side rear door on the pole, the small four-door continued in a second 180-degree spin, coming to rest close by. Three silhouettes moving in the car were a good sign; at least that was my first impression.

The radio speaker in my left ear began to broadcast a second transporting unit's dispatch as I approached the wreck carrying some equipment. Setting the kits on the car's trunk, I started a walk-around assessment, beginning at the damaged door. Bad news, the rear seat occupant was slumped over, unconscious, with part of his head hanging through the glassless opening. Blood ran down the outside of the car, already freezing to the painted surface.

The driver assumed the position of official spokesman for the small group, the only occupant capable of speaking now. He explained over his shoulder; he realized too late that they were approaching the top of a hill that would be slippery. Sounded like a case of braking too heavily and no traction. The driver was ok by his admission, though I could see blood on his face. Maybe not so ok; he was still behind the wheel.

The front seat passenger was awake but not speaking. The impact came from the side of the car behind him. The glass in his window was intact, but I bet he still had his bell rung. Probably not the medical description you wanted for a primary assessment. There was no blood to see.

Dispatch was not pleased to hear the request for a third ambulance and rescue. A pumper crew was already on the way, but it was no time to be shy. Cancelling a rescue crew early on is always easier than tacking ten minutes onto a response time by calling them after the fact. The car was bent like a pretzel; neither passenger's side door would budge.

Gagging slightly on the oral airway as I slid it past blood-covered lips, the early twenties male accepted the plastic tube for the moment. His teeth were not clenched, often an early sign of a severe head injury. He would probably pull or spit the piece out when he came around. Grabbing the oxygen kit, I could barely pull the Velcro holding the cover on the cylinder.

Have you ever cut yourself or smashed a finger experiencing a delayed pain reaction? That pain that creeps up behind you then hits you right between the eyes. Before joining EMS, I worked in the lumber industry. An outside job, the cold was brutal handling building materials in the winter. I experienced frostbite in several fingers. The ordeal continued to provide a lasting memory when cold weather hit.

Numbed fingers throbbed beneath the thin blue gloves. Fumbling with the parts, connecting a brittle plastic mask to the outlet was difficult. The easy part was turning the tank valve wide open. Litres per minute did not matter now; a hiss escaping from the mask would have to do.

The non-rebreather mask too stiffened from the cold to mould to his features, hung crookedly across the patient's blood-streaked face. After filling the reservoir bag, it refused to inflate and deflate with the patient's breathing, only crackling in the night air. A curled supply hose would not relax, pulling the mask further away. The compromise was better than no oxygen.

A collar was next for the unresponsive fellow. Splattered blood covered the back of my gloved hands and the reflective cuffs on my coat. Impressed with the stiff plastic neck support, the hard shell didn't crack, moulding the brace around the patient's neck, inside his heavy jacket.

The driver was babbling now about not being drunk. I couldn't tell if he was drunk or not; the cops could figure it out. The front-seat passenger to my right was starting to moan and talk; the response was an improvement.

There was not much more I could do until help arrived. It was time to focus on the smashed head. The impact on the patient's door likely injured the victim's neck, sharing the force with some internal organs.

Reaching around holding each side of this young victim's neck, sticky, freezing blood oozed from several head lacerations covering the gloves. It was easy leaning in to stabilize the patient's head and neck. The car's roof was pushed in almost two feet with the impact. The vehicle had bounced back, several feet from the pole.

Finally, the first ambulance, its lights flashing, coming head-on up the hill. My back was to the approaching Trafalgar Street engine company number 10; their grinder siren wailed in the distance beyond the top of the rise. Adjusting my hands to support the victim's head, the urgency of the cold struck me. There was no feeling left in any fingers now.

Flexing my forearms to control the stiffened hands, my fingers were no help. Shifting my arms to maintain a grip, the gloves moved, revealing another hint of the dipping temperature. Frozen blood stuck to the vinyl medical gloves, flaked off of the fingers in the shape of small pink chips, fluttering away in the frigid breeze. The pale light cast from the side scene lights on the SUV highlighted the flying, solidified body fluid. Drops of blood froze then flew off the patient's hair as he shuddered from the cold and pain.

The action hit fast forward for an instant. An ambulance, the first fire crew and a police supervisor arrived. Seeing the scene, the first medics dove in. Sharing the care for the two other victims between them, more collars, some bandaging for the driver's head wound, then progress came to a stop, nothing.

The captain from the engine company offered an update after a brief look at the mess. Rescue would be a few minutes after clearing from a general alarm in the city's core.

The car bulged on the driver's side from the impact transferred through the frame. None of the vehicle's doors would give in without a small fight. The firefighters deserve credit; they made an effort. The pump crew's Halligan tool, a crowbar, was no match for the pinched steel. There is no substitute for heavy hydraulics; the rescue unit rolled up a minute later with two ambulances on its heels.

Time seemed to stand still again; fingers stopped aching just after the forearms took over. I was a mess. The hands gave into the cold too soon, a spinoff from the old injury. Some of my grief was likely age-related; that was difficult to admit. Then there was that voice in my head, coming from the radio earpiece, actually.

Dispatch called me several times; the bloodied and numb hands providing traction to the victim's neck were a distraction from attempting to answer. Besides, it was probably an update. The gang was here now; what pressing matter awaited.

Rescue made short work of the doors, only opening the driver's side. Releasing the passenger's doors would have delayed the extrication of the unconscious lad.

Handing off to a fresh crew, the look on my face probably spelled he's lost the edge. I withdrew to allow a medic kneeling on the rear seat to stabilize the unconscious victim's neck. My fingers were frozen in place, hands paralyzed from the cold.

Returning to the SUV, luckily, the door was not locked. The Anti-Theft system was engaged, leaving the ignition on, lights flashing and the interior warm. Fingers went around the door handle; there was no response to grip the latch, just to pull.

Sitting in the warm cab, a burning sensation spread through the gloves. It would take several minutes before the pain eased to return some feeling. Anyone looking my way would wonder why I was sitting motionless in the vehicle. The white hardhat was still on; there was no typing on the computer or talking on the phone. Over the years in EMS, my hands were reminded of the original frostbite insult; this was by far the worst refresher on pain.

Finally, able to peel the gloves off, the last flakes of freeze-dried blood flew onto my lap. The hardhat tossed over my shoulder bounced off the kitbag on the seat, landing on the floor. The aching peaked, trying to clench my fists in an exercise to regain their use. Gripping the radio microphone felt clumsy, like an unintentional motion.

Dispatch put me off when I called, suggesting I contact another communicator on a landline. It couldn't be urgent; the dispatcher would have relayed a message through a medic to check on me at the scene.

Pushing buttons on the cell phone was never more frustrating.

There was a hesitation when Louise answered my call. Wanting to whine about aching hands, her words left me speechless. "Make your way to Vic ER; your nephew just arrived there with a crew. He was stabbed at a club downtown."

My oldest nephew worked the front door of a licensed establishment and was there tonight; I spoke to his mother earlier. The clock ran for a minute while I collected my thoughts. There were lots of death notifications in my past. There were even a couple of times greeting a distraught visitor at the doors to the ER, leading them to their ill or injured kin. Being on the receiving end of bad news tonight was a first.

Calling my sister ranked right up there with the worst assignments on the job ever. Dispatch offered no details; I missed the call and radio patch to the ER. The drive to pick her up was not on the official "ok" list with my superiors. That would get sorted out in the morning.

Our drive to the hospital went off with few words. Usually, I would have an answer or guess for everything. This was a departure from the normal me. Pulling up to the hospital, sis two-stepped it in through the ER's front doors before I could park and go in through the ambulance entrance.

As it turns out, my nephew and another doorman tossed a few patrons out during the evening. The group was from Toronto, branded "bad guys," according to the cop as he walked away from interviewing my nephew.

With the bar closed, the staff teamed up, cleaning the place for the next night. One of my nephew's jobs was to walk the pile of garbage out to the steel bin behind the club. Things went sideways after a couple of trips.

Confronted by the ousted group, he retreated to his girlfriend's unlocked car in the lot. She worked at the club as well, serving tables. Taking sanctuary in the car sounded like a good plan.

That's when one of the bad guys reached back into his car and pulled out a machete. Sitting in a locked vehicle works sometimes. When the sword-wielding guy took matters into his own hands, the gloves were off. Systematically walking around the car, the swordsman proceeded to remove all the glass that would shatter.

It must have been a sight. Finally, unable to outpace the aggressor as my nephew moved from seat to seat, then climbing from front to back, the machete his its intended target. Causing multiple slashes more than stabs, his screaming attracted other employee's attention at the back of the building. The unwanted onlookers drove the crew back into their car, departing for the GTA.

As bad as the injuries looked and the number of stitches needed to sew him up, it could have been worse. The blade's wounds were superficial. My sister held up well seeing her kid in the ER. I was thankful. Fortunately, the injuries were not life-threatening, though the experience scared the shit out of him.

The rest of the shift was a blur.

Medics, or for that matter, all responders, serve without reservation. Able to work on others as if immune to their suffering, call it professional camouflage. When it comes to a loved one or a friend receiving the attention, the gloves come off. We cry like the next soul.

Pickup sticks

Having worked for a lumber company for a couple of years before joining the ambulance industry, the irony in this call left its mark. The highway was ice-covered, an excellent day to be sitting inside, wishing you were out there, decidedly not the opposite.

Despite the slippery road, stalwart truckers were pounding down the highway. Slowing for accidents that blocked or slowed their progress, they attempted to drive at the posted limit. It was way too fast.

Called for a transport truck that collided with a van, we travelled east of the city to get behind the accident. Riding with Dennis was always a thrill or frightening, depending on how you looked at it. He was a shit disturber. Enjoying practical jokes, he was predictable.

The drive was harrowing enough to slow Dennis down to just below the posted limit. If it weren't for the small red and white light on our roof, trucks still on a mission would have passed us. Dennis stole the road, placing the Ford hood emblem on the centre line.

Overtaking vehicles, some chose to slow as we passed to their left; others pulled over. One car spun slowly, almost lazily, into the ditch when a front wheel hit something on the shoulder. It drew a devilish laugh from my chauffeur.

Arriving at the scene, Provincial police marked the perimeter with red safety flares along the shoulder. Only slowing traffic for a moment, the wintery hazards did not end when you arrived at the scene.

Passing vehicles still focused on their destination, continued cutting it too close to all of us walking around the minor disaster. Well off the road, you could be hit today if a driver spun out and sailed into the middle of our accident field.

Strewn onto the highway's right lane and well into the ditch: thousands of spruce two by fours. All lengths of framing lumber flew off the truck's platform. The rig lay tipped up on one side. The force of the crash breaking the heavy straps holding the lumber secure before the upset.

Traction from more than a dozen tires travelling sideward left furrows in the soil once covered by fresh snow. The cab and trailer came to rest on their side. But not before catapulting the load. It looked like a giant field of the old game of pick-up sticks.

Burrowing into the soil, the driver's side of the cab's roof scooped dirt like a large excavator. It would be the death of the driver.

There were two vehicles involved. Our other ambulance responding was caught up in the mayhem a few miles away. Dennis and I split up; I headed for the cab towards an investigating police officer.

Dennis walked to the panel van ahead, still on its wheels. The damage around the roof and sides had me thinking it rolled then righted itself. I lost him when he walked around to the driver's side of the van.

The officer squatting by the eighteen-wheeler's cab's front windshield pointed to the snow and dirt mound pushed ahead of the bulging roof. Caught up in the debris was the exposed head of the driver of the rig. Leaning in to check the trucker's pulse, the injury to his head aligned with being thrown around the cab.

That included striking the roof as the cab filled with snow and dirt crushing him. Pulseless, this victim had been there for some time. There was a mean twist in his neck, likely the most significant contribution to his demise.

Turning to the officer, he confirmed the fellow was pulseless when he arrived. It would be up to the rescue squad or a tow truck to get him out. I walked away, telling the officer I was going to the other vehicle. Looking back, the constable had that thousand-mile stare. The kind you get when a call strikes a nerve.

Heading back to the panel van, the painted sign on the side was for house framing. A front wheel was bent out at a precarious angle. The sides of the vehicle meeting at the now peaked roof were pinched together from rolling.

Lying crisscrossed around the vehicle were thousands of pieces of lumber. Narrow black metal bands snapped under pressure releasing the bundled lumber, leaving sharp exposed edges. The area was a minefield.

Approaching from the passenger's front corner, Dennis stood motionless at the rear doors. Rounding the back corner of the totalled van, Dennis had opened the doors with a police officer's help. Our crowbar leaned up against the partly open door. I wasn't ready for the scene inside.

The van served as a supply vehicle to framing crews building the skeletons of new homes. It also worked as a crew hauler. Behind the front seats was an upholstered tub chair from the sixties. Turned on its side, the worn and dirty furniture partially hid its lifeless occupant.

Lying behind the chair was another victim. Covered in tools and fifty-pound boxes of nails, he was pulseless when I climbed in and checked. The fellow under the tub chair was also pulseless. Dumbfounded, I turned to Dennis to see his reaction to the scene. The returning grimace from my workmate spoke volumes.

The victims were nailed. Loose spiralled ardox nails, airborne in the rolling van, struck and penetrated both men. Pushed into their bodies, now looking more like porcupines, the spikes stuck out everywhere. There were also holes where nails penetrated the victims then fell out. Blood sprayed everywhere with the rolling motion of the crash.

Climbing over piles of debris towards the cab, a third victim, the driver, was thrown sideways from his seat. A crushing head injury claimed this fellow. One of the men, likely the front seat passenger, had been thrown back past the upholstered chair. No one had the benefit or protection of seat belts.

Returning to the rear doors, the smell of coffee with cream and sugar hung in the air. On the floor lay a crushed thermos bottle that once held the warm drink. A lunch pail burst open from a flying box of nails revealed a wax paper package, likely a sandwich. The entire framing crew wiped out on their way to a construction site.

This accident scene required a coroner and a squad of police with cameras and tape measures. There were no direct witnesses to tell their story; it would be up to other passing drivers to paint the picture.

Hearing a horn honk from the second ambulance, Dennis gave them the wave off. Getting out of their vehicle would only serve to add two more rubberneckers and more paperwork. Glad to shut their lights down and drive on, we would catch up later to share the tragic scene.

There was still a lesson to be learned here. A heavy tow truck arrived from the city's largest towing service. Directed by the police to lift the cab to release the driver, the operator had help from another hoister. Raising the heavy cab, you could see the victim, who now could easily be freed.

Thinking I was bulletproof and ten feet tall in the rescue business, I ventured in under the cab as it was suspended. I could just yank on the partially released victim; it would be easy. It was still a few feet to reach the victim. Short of the target, I started to lean in further. There was a blood-curdling scream from behind.

The tow truck operator lost it. My carelessness scared the bejeebers out of him. Pulling back to a safe distance, I apologized. He directed the other operator to stop his winch first. This left the cab to sit off at a safe angle.

The muddy and snowy contents of the cab dropped clear of the rig exposing the driver. It was safe to pull the victim clear for the responding coroner.

I went on to meet the tow operator who owns the firm to this day. The service is still under his direction. Three generations have run the operation known far and wide for its recovery expertise. A reality television series continues to reinforce his team's skills.

The professional knew what he was doing; I was just a rambunctious kid, luckily hearing the scream. I was embarrassed but recovered without so much as a bruise.

The call was no test of medical prowess, rather good preparation for future accidents. Seeing terrible sights and having the ability to re-focus on the injured and live victims is a bonus. It is no shame to react strongly to death and severe injuries. It's a normal reaction to abnormal circumstances.

Returning to the office following the call, the drive back was full of loud descriptive recollections of the scene. It was like a post-call debriefing. Dennis was a good listener; his police experience made sure of that. Today medics receive peer support. I was fortunate; I got the early field version.

Had enough?

There are hundreds, possibly a few thousand, crashes in my repertoire, all providing distinct experiences. Sounding like bragging rights; it's not intended to be. The collective experience left its mark. There have been some dandy crashes purposely left out with good intentions.

Thankfully, most incidents were much less severe. Automotive construction and safety features, the standard for current vehicles, spare their occupant's the devastating trauma earlier drivers endured and, in some cases, succumbed to.

To this day, the human factor still creates most of our accident work. In the extreme, poor judgement and carelessness are our job security. You can always throw in some inclement weather for good measure.

Medical emergencies remain the bread and butter of paramedics; accidents change up the day. Most medics I know perk up at the chance to respond to a crash while dodging others in poor weather. Cold, rain, snow and so on…. letter carriers we could have been.

12

Guns and Knives, Good Grief!

Watching westerns as a kid, I never questioned; who really shoots or stabs another person? Looking back to my youth, there was no entertainment value in violence. Dad fought in World War II. He spoke sparingly of the details when I was an adult.

When it's your bread and butter, responding to a penetrating trauma call is not entertaining. It is more like another thing to get your head around. As callous as it might sound, violent incidents have become "another day at the office." Paramedics are not involved in the prevention and control side, like our friends serving in law enforcement.

Can't say as I even remember reading about shooting or stabbing in the paper or watching a report on TV news before EMS. The exception would be a couple of famous assassinations in the sixties south of the border. Once you are in the profession, it's only a matter of time before you run smack dab into both forms of trauma. Compared to the media's dramatic portrayal, it's never pretty in person.

Seeing the damage caused by weapons was a life changer. Accidents are one thing: poor judgement, weather and human error often the cause. Few stabbings or shootings are "accidental." Seeing an intentionally administered hole in a chest, head or anywhere is a frightening experience.

Playing with my original cap gun as a kid, the silver weapon held a red paper strip with those explosive dots. Pointing and shooting was a novelty that wore off quickly. Soon, I was smacking the paper dots with a hammer on a concrete step. It was the source of more laughs than excitement with my pals.

Dad introduced me to guns and target practice as a teenager. Crazy as it might sound, we built a target range in the basement. Education and safety were permanently embedded in his chatter. Friends and I in our teens took a gun safety course and would go out hunting groundhogs. Even that wore off right after high school.

In a non-fatal experience years later, several medics went out to experience paintball. The organizers split our group into two teams. Available in a rainbow of colours, my choice of the projectile was red for blood. If you ever wanted to change your mind about using a weapon, choose red to mark your results.

The opposing team neared our fort, where we protected our flag. Cathy, the only female medic out for the adventure, stuck her head and shoulder out from behind a tree. It was a fatal error on both our parts; headshots were not permitted. The red round was intended for her shoulder.

Instead, the pellet hit just above her protective goggles and right between her eyes. The resulting red "V" ran upwards into her hair, startling me. Dropping the paintball gun, I stepped back; we just looked at each other. Realizing she was ok, the shot didn't count. We carried on, but I never felt the same about guns again.

I have had the opportunity to go to an outdoor range with a police tactical team shooting various weapons. It was an eye-opener shooting a submachine gun. Any thoughts of voluntarily defending my country evaporated with the adventure.

My second experience was at an indoor range. I stood and watched as another group fired at military silhouette targets. Choosing the traditional bullseye targets was enough for me. The afternoon with handguns still has me puzzled as to why people shoot each other.

Hip cannon

After completing school homework, Sunday nights were reserved for TV. The Ed Sullivan Show, Bonanza and the like. The western drama had its fair share of savagery, though not overly dramatic compared to the wild west on our city streets. Today, the evening news from both Canada and the United States hardly misses a night of shootings.

Working a Sunday evening, the TV at the office was tuned to sports. Howard ducked back in the radio room to answer a phone. Still holding onto the handset, he rolled out to announce the assignment.

Most dispatchers would have grabbed a dispatch form first. Times are everything to the government. Looking at Ethan, the one-liner belted out for a "kid's just been shot, *plece* are on the way." That's right, *plece*. Howard was an east coaster; you got used to the pronunciation for the police.

Bounding out to the garage, I was already going ten over the speed limit. That was the grace we were given when driving with lights and sirens. Ethan was last to get into the Ford. My head stuck through the window into the cab, waiting for updates on the radio; there were none. Way too eager, huh!

Arriving at the scene, I don't know what I was expecting. Gunshot victim(s), lots of cops and flashing lights? You learn early; the police always know more than they give us to go on. When they are running around, it is usually a sign of tension and high drama. There was no running tonight.

Two black cruisers sat out front, red lights idle. There was no sight of a melodrama in progress. That's not to say there was no trauma. Neighbours absent from their doors and windows missed the excitement inside the single-family home.

The scene inside began at the front door with an average-looking household, clean, well decorated. The voices from the dining room were frenzied; crying was audible. A police officer stood in the front hall with a shiny silver revolver in his hand.

The rotating cylinder that once held six bullets was open to prove its safe status. The constable's other outstretched hand held a couple of brass cartridges. The constable's glum expression drew the first brushstrokes of the bigger picture.

Leaving the stretcher in the small entrance, both hands were occupied with the first aid box and oxygen kit. We rounded a corner and passed through an arched opening into the dining room; a large table was pushed awry. Ethan was just behind me, looking over my shoulder. A white tablecloth wrinkled from being pulled sideways was sprayed red, resulting from some high-velocity trauma.

A second officer knelt next to our victim, his hands holding a blood-soaked head steady. A teenage boy stood close by, crying and speaking in gasps, exhausted from emotion. The air in the room was heavy, with the smell of gun powder. Asking if there were more victims, I imagined from the smell that there were others close by in adjacent rooms.

With a simple shake of the head, the officer's gaze returned to the child on the ground. Kneeling next to the young victim, I was unsure if the teen was old enough to drive yet. Two other boys stood silently by their sobbing friend, just steps back from the motionless victim.

The kid had blood coming from both sides of his neck. The hardwood was red from the gushing soft tissue injury. We passed by the gun's enormous barrel on the way into the home; the hole admitting the bullet on the patient's neck seemed surprisingly small. The officer moved his blood-soaked hand away from the other side of his neck.

There was a crater, the exit wound. Below the ear was an irregularly shaped opening with flaps of skin burst out or cavitated from the passing projectile's force. With this much damage at the exit, the internal trauma must be catastrophic.

The young boys stood still; they had the thousand-mile stare. Watching silently as their pal lay gasping on the dining room floor, they were helpless. What was their story? It would be helpful for the ER staff. There was time for that yet.

Ethan slipped away, following his over-the-shoulder assessment. We talked earlier on the way to the scene; I knew he was going for a backboard. The victim was breathing but unconscious. He took an airway; it was a mess. Blood was effervescing from his mouth.

It was difficult to tell which had been penetrated; his airway, esophagus, or both. The oxygen mask hissed as I covered the kid's nose and mouth. Oxygen was the standard of care. By turning the green plastic face cup off centre, I could suction. Blood continued to escape from his draining wounds.

Suctioning with our pre-historic manual portable suction unit was not making much headway. I kept it up, though. With the possibility of the patient's neck being injured, he could not be moved. Until his spine was secured with a collar, suction was my only option.

Covering the holes with bulky dressings, it was impossible to go around and around the neck with a roll of Kling. We used stretchy gauze to secure bandages. Our white, adhesive tape would never work with this much blood.

The universal solution was a triangular cotton bandage. Once around the neck, the band of starchy cotton cloth could be tied off at the side. Knotted over the exit wound, the pressure was put to good use to control the bleeding. Would it even be possible to stop the bleeding? You couldn't bear down too much around his neck.

My bare hands were sticky, covered with blood. So were the discarded paper wrappers from several dressings. Blood in large quantities smells when it is drying. Both knees and lower pant legs were dripping as I returned to a squatting position from kneeling.

From behind, I could hear furniture dragged across the floor. Ethan was on point, moving a chair out of the way. Enlisting a kid, they dragged the long dining table off to the side of the room against the wall.

The cop saw his opportunity to help. The backboard was leaning against the wall. Setting the edge of the board beside the patient, he was ready.

Bonus. My experienced partner covered my missed opportunity to request a cervical collar to protect the victim's neck. Throwing it to me over the corner of the table, it was a lucky catch. Sticky hands saved it from falling on the kid. It would have only added a slight insult to his injury.

Covering the dressings, the neck brace supplemented the support for the damaged structures beneath. What would the x-ray look like?

Rolling the kid up on his side, Ethan held his head. I took the opportunity to look at his back. There were no other injuries visible, despite the sizeable blood puddle now congealing. Formed under his shoulder and back from the massive hemorrhage, the red mess fell off in jiggling shards onto the stained floor, so much blood from one bullet wound.

Gravity did its thing. It was a brief chance to drain the brighter red blood from this kid's mouth and airway. The suction in the truck would do better. With the board shoved against the victim's back, the darker jelly-like congealed blood gathered in a ridge on the floor. A small towel around our pillow dried off our sticky hands for the lift.

The second officer came into view under the arched entrance to the dining room. Another voice accompanying him, a sergeant with the chevron stripes on his epaulettes, distinguished the rank. It was time for the story. The police supervisor would stay with the witnesses while asking the original cop next to the patient to come out to the ambulance.

Ethan was as interested as I was to hear the history of the incident. The officer with the gun behind his back also followed us out as the Sergeant took charge and guided the three boys into the living room for a talk. It was an unusually calm scene as we rolled over the threshold through the front door and out to the ambulance.

Ethan could have taken over. He knew the one officer and was the senior medic between us. He looked at me as if to say, what are you waiting for? Checking around almost nervously for neighbours or gawkers, the darkened yard was silent save and except the puffing exhaust from our waiting ambulance. The officer that greeted us at the door secured the weapon in the trunk of his car.

Announcing to the caregiving constable, I had two questions, the officer at our side was expecting both. His first tidbit was a .357 magnum; he called the revolver a Python. It meant nothing to me; it turns out it was a real hip cannon.

The second question; the kid's parents were out for the evening. The homeowner's son, the crying pleading friend, brought dad's gun out. Having been previously shown that there were blank rounds in the house, he demonstrated the weapons deafening discharge.

There were multiple seemingly harmless rounds fired in the room, hence the cloying odour of gun powder. After several shots, the gun was passed to a friend and reloaded, with tragic results. The kid that replenished the firearm was not familiar with weapons and ammunition. A bullet casing minus the projectile looks different than a live round.

There is a crippling difference between the two types of brass casings. The blank round had a crimped brass end and no bullet; the live one was filled with a lead projectile protruding from the brass. It was a detail missed by the inexperienced loader.

As bad as it was to point a gun and discharge it towards someone, they were lucky. The group initially beat the odds of causing hearing damage, burns, or blast injuries from the gun's muzzle. The distance between the gun and the kids must have played a considerable part.

We had enough; leaving the two cops in the driveway, we were off. The drive to the ER went off without a hitch as I suctioned the kid. I was barely six or seven years older; it hit close to home. The light green plastic oxygen mask was covered in frothing blood before the halfway mark to our destination.

Trading the passive oxygen mask off for a bag-valve-mask ventilator, it was time to take charge of his breathing volume and rate. The patient's respirations were shallow. The patient could not wait any longer for assistance. Strapped to the board, head taped in place, I turned the board onto its edge to drain the victim's airway. The suction in the ambulance was not keeping up.

Staff waited inside and outside the resuscitation room as we rolled down the long hall to the ER. Stepping in, the doctor needed no report to see the distress. The one-liner of calibre and the entrance and exit wounds did not distract the practitioner.

Suction and a light down the airway, and the patient received a secure airway in less than a minute. We pulled our dripping stretcher back from the room. A portable x-ray was summoned.

We retreated to the ramp in front of the ER to clean up our truck; what a mess. It was a two-person job to mop up blood from the floor and the side of the bench. The suction would have to wait for the sink in the slop room at the office.

With all the sputtering, Ethan pointed out that my powder-blue uniform shirt was splattered with red spots. What did it matter? The dried blood on my knees and lower pant legs had already taken on a dull sheen.

The contaminated clothes would mean a trip home to change, though it was near the end of the shift. Maybe I could bail a few minutes early. Back in the day, stains on our uniforms could be cleaned in the ER with hydrogen peroxide. A clear liquid that foamed when applied to blood, this showing was way beyond spot removal.

At the office, diluted blood ran down my pant leg and over my boot onto the concrete floor when a poorly aimed rinse passed over my shin. I was in for a major clean-up when I got home. A green garbage bag stuffed into my pocket would bag up the evidence for the dry cleaner tomorrow morning. Mom would shoot me if I made a mess cleaning up at home after work.

There was no news waking up the next day. Arriving for the afternoon shift, the results were fatal. Surviving some initial surgery, the kid succumbed to the injury.

Fortunately, I did not have to look the victim's parents in the eye; what a relief. The police arrived before us; court time was stroked off the follow-up list. The scene, then the kid sputtering in the back of the ambulance on the way into the ER, was enough.

Little heroes

Domestic abuse has been around for time immemorial. Never a witness to the subject before working EMS, my personal experience was a home life where a raised voice was a rare exception. Initially exempted from conflict, the sights working EMS of bruised women and scared kids in a home left me with questions.

There have been one-sided fights and a push down a flight of stairs. Injuries have often been explained away as "falls" by both victim and aggressor. Choking remains one of the most barbarous acts inflicted on women. It frightens and injures in an instant. The police have training in reading the signs. Paramedics were undertrained and overexposed to the result of some terribly violent acts.

It will never get any easier to see the effects of domestic violence. Hearing activists speak on the topic takes on special meaning, having witnessed the results. Thankfully our local police service has taken a leading approach to the issue in concert with some local mavericks for the cause. Despite their diligence, a shift rarely passes without hearing another hail for EMS to assist a victim.

Mike and I just cleared from a return transfer to a nursing home following an ER visit. These assignments were the bread and butter of EMS in the early years. Emergency calls represented less than forty percent of our call load. Being sent to an emergency was a given. Routine calls paid the freight, "hot calls" were the real reason we were all out for the shift.

Sitting back in the tiny radio room, Kelly cleared his throat as he started to transmit. The last part of the throaty sound was the opener for the hail. Assigning us the call for a reported shooting, you could hear the envy in his voice. He was a medic-turned dispatcher.

Call details described a head injury. No mention of suicide? Kelly paused as he added that a young male made the call for help. Advising it had come via 911, the kid was current with the community's change. I wanted to meet this child. He must be in shock or as cool as a cucumber.

The recently instituted 911 program offered a unified three-digit solution for calling in an emergency situation. It was a sign of progress compared to the previous seven-digit emergency telephone number each separate service had in the past. It would prove to be a real asset.

Answered from the police radio room, one feature allowed the communicator to lock in the line. Silently denying the caller a hang-up, the line continued to pass information to a call taker. The dispatcher or a supervisor could also listen in on a muted line to voices or background noise coming from the scene.

With no updates during our three-minute drive, Mike asked if there was any more information. Kelly had nothing to report. Today paramedic crews would stop short and wait anxiously down the street out of sight. Staging for a potentially dangerous scenario, we now defer to the defensive stance preferred by police and medics alike. This was in the old days.

Sent to a subdivision I drove to several times in my lumber yard days, it was easy to direct Mike to the crescent-shaped road. Lined with semi-detached homes, it was full of hard-working families. Homes were well-kempt and not ostentatious. A couple of kid's bikes and a wagon sat abandoned on front lawns in the late evening.

Stopping in front of the dwelling, the driveway arched up abruptly from the road. The kind of lane that would catch a rear bumper in a rush to pull away from the scene. Parking on the street kept things simple.

Turning off the emergency lights for the last couple of blocks, Mike was coaching me. I was not driving regularly yet. If it was a suicide call, privacy for the caller and relatives was assumed as a non-verbal request. Besides, we did not need an audience if we were to have to walk out the front door carrying a patient with a head wound.

Not waiting to haul the stretcher up the sloped driveway, I grabbed the oxygen kit and first aid box. Thinking it was a good thing the surface was dry tonight, I jogged up the incline.

Arriving at the front entrance, the aluminum storm door was latched. The inside door was ajar, revealing a dimly lit hall. Tapping lightly on the frame, the resulting rattle was intended to announce my arrival, not startle the already upset residents.

In seconds, two small boys appeared at the door. The taller of the two reached up, releasing the lock. Fighting the assumption that this was a suicide scene, I paused. Holding the door from opening more than a few inches, I spoke to the older kid and asked what happened.

Looking up at me as I leaned in to hear his subdued answer, his reply was shocking. "Our dad just shot our mom." In disbelief, I asked him to repeat the statement. My hand now firmly on the door handle, I hesitated while deciding whether to close the door or yank it open. "Dad shot mom in the den."

I pulled the door open and set the equipment down. Reaching out, I placed a hand on each of the kid's shoulders. Crouching, studying the boy's eyes, I asked where their dad was. A sound from the end of the corridor distracted me.

Walking up the hall, shoulders rounded in a defeated posture, a man approached the three of us, still lining the front entrance. Standing, I kicked the equipment to the wall wanting an unimpeded escape route. The youngest boy spoke up, "that's our dad." Staring out the door into the front yard, his hands were empty.

Where was Mike? Stepping to the side, the fellow passed wordlessly, opened the storm door and walked out without so much as a look over his shoulder. The kids headed up the hall. I was defenceless, no portable radio, and I don't think I could have mustered a scream if I wanted to.

Picking up the two bags, I called for the boys to show me where mom was. Walking calmly down the hall, they stopped at the end, turning, both pointed to their right. As I reached the end of the passage, there was still a slight haze and the pungent odour of gun powder in the air.

Looking to my right, a woman lay reclined on a short couch. Head resting on a pillow at the far end, her feet were propped up on the arm hanging over the end of the green upholstered furniture closest to me. The wall next to her head was spattered with blood. Some hair was dangling from a larger piece of tissue suspended below the spatter.

Conscious but unable to reply to my questions, she could not blink her eyes when I asked. She squeezed my hands with hers when commanded. It was a job to talk in a quiet and calm voice. I wanted to yell down the hall for Mike.

Looking at the side of the victim's head, it was a grisly sight. Just behind her left eye, you could see her brain, exposed there was very little blood. A long trench-like avulsion cleared out the scalp, skull and surrounding tissue. She looked frighteningly calm.

Although she showed no distress, I opened the oxygen kit and sat a faintly hissing oxygen mask on her face. The elastic head strap at the mask's sides would have to wait until I dressed the wound. I dropped the tin top of the first aid kit when I heard the front door open.

Standing, I did a counterclockwise turn to go to the hall. Goosebumps preceded weak knees when I panned around the room. Lying across the arms of a chair, a few feet away, was a rifle. Completely missed entering the den; it jumped off the page now.

Looking like the "Rifleman" just set it down; the short carbine style gun had a long-rounded handle on the bottom by the trigger. Having watched the western drama, a willing hand could effortlessly cock the steel loop downwards, returning it to reload. I only ever watched the show in black and white. This was a nightmare in living colour.

I turned to tell Mike we had a live victim and needed a backboard; I was in for my second shock of the night. Dad walked silently up the hall towards us. Walking towards him, I blocked his entry to the room.

Looking back, I think I intended to prevent him from picking up the weapon to finish what he had started, or worse. Wanting to block his access to the gun, I also pushed one of the boys behind me. It was a good thing my bladder was not full of coffee.

With as much of an authoritative voice as I could summon, I looked straight into his eyes and warned him to turn around and leave. Wishing for an instant that I was a cop, they always have a plan. I was impotent at the moment.

Without hesitation, for some reason, the man did an about-face and left as silently as he had arrived. Walking over towards the gun, I noticed a phone on a side table. For the first time in my life, I dialled 911.

The emergency call taker issued her greeting, "Police, Fire or Ambulance, what is your emergency? Now, I am not known for brief conversations. Ask me the time, and I will give you the story of the Swiss watchmaker's struggle to build the timepiece. Giving the address, I asked why the police were not inside with us.

The communicator was taken aback. She was sequestered in the radio room at Dundas and Adelaide miles away. Why should she know I might need a diaper at any moment? She advised that the officers were waiting down the street for a Sergeant to arrive.

In the politest response I could string together, I told the woman to send help. Adding that, the constables should watch for the man who was somewhere outside. He was probably wandering around aimlessly if his demeanour moments earlier was any indication.

Hearing the door again, I spun around, expecting to have to block the hallway a second time. Mike was high stepping it up the corridor; he knew something was wrong. Relaying to me that the man approached him outside then stood silent and stunned. When he blocked the sidewalk, Mike returned to the ambulance. Suspecting that the fellow might be the shooter, he called for assistance by radio. Mike was unaware of what I had already done.

Asking for a backboard and a collar, the lanky medic disappeared and returned within a minute. I jumped as I looked up from the patient when he bounded in through the door. The sound of the metal latch had me rattled.

During Mike's absence, I covered the head wound with a moistened dressing. The bandage was to keep the injury covered, not to control bleeding. There was less than a teaspoon of blood running down to her chin.

After loading, then strapping the woman to the backboard, the cavalry arrived. Guns were drawn in defence of the reports of a shooting. A day late and a dollar short, as dad used to say, they were still a welcome sight. The boys seeing us talking to the police came away from the wall. They were too frightened to speak while we worked on mom.

Reporting that the man walked right up to the sergeant, one of the constables advised dad was safely in custody. It was a relief knowing the surprises were over for the moment. Seeing the weapon on the chair, a constable positioned himself next to it and began to write in his notebook. Looking at the other cop near the hall, he proclaimed he had a .444 Marlin.

There were lots of hands to carry our victim out to the stretcher on the sidewalk. Turning to the oldest cop in the group of three, I asked him to look after the two boys. Moments later, they walked out of the front door to the next unit.

The silhouette of a curious neighbour waited inside, nose stuck to the glass. Unaware of the incident, the woman's innocence would help the kids. The door opened slowly at the beckoning of the officer. Their brief conversation ended with a gasp, both youngsters disappeared behind the door.

Loading then transporting the woman to the hospital, I was left with lingering thoughts of the kids on their own with the neighbour. Some anxious grandparents would race to the scene, hearing of the incident with any luck at all. The boys would need professional help to come out of the other side of this experience.

The woman did well. When we left the ER, doctors stated she was millimetres away from a permanent brain injury or worse. She would be in for a lengthy stay at the hospital to have some work done to replace the missing bone from the side of her head. Someone was on her side that evening.

Waiting in the emergency department's back hall, two officers in plainclothes showed up to take our statements. I gave too much detail. Backing off, I related how both boys, in succession, stated that their dad had shot their Mom. The clincher both pointed the male out at the scene as their dad.

We were never called to court. Mike and I guessed that the fellow admitted to the incident or that his actions resulted from a mental illness. Despite being at the scene first and describing the experience, someone else closed the evidence loop. Good enough for me.

Big mess

Every suicide event, attempted or successful, is a saddening ordeal for me. As a young medic, the experience was only worth the face value. I never looked beyond the obvious. As time wore on in the industry, I began to look at the scenes and wonder; how lonely it must have been for the victim to be alone just before taking their life.

Attempts, experts say, are a call for help. Reaching out early for a willing ear or a ride to the hospital before going too far, there are still options left. Serious contenders have run out of options or see none. Pushed beyond their limit, the feeling must be mind-numbing.

The jumper standing, looking, then going over the edge. Someone with a rope tightening around their neck as they stepped off a chair, ladder or table. A shooter, starting to apply pressure on the trigger, never hearing the click. Sitting in a car, motor running, an extension to the exhaust taped in a window as consciousness fades. Consciously feeding yourself pill after pill, then drifting off. There are lots of ways to do it.

This evening, a sick man sat on the edge of his bed. Stricken with a breathing illness, now relegated to his room. Always short of breath, unable to endure walking around his own home, he wasted away, helpless.

With all that time to ponder his situation, he formulated a plan. Pull his loaded shotgun out from under the bed and reach into a drawer for a ruler. As relatives sat at dinner close by, he could not join them to eat without gasping for breath. His portion sat cooling on a table beside the bed. Wanting someone to be there for his spouse, he purposely chose this time.

Sitting in the lounge at supper time, our shift started at four in the afternoon. We were only a couple of hours into the tour. Nicholas and I relaxed watching the local news. We were up next, the only crew at the base. The other units were out and around; who knew or cared where they were.

Howard slouched back in his rolling chair in the radio room. You tend to get drowsy after single-handedly inhaling a whole pizza. It was not the first time ingesting a behemoth deluxe left us wondering how he did it.

Answering the phone was not usually a timed event unless you are a dispatcher. We all hoped Howard would not fall off the seat in his haste. Howard did not get to the door to announce our assignment. His booming voice blasted from the desk that we were responding to a shooting, likely a suicide. The only specifics: "sounds like he is gone."

Working with Nick, I usually drove. The choice drew no argument from me. It was a ten-minute ride to a familiar area. The police rolled up just as we got to the back doors of our van. Two officers exited their patrol car approaching us in the driveway.

I wondered how two uniforms were working together. A discussion later revealed they had both been at their detachment when they were given the call. They decided to ride double since they were going to the same scene.

Reaching the front door, there was no room in the hall for our stretcher. Carrying the oxygen kit, Nick entered behind the first officer, his hat in hand. I followed with the first aid box trailed by the second constable. Sitting in the living room was the patient's wife, crying as she was introduced by her sister.

Introducing himself as the brother-in-law, our greeter led us to a bedroom. Ready for almost anything, I opened the door when he hesitated. The man indicated he looked earlier after the group heard the gunshot then quickly closed the door.

Lying back across the bed was an older man. Feet stuck out almost straight towards the door; he was motionless. The room emitted that smell of a permanent resident, like a nursing home. Poor ventilation, the result of a normally closed door, sustaining the odour.

Between the victims, outstretched legs sat a shotgun. The weapon slipped down following its discharge, with the trigger facing the ceiling. The gun's 12-gauge muzzle lay right on the fellow's crotch. An old wooden, foot-long ruler discarded on the floor looked like it had fallen out of the victim's hand as he collapsed on the bed. The same hand hung palm down just above the wooden stick over the edge of the soiled mattress.

Taking the lead, the officer reached inside and turned on the room's primary light on the ceiling. It was a dated square fixture with whitened glass. Within a second, I wished it had been left off.

Why do we look up at a light when we turn it on? Is it in anticipation of the bulb burning out with a sudden flash or not working at all? Once illuminated, its partially obscured beam revealed a stained ceiling. The glass fixture and the painted surface were showered in an area four times the size of the glass with brains, hair and blood.

Shattered into small pieces, human shrapnel clung to the walls and ceiling as if ordered there by the gun. The smell of blood and body fluid hung in the air. There was an ominous feeling, standing surrounded by the elements of death.

Nick walked over to the bedside surveying the scene. Turning as I walked up to his side, the sight was a first. The victim inserted the gun's muzzle into his mouth before using the ruler on the trigger to discharge the lethal blast. The deduction did not require detective skills.

At the time, I assumed it was always the bullet or pellets that did the damage. It was a naivete soon to be shattered.

Following the call, a constable on the police forensic unit cleared up the ill-conceived assumption. With any gun's discharge comes the energy or burst behind the projectile once it has cleared the muzzle. As if the bullet or pellets were not enough.

Shot at close range, the accompanying blast compounded the damage inflicted by the passing projectiles. Taking a closer look, I was glad I had an empty stomach. Looking down into the patient's face, it was missing.

The blast's force exploded the victim's head. Propelling the entire cranium upwards, it blew the contents up and out. The sides of the fellow's head, including his ears, were draped outwards onto his shoulders, peeled back touching the bed. The face and skull shattered from the blast were missing but looked to be evenly distributed about the room.

Bits and pieces of cranium lay on a nearby dresser. Tissue dangled from table lamps, sat on picture frames, and littered the exposed parts of the floor. Still, more melded into patterns on the carpet seeking out every nook and cranny. There was not a single chunk visible, larger than a dime. As the mortal debris dried, some smaller bits could be heard falling onto a long-outdated newspaper lying close by.

Our patient died from the bloody obvious. Then there was his heart. The beating organ continued to pump out every available drop. Coming through major vessels torn apart by sheer force, volumes of the warm red body fluid ran onto the bed. It exited through the open cavity that had once been the bottom of the man's mouth and neck.

Blood sprayed onto the wall behind the victim until the current ebbed. Overflowing the mattress, red tracks ran down the wall behind the bed to the floor below. Darkened with time and missing the life-giving oxygen, the liquid now resembled a pool of dark syrup.

Nick worked EMS for a couple of years longer than I. He was non-plussed with the sight, and now with nothing to do but the paperwork, he turned to the officer and quietly announced we would be leaving.

Following us out the front door, the young constable acknowledged it was his first time on a shooting suicide. With the door safely closed, I agreed with his obvious suggestion the next move was to call the coroner. Despite being very sick, the method of death would likely result in a trip to the morgue.

I knew the other officer who was still inside the home talking to the relatives. Using the in, I quietly suggested to the constable that if the family required the mess to be cleaned up, they could call me through our radio room. Nick looked at me like I was insane.

Howard and Sam had been doing "clean-ups" for years. Listening to the dispatcher and my supervisor for my short time in the business, passing up the job was a lost opportunity. I had never done a clean-up. How hard could it be?

The boys made it sound simple, with some elbow grease and a strong stomach. I listened to the list of chemicals they used. Pricing the job was like pulling a rabbit out of a hat. There was no disaster clean-up company in the phone book then. Offering the service was done through word of mouth.

Returning to the office, Nick was silent for the drive. Once in the lounge, he lit up a cigarette while he did up his ambulance report. Howard listened as Nick narrated the highlights. Giving up the secret, my offer to the police for the clean-up drew little response.

Thinking Howard and Sam sitting in his office nearby would be mad losing some business, I waited for the backlash. Sam strolled out to his door, coffee cup in hand; he smiled at Howard. These two were betting I would miss the mark, and they would get the call to complete the substandard job.

An hour later, Howard rolled the squeaky chair backwards out of the radio room. Handing me the green telephone handset on the end of a mile-long coiled cord, he smirked. Checking his laugh, he said, "it's the cops."

The constable I met on previous ambulance runs spoke up now and asked how much I wanted to charge for the task. Pulling the number out of my hat, I quoted four hundred and fifty, including materials, labour and to haul away the mess.

Without so much as a pause, he asked when I could do the job. Reeling now from the surprise, I explained I was off at midnight and could start right after. The mess would be easier to clean the sooner I got to it.

I was to find the front door unlocked and could let myself in. The only instruction was to clean up the artwork and furniture and place the personal jewelry in a plastic bag outside the room. Everything else could go to the dump.

Stunned at the prospect of staying up all night, I sat down and pencilled in a list of supplies. Looking on in silence, Sam was probably pissed that I spoke up for the job. It was beer money for him and Howard.

Both Sam and Howard shared story after story of cleaning up the worst messes around the city. They made good money since it was such a macabre task. I innocently paid attention to the details, asking questions on their methods and supplies. This was my chance.

The rest of the shift was a shutout. We cleaned and counted supplies in a couple of ambulances with the slow night. Taking the cleaning assignment personally, I thought it was a lesson from Sam for taking their beer money. Nick thought I was crazy to do the first clean-up job on my own, not deferring to their experience.

It was a quick trip home and into a worn jumpsuit from my fire service in exchange for the uniform after work. A change of clothes stuffed into a bag was the backup plan. Making less than six dollars an hour working EMS, I would find out tonight if this was a good plan or a curse.

The guy at the 24-hour variety store probably thought I was cleaning up after a murder. Carrying a mop, garbage bags, a couple of bottles of that strong liquid orange cleaner and several rolls of paper towel and a short roll of duct tape to the counter, I got the stink eye. I looked back as I left. He did not look out the door to get my license plate number.

It was quiet; the streets were empty as I drove into the subdivision. The neighbours probably didn't know yet. If they were looking outside during the incident, they watched the ambulance come and leave, then the police and the body removal wagon. The patient was sick; it was sad but expected.

The big secret was on me. The assignment: do the clean-up and get out of Dodge before the neighbourhood woke up for their Monday morning coffee. As I crossed the threshold, I was thinking had I bit off more than I could chew…hell no! False bravado?

Gathering up the convenience store supplies, a plastic drop sheet leftover from painting a bedroom, and some 100-watt light bulbs, I was out of hands. It needed to be a single trip into the house to avoid attention from curious eyes if someone was still up at this hour.

The silence was deafening throughout the house, occasionally creaking as I made my way to the bathroom. I needed a cleaning room and a large basin, aka bathtub. After the fact, cleaning the tub and floor would be less work than using just the plastic bucket I scooped from my place.

Closed in now, it was an uncomfortable feeling returning to the scene. The empty house and room would never be home again to the departed. The returning family would surely be permanently scarred from the experience and memory. Maybe they were a step ahead, and I was helping by doing the pre-sale clean-up?

Opening the bedroom for a second time, there was no surprise behind door number one. The potent smell of drying body fluids and scattered human tissue ruled the room, in addition to the institutional "sick person smell" that hit me on the first round.

Turning on the light, it would not be bright enough. Emptying the supplies out of the rigid plastic bucket and flipping it upside down, I stood on the five-gallon container serving as a makeshift stool.

Removing the white glass lampshade, its contents surprised me. Bits and pieces of tissue and hair covered the lens's face and one corner inside the light. The latter debris launched over the edge. The thin glass miraculously escaped flying pellets earlier.

The fixture was equipped with two bulbs at some point. I removed the remaining underpowered light and the second, long burnt out. Replacing the two with bulbs brought as a contingency plan, they sprung to life. Working in a brightly lit operating room was not how I originally envisioned the wind down from an evening shift.

Seeing clearly now, what I missed earlier was a mistake. Every inch of the space would have to be cleaned. There was some junk removal to do first. Living in a single room can make one very self-sufficient.

The empty bed, mattress covered in dark hardened blood, was high on the list to toss. Removing it early would give me more room to work. Open drawers in a chest exposed the most intimate details of the owner's passing. Now covered in biohazards, some of the contents would have to go.

Every square inch on flat surfaces around the room was covered in dog-eared magazines, empty plates and cups. A TV table set up as a work stand supported now unnecessary health care supplies. Leaned against the walls were projects past. There were boards covered in puzzles and books totalling thousands of pages. It all went into the giant green garbage bags bought at midnight.

The lineup started just inside the front door. Doubling up the bags, it was no time to add to the mess. Clothes and magazines in bulk were next.

The drop sheet was an invaluable bonus. Thinking I would spread it out to avoid drips of body fluid on the floor, its importance was underestimated, and purpose reassigned when tackling the bed.

A blood-soaked mattress can hold litres of the red stuff. Insulated from drying in the hours since the fatal shot, the trapped fluid ran out and onto the floor, standing the worn and flopping bed on its edge.

The drop sheet found its new home. Wrapped a couple of times around the mattress. I dragged it out of the mess before going around it the final time.

Tucked in at the ends, duct tape sealed the deal. In the darkness, the package made its way past the garbage bags to the darkened porch.

Returning to the bedroom, I smelled my hands as I passed through the hall. This was in the days before gloves. Glad for the privacy, I looked forward to a long hot shower later.

Hidden under the remaining box spring was a treasure trove of goodies. Cutting the cloth off the box spring, it could not drip its way to the door. There was no more plastic. Note to self, think this one through next time.

Secreting food under a bed was a trait fit for a kid. The owner had long forgotten his supply of treats. Cases of the shortlist of favourite chocolate bars were years beyond their best before date.

Although not labelled with an expiry warning, they were hard as a rock. Broken open, milk chocolate and peanuts turned to dust. Don't get the wrong idea; they were heading for the green bag next to me. Honest!

The next trip down to the temporary dumpsite delivered the box spring, followed by another full bag before returning to the bedroom to survey loose ends. Perched on top of the remaining case of hidden treats, to use the term lightly, was the final surprise.

Sitting in a sheltered space that was barely four inches at the time of the shotgun blast was some bone. An irregularly shaped piece of the very top of a cranium rested upside down, stuck to the cardboard. I vowed never to eat that brand of confection again. Lifted out of its anatomical position, it most surely ricocheted travelling here.

About the size of an ashtray, it went right into a green bag. Typically, when doing a body removal, you include every piece of human tissue recovered with the remains. The victim was long gone. It would have been worth the price of admission to witness the bones path from owner to resting place.

There were personal items to bag up; it was a shortlist. Some jewelry and papers, there wasn't much. The worst was yet to come. Now, with space to move in, some warm water and cleaner, the work began.

Pictures lowered off the walls were wiped down several times. Dresser, chair and bedside table scrubbed; there was human debris everywhere. With the water came the re-activation of the odour of human tissue and bodily fluid.

Hair and tissue hung from the hidden wire that once supported a large painting. Several feet away and above the patient, nothing, including the artwork, escaped the shower of the victim's remains. Hearing the vivid description of several clean-ups sitting in the lounge back at the office was a far cry from this experience.

I was sweating from the exercise in the small room. Perspiration ran off my head and into my eyes. Too afraid to wipe my brow with a bare arm, a paper towel served the purpose. Thrown to the floor, the discarded wipe mixed in with the mess for a future volley into a garbage bag.

The top edges of open drawers showed signs of splatter. Wiped clean, the furniture made its way to the hall just outside the door. There was no rearranging this room at the end. It would be missing too much.

Soapy water in the bucket became brightly tinged. Pouring the lukewarm contents into the bathtub, hair and a couple of pellets sat around the drain. It took another half a dozen buckets of fresh soapy solution to clean the ceiling and walls.

The gypsum board ceiling suffered scars beyond a simple wipe down. A few dozen pellet holes and dents from flying bone marked and penetrated the surface. The repair was beyond this midnight visitor's reach. Following a second cleaning, the wall was faded but sanitized.

Warm dirty water and cleaner streamed down my arms into my pits. More drops of something ran into my eyes over the next two hours. Hands wrinkled from the continuously wet skin and irritated by the liquid cleaner set me to thinking. Was this a good idea?

The whole plan sucked for the moment until I could fold the results in half and put it in my pocket. Maybe it was time to reward me, a selfish treat. A new propeller for the ultralight airplane, my current hobby? Some would look at the fee for the service as an attempt to take advantage of grief-stricken relatives. With all the details required to address the mess, I thought not.

Working my way out of the now medicinal smelling room, a row of garbage bags blocked a quick escape. Cleaning up the washroom, it looked sparkling bright. There was a chance now for a new normal with enough time between the previous evenings' events and the resident's return.

Cleansed furniture returned to the room, leaned against the wall, and a ceiling peppered with tiny holes was the marker that something sinister happened. The missing box spring and mattress set could be replaced after some patching and painting. Memories would fade. At worst, the home could be sold off. The future owner would be none the wiser.

Emerging from the creepily quiet workspace, the early morning light was still partly hidden by a residence at the end of the street. Bags of nasty refuse in each hand, I loaded the old grey four-door. Oh God, I hoped there were no leaks. The upholstered seats would stink.

Several trips and the rear seat and trunk were full. Years of monthly magazines describing faraway places, others journaling historical events, filled the back of the car. Old, soiled clothes and bed linen dripped inside the confines of other dark plastic sacs, doubled for safety.

Finally, a couple of trips to get the mattress and box spring to the driveway were awkward. A bed is difficult enough if you carry it on your shoulder. To nurse it out and onto the roof of a car without tearing the plastic, a tedious chore.

Tying the lot down, running the ropes in one door and out the other, the load was secure. I made it this far in a macabre journey; what next? Returning briefly to clean the sink for the last time, then my arms and hands, I thought the experience was over. The sun was coming up.

Closing the doors on the lines was the last step. A few seconds after slamming the front passenger's door and seeing the mattress jiggle from the added tension on the old rope, a trickle of red ran down the window. The grey four-door looked like a mobile horror show. A quick getaway was in order.

Driving through the early morning sunshine to the landfill at the edge of our city, I recalled previous trips to discard junk from Mom's place. There was a checkpoint to drive through. You had to produce a driver's license to confirm your municipal lineage.

Blood ran down both sides of the car now; it streaked backwards from the wind. I would indeed be arrested for concealing a crime. There was still time to turn around to rethink the disposal.

Approaching the metal-clad hut, the inside of the car stunk from drying body fluid. It was an unexpected bonus for all my hard work. Now I really must look guilty with the wrinkled-up nose.

The fellow inside did a double take. Trickles of the red stuff down both sides of the car dried firmly to the glass from the drive. Ropes holding the bedding down wore through the covering, loosening the load. With a teaspoon of courage, I rolled the window down and began with, "a real mess, huh?"

Before he could dial the number, I chased that gem with, "I have been up all night cleaning up a scene of death, feel free to call constable (I actually gave his name and the number for the detachment)." Dad always said, "Curly, tell the truth, and it will set you free."

It must have been my honest face. Without hesitation, the city worker returned my license and waved me off to the steel bins behind. The fellow would have a tale to tell the guys in the lunchroom today. Maybe he would even drag them out to view the mattress now swimming in darkened blood beneath the plastic.

Like a race car pit stop, I unloaded the mess. Thankfully, the rooftop cargo was the only package to leak. Ropes and all into the awaiting bin, I slammed the doors and departed into the morning sun.

On the ride home, I collected the reward. At the time, looking a relative of the departed in the eye, there was no hesitation in accepting the fee.

It was more than an ambulance attendant's standard wage. Considering all the details, physical slugging and missing a night's sleep, it was a fair settlement.

Put to bed, the only inquiry from Howard then Sam a few shifts later was an echo. "Were there any callbacks to touch up the job?" I shared that there were no calls, and with a clear conscience, thanked them for their instruction. Despite some surprises, being armed with their idle chatter was the ammunition needed to tackle the job.

Self-inflicted, kind of

Being randomly shot as an innocent citizen changes a person's life. Did that even need saying? Without warning, you are injured, frightened beyond belief and worse. If you survive, you also carry invisible scars only a victim can relate to. That's on top of the physical leftovers.

Paying someone to shoot you, as incredulous as the request might seem, was supposed to make this next person's life better. No, it was not a cry for help with an assisted suicide. Knowing someone would shoot you at a prearranged time and location, you would think the anticipation would be paralyzing.

Sitting at a freshly opened station, Cathy and I watched the small television on the table at the side of the lounge. One of the first colour TVs at an outlying station, the attraction was still a novelty. The ebb of calls on the evening shift got us safely to the mid-point.

Bored with the pace of weeknight entertainment, I stood to go next door to the variety store. With perfect timing, the shiny new red dispatch phone jingled a few feet from my chair. The clock just passed eight PM.

The hail for reports of shots fired has never been taken lightly by our medics. Thankfully, we don't do enough weapons calls to have the variation on a trauma call fail to pique our interest. "All hands on deck," we jumped into our also new high-rise van ambulance. The Omaha orange stripe down the side was a recent change across our province to squelch the outdated blue and white busses.

Responding to a high-rise building in the city, no apartment number was given with the details received over the hotline. Asking for overlooked directions, Gail, our dispatcher, updated the call information advising our victim was out in front of the building.

Was the patient shot somewhere else, then dropped off? A few shooting and stabbing victims over the years were deposited at our ER's front doors. The move was an attempt to conceal the crime scene and protect friends and suspects, sometimes one and the same.

Arriving to find a car parked in front of the building, police with better call details pulled up before us. Still responding right to the patient in the day, the safer and revised method is to "stage" until our law enforcement friends advise the area is safe. Paramedics then rush in protected by the police, who have hopefully secured the weapons and suspects, and paved the way for a trauma call, no surprises.

Cathy, taking the attending role, walked right up to the constable standing next to the car. Sitting on the passenger's front seat with his legs swung out, the victim was chattering about getting to the hospital quickly. The scene was secure; what was the rush?

Looking at me, rolling his eyes, was an officer I befriended earlier in my career. The sarcastic visual for my eyes only spurred an already overactive curiosity. Getting the high sign from Bill, he wanted this guy gone from the scene. The story would come later.

Hearing Cathy's questions, neither of us could see the bloodbath often resulting from a gunshot wound. Our patient was strangely calm for having been shot. Or was he?

There were responses to care for mental health patients, victims of stabbings and shootings. Looking for a massive police response and the attention of many, patients often wound up suffering delusions or imagined injuries. Tonight, with the stretcher nearby, Cathy's request for the patient to stand up produced the first evidence of a misadventure.

Leaving a noticeable red smear behind on the lighter upholstery, I looked more for a gun left behind than blood. I'm not scared of blood. The finding alerted Bill, Cathy and me to the possibility that this was more than a mental health call.

Involuntarily it seemed, our victim leaned over and squatted down as he transferred under his own power to move to the ambulance. The patient spun to his right, ending up chest first over the trunk of the car on his forearms. It was unplanned. He looked a little worse for wear, pausing to regain his composure.

In a strange request for a victim, he asked to be handcuffed. Not to be outsmarted, Bill honoured his wish. Ratcheting the bracelets firmly around his wrists, our victim paused as he stood next to the stretcher. We took the time to examine his injury.

Speckled through blue jeans were red dots, proof of being on the receiving end of a shotgun from some distance. The pellet holes covered his butt from side to side, probably hurting a lot; the wounds looked shallow.

The patient, wanting to speak in the back of the ambulance, beckoned for all to climb in. Other officers pulled up to the scene, the late arrivers in darkness, no red lights. Did they have the story we were thirsting for?

Our victim opened like a tap, pouring out a story I could not conceive of. Shot from a distance, who was his accomplice? Then call the police on themselves; it took a plot and some help to arrive here. I forgot for the moment. Not my problem; I'm a medic.

Begging Bill to call another officer he named, the victim admitted to owing money to a criminal group while serving the dual role of working with police as a snitch. According to him, he had just been found out. In a poorly conceived coverup, the man paid a cohort to pull up in front of the building at a prearranged time.

Bending over at the door of his car, the victim waited. The shooter was compensated to aim the gun from his vehicle and fire at a harmless target to make the tattler less suspect. He was convinced the "bad guys" were watching him. Seeing the wounding was supposed to cover his defence. Sucks to be you, buddy.

The blast could have really hurt him. Luckily our patient suffered superficial pellet wounds. The distance and angle were his friends. Safely lying on our stretcher, the victim explained that he hoped the staged event was witnessed to dispel his opponent's suspicions of being a rat.

Leaving the scene, the patient asked for his cuffs to be removed. Fooled once, Bill was not about to be taken advantage of again. The patient rode the rest of the way in the bracelets while Bill recorded his notes. Some names and places needed to be investigated.

Cathy's job in transit was simple; the patient was distracted by the inconvenience of it all. He stopped complaining of any pain, and there was no measurable blood loss to deal with. With a quick chat in the ER, the receiving nurse pushed us through. Our arrival went unnoticed by all but a few in the hospital.

Plainclothes detectives waiting patiently inside the department followed the patient to a pre-assigned room in the back hall. Bill held back, hardly noticed as a guest in our ambulance, the incident would be in the detective's hands. We cleared the call, wondering if we would be called to court over the unusual hail for a shooting.

Last resort option

Standing in the downtown ER waiting for your partner to clear, you were sure to get an eyeful most evenings. It was a real show provided by patients and relatives in the waiting room ranging from yelling matches to fighting or merely acting out. This night was no exception.

A couple were having a domestic here and now. Already sporting a small cut over an eye, the vocal patient was waiting for his treatment. He was getting an earful from his partner for some unspeakable transgression. Another couple across the floor turned away as the pitch increased; an orderly leaned out to quell the sound.

Before the days of in-house security staff, orderlies kept the peace. Many tasks fell into the laps of the fellows' wearing the white pants and tops. Often referred to by mental health patients as "the white coats," orderlies worked hard and were seldom thanked for their challenging and sometimes dangerous work.

Today, specially trained men and women staff the ERs in an expanded role. Known as Emergency Department Technicians, some are actually paramedics. Their profession is invaluable. Security officers representing the hospital are also a permanent fixture in the department. There, enough history.

Two stepping out through the department's door, Peter only briefly paid attention to the loud couple as he passed. He was on a mission.

Together, we stuffed the rolling cot through the van's rear doors; he waited for the cab door to close before announcing our assignment. There's been a "police shooting." Rolling down the road, we really didn't discuss a game plan. Peter had worked part-time for a couple of years. We didn't really know each other's style, creating a challenge for unusual calls.

Arriving at the scene in a couple of minutes, it was late evening. Adjacent to a roadway, a tall, dark apartment building loomed in the background. It was more like working a motor vehicle collision scene in the darkness.

On a berm beyond the road's edge, a man lay motionless on his back, a constable knelt beside the patient. The scene quieted as patrol cars arrived, doors slamming nearby. Rolling the empty stretcher across the soft earth, I sensed the patient's weight on the return trip to our ambulance would be a test. The ground was damp as our knees pressed into the soil below the smell of freshly cut grass.

Our equipment set down around us, my flashlight shone across the turf at the victim's side. Peter asked the officer what had happened. A quick look with a flashlight revealed blood around the quiet victim's upper chest and shoulder.

Without hesitation, the officer in a light blue shirt and dark pants with a red stripe along his leg that straightened as he stood stated, "he's been shot." Pete, attending the call, reached out to feel for a pulse. Checking the wound, I pulled the victim's shirt aside and, using the light found one small, darkened round hole, likely the entry wound. Pete spoke up to share that the patient was vital signs absent.

Starting CPR in the dark, we shared the duties. The officer stood quietly, watching us work the patient. Looking up into the darkness, I asked if we knew the bullet's calibre that wounded the patient. The abrupt reply "a .38" broke the silence.

Sensing the answer to the next question, I was still thinking about our safety. Cautiously looking the officer in the eye, I asked, "do we know who shot him?" "I did," the officer stepped back and surveyed the scene. Listening to Pete counting my compressions, I lost track. I went back to work.

Seeing the beams of approaching flashlights, more officers converged on our dark workspace. A Sergeant spoke to the officer at our side, and they left quietly together.

After a couple of minutes of CPR with no positive results, there was no use in continuing the resuscitation at the scene. If there was any hope, continuing CPR and quick transport to the best hospital for trauma were the moves to make and now.

Announcing our intention, an officer assigned to accompany the patient picked up our extra equipment. A quick transfer to a backboard, then to the stretcher, and we were off to the waiting ambulance. It was a short trip with a lighted police vehicle following.

The three-liner radio patch to the nurse was simple; it was over quicker than a muzzle flash. We were on their doorstep in a couple of minutes; care was limited to basic life support only in the day.

Following the call, we were approached by a constable and asked for a brief statement. Returning to the front entrance of the ER, it was a quick clean-up. I felt disturbed by the call.

Knowing the officer from several previous runs, the concern on his face told me it hit him hard. Tonight was one of the calmest scenes at a life-threatening call that I can remember. We cleared the hospital, hearing that the results were negative after attempts to resuscitate the young man. It was no consolation tonight that everyone did their best.

The word later was that the incident started out as a domestic incident; it turned sour when the officer arrived. The male was reported harassing a resident of the building behind our scene, approaching the cop in a threatening manner. The officer went on to take the appropriate action. His actions were validated following an investigation.

There was never a single reference to the call in our future when we met on the job. My heart went out to the constable; exercising the last resort option is a mammoth burden for any police officer.

All the way

Starting early in my career, the theme of domestic violence planted its roots with this call. Working with Dale, this incident took place around the one-year mark for me. We sat idle at the office for a couple of hours this evening.

Not being a sports fan and easily bored, I would often sit in the radio room if certain dispatchers were working. Football was not my thing, and Steve was a great mentor. We talked shop.

Putting in his early years with the London England ambulance brigade, Steve was brimming with tales. His brother was back in England, working the front line in their EMS system. The other London across the pond boasted a population of millions. The calls seemed different, or at least entertaining.

Following Steve's rendition of a call to pick up a fellow who threw himself in front of a subway car, he turned to catch the radio. No sooner had he rogered a car at a hospital than a phone line sparkled to life. LPD, the London Police Department line, came directly from their radio room.

A new building at Dundas Street and Adelaide Street, the London police headquarters boasted the latest technology to provide the service we take for granted today as 911. There was no gloating about the radio room at our ambulance headquarters, an eight-by-ten-foot passageway, a desk along a wall and a door at each end.

Our ambulance communications hub doubled as a hallway to come from the front office to the lounge. The technological resources at the dispatcher's fingertips were a real attention grabber. The small cassette recorder on the desk next to the phone could replay calls when details were missed. *Ooh, ahh, oh crap*, it was a sight.

Hanging up the phone, Steve shared his last story for the shift. Pushing me out of the way, he wanted Dale to get the scoop, so he didn't have to repeat himself. Dale was driving. Heading to a home in the northeast, we were dispatched for a stabbing.

Dale was not in his happy place. Considering himself a couple of steps above the crowd, he liked to attend with his experience and expertise. You only had to ask him. He drove tonight to avoid being critical of my driving. Dale did not like being chauffeured by a junior employee; and told me so. That much was clear starting from the vehicle check going forward. Dale would be in charge.

Heading out, he knew just where the place was. Issuing direction on how the situation would be handled, his grumbling ceased. A couple of blocks later, he started again with how we would manage the patient if they were hurt here or there.

His ego had worn thin on others. I was too junior to step up and push back. It would be another year before I grew wings and really took charge of calls. He would leave the industry by then.

Arriving at the scene, we beat the police. Dale figured the "bad guy" already left, given the street we were on, walking up to the home. Boy, was he wrong!

The front door was opened in a matter-of-fact motion. The woman who greeted us was calm. I could hear kids in the background, their tiny voices muffled. The faint odour of supper hung in the air. How could this be the scene of a stabbing?

Dale asked if she called the ambulance, the woman answered with a quiet yes. We followed our caller to the kitchen. I was attending; the task of carrying the oxygen kit fell on my shoulders. Branded the junior guy; I guess it was also my job to bring the first aid kit.

Shown into the wartime home, the small kitchen was barely large enough for the little table off against the wall. Stepping out of our way, the woman introduced us to her common-law spouse. He lay motionless on his back on the linoleum floor.

There were some stabbings in the first year, bar calls and fights; I missed the domestics. My number was up this evening. A "twofer" tonight landed me the combination of a two for one, a stabbing resulting from a domestic disturbance. Oh, and throw in murder to make it a trifecta of trauma.

Sticking straight up out of the man's slightly built chest in perfect alignment with his heart was a knife with a blade measuring at least a foot long. The handle and an inch of the edge stood poised above the victim's ribs. It looked like the tip bottomed out, striking the floor. A quick roll of the patient to check, and our assessment was spot on.

A small spot stained his shirt and the floor below where the tiny point of the blade exited into the solid linoleum surface. Left inserted through his thoracic cavity, we did not touch or move the weapon. Checking the victim's carotid pulse on the side of his neck closest to me, his heart had stopped entirely. There was no breathing.

So, where were the cops? I'm thinking in the circumstance, they should have strode in guns drawn a long time ago. Not sensing any imminent danger from the patient's spouse at this point, I wasn't about to panic. Thinking more about the kids now, I asked if they were "ok"?

Receiving the affirmative and that they were safely in the other room, Dale took the lead. Asking what happened, I sensed that we were looking at the person responsible for the patient's condition. Still no emotion.

The woman, in brief sentences, explained she and her partner argued during the evening. When he attempted to attack her, it was not the first time in their relationship. She decided it would be the last. Surprising him with the blade when she turned to confront his assault, she buried the knife in his chest, sending him to the floor. The stabbing motion was accentuated with a second shove to its final resting place.

For some reason, this was not enough information for Dale. He inquired when the incident happened. Surprisingly the woman answered that the final blow occurred nearly an hour ago. Was she waiting until he was good and dead?

In a move seen only once in my career, Dale brought his pencil to bear. I checked the patient's vital signs; the victim had none. Dead in my books, I was seconds from phoning Steve in the radio room to advise him and ask where the police were. Something my senior partner should have done.

Dale turned the pencil sideways and placed the lead lightly across the victim's cornea. What was he doing? Surprised, I asked what he was looking for.

Dale explained in a calm tone if there had been a cessation of circulation for a length of time, the pencil should leave a dent in the cornea. If the intraocular pressure was still present, indicating a more recent cardiac arrest, the tissue would rebound. The test wasn't in any book I was assigned to read during the month-long training at camp Borden.

From behind us now, there was a loud tapping at the front door. Exclaiming the police arrived when our greeter opened the door, the officer in a British accent called the woman by name. With his personalized salutation, I suspected there was a history associated with this address.

Asking if the children were ok, she answered in the affirmative and led the two officers to us, still kneeling on the kitchen floor. With a quick look at the scene, the Brit led the woman off to the room, where the children sat quietly.

We explained to the second constable that we found the patient in his current condition. He was deceased, and if you could trust Dale's statement, he had been so for some time. We left our names and had a talk with a couple of detectives at the office later that evening before going home.

The most puzzling event of the evening still begged the question. Where did Dr. Dale learn the medical test that he carried out? Asking him in the garage while cleaning up our ambulance, he replied he witnessed an emergency physician do it. Adding it was a VSA patient that he recently transported to the department.

The doctor wanted to confirm with the examination that the patient expired some time ago. Dale acknowledged that tonight was the first time he tried the procedure. Note to self; if it's not in the manual, keep your hands in your pockets.

The woman was the victim of record on so many prior occasions that the court never convicted her of a crime following this evening's events. Exonerated of the accusation, our paths never crossed again. She was my benchmark for "the victim," I have thought of the kids several times. They never entered the room during our call.

Despite the training and mental preparation for the calls depicted above, the men and women that serve and protect the public are under-appreciated. Thank first responders for their service the next time you cross paths with one or a crew. Buy them their coffee if you are near them in line at the shop. They will be genuinely surprised and shy when receiving recognition.

Appreciate that they have accepted the responsibility of protecting and serving us. I have witnessed the same public expression when visiting the United States and often wondered why we don't offer our thanks at home. It's a missed opportunity to respect a responder.

13

A strange but true collection

A respected colleague often mocks me after relating a tale. Repeating my introduction, "You can't make this stuff up," Vince smiles, then laughs. I'm not sure if it is with me or at me. It's about the most accurate rationale of our profession that has passed by my ears.

Paramedics often raise the topic of human behaviour and their experiences with colleagues, family and friends over their career; mine has been no exception. Some stories from a life of working for the Emergency Medical Service just don't quite fit the routine categories. The central theme; an apparent or perceived medical calamity.

Responses detailed here represent some serious, life-taking and other life-threatening events and circumstances. Yet, other calls have an element of humour amidst the sometimes sad nature of our business.

One thing for sure, you never know when you climb in an ambulance just where you will wind up or what you will be called upon to do to assist the public. Heading out for one call, your course can change in a heartbeat.

Don't give me your lip!

I love the melodramatic preface to some stories; "it was a dark and stormy night." So much for the 1800s. Paramedics respond to more calls on clear sunny days than the setting above. This call was no exception.

Artie and I were heading out to stand by at a station that was a hovel. It was not the host location to our "cock a roach a thon" but ranked a close second. This room was too hot, winter and summer and claustrophobic to many who roosted in its dated confines. Any out was a welcome relief.

With only a minute to go to our post, the archaic tube-style two-way radio spat out some static with a message. The request: respond to an address for a "pop can stuck to a face." It was a "code three," an emergent call without the pomp and circumstance of a full-on crisis.

After a couple of laughs and the thought of a soup can stuck on a skunk's head on a card that I gave mom for her birthday, we focused on regaining our composure for the patient. It would not be acceptable to roll up on the scene laughing out the window. No matter how much we wanted to, empathy 101.

Met on the front lawn by a distraught father, he led us to his backyard. The incident this afternoon interrupted a BBQ. Like a good medic, I always assess the food situation; the burgers had been turned off on the now fading grill.

Sitting side-saddle on the plank seat at the table was a young teenage girl with a panicked look in her eyes. It was easy to see why. Perched on her face was a ten-ounce pop can. Tilted upwards, the can was supported by a consoling mother also sharing the panicked gaze.

Looking at each other, Artie and I shared imaginary bursting shirt buttons begging to see the humour in this predicament. Alas, there was work to do. It was time for some backyard surgery. Speaking calmly to the small gathering, I explained that a trip to the ER would only bounce the can around and aggravate the situation.

Asking for permission to operate here and now, the father could see our point; the young lady was in no position to argue. She blinked, he nodded in approval. Like boy scouts, we brought our newest instrument to the lunch.

The "lifesaver" was the shiny set of shears in the small holster on my belt. The tool was an addition to our craft from its Austrian designer, the lightweight but heavy-duty scissors could cut pennies if called upon. Leather jackets and zippers were a higher likelihood in our profession.

Planning as we went along was a strength Artie and I shared and enjoyed. Paramedics can train all they want, but out in the field, every call is a slight variation on the original theme we received training and instruction for. This scenario was not within our scope of emergency patient care skills. Yet.

Sitting facing our patient Artie was calm as he instructed the young lady to sit still. The burgers smelled enticing as we assessed the hungry teen. Mother spoke up now, providing the circumstances of her daughter's entrapment.

The brand-new style of drink can was a recent innovation. Designed to eliminate the need for an outdated punch style opener, it streamlined the consumption of your fav beverage. Pulling a ring tab forced a small oval section to separate from the top, opening the container.

Have you ever tipped a drink up and sucked the last drop out of the inverted can? In the beer-drinking world, it's referred to as "shotgunning." This kid did. Then, she moved her lip further over the tear-drop-shaped opening. Suddenly the soft and vascular tissue was drawn into the vessel by the remaining vacuum on the inside.

Suction drew blood into the trapped tissue, swelling it and preventing its escape past the sharp aluminum edge. I would have looked panicked too. Keeping our victim calm was half the battle.

It was a good thing the high-tech can still had an old-fashioned crimped rim holding the bottom on. The metal edge gave a solid starting point to begin the delicate procedure. Mom supported her daughter from behind and spoke quietly as Art sat patiently, steadying the container.

Standing at the patient's side, the shears, not me, performed their magic. Turning the scissors around in a less than ergonomic fashion, it took short bites at the can's bottom edge to release the disc. There were some worried looks as the tin moved slightly with each cut.

Looking up into the can, Artie described the crimson blossom that the entrapped lip had taken on. Entrapped conjures up the term firefighters use to describe accident victims stuck in their mangled vehicles. This was no place for the Jaws of Life.

Our next hurdle was to remove the side of the can. Suggesting that we spiral up the side was a better plan than mine. Artie hit the nail on the head. I thought about going straight up the side. That move would have required some wiggling to turn the scissors sideways under the lid.

Like peeling an apple with a paring knife, the side of the can splay out from its original shape in an unwinding motion. Artie's hands moved slowly to support the disappearing drink container. Lots of encouragement from Mom and face-on reminders from Art, and we were left with the lid and a sharp edge, well away from the patient's lip.

Our victim's family and her friend gasped when the purple bulb was exposed by the missing tomb. We were down to the final steps. Luckily the oblong opening in the can's top did not completely admit the lip. Near the center of the disc was some daylight.

This was the point that had me squirming. As successful as we had been, a slip here could cut the girl's lip with the thin edge exposed by the missing ring top. Cutting the thick, crimped edge of the can could snap it sideways when the shears passed through.

It was a lot of fear for nothing. Holding the lid solidly, Artie's hands were braced against the young lady's cheeks to support the shiny disc for the last cut. The look on the girl's face told the tale. Another roadblock popped up with the first attempt to gently twist the lid open.

Stalled by the possibility of the sharp edge inflicting some pain or further injury, even with small clipping moves, a final maneuver was still necessary. Cutting through the rim on the opposite side below the teen's lip, the lid opened by spreading the top of the can sideways. In a move looking more like a reverse Pac-Man, the un-chomping action opened the disc, quickly releasing the swollen upper lip.

There was no cheer when the patient escaped. A nearby cloth, some ice water and a couple of cubes from a cooler started the rehab process.

Giving each other "the look," Artie and I packed up and left the thankful family. Embarrassed at the prospect of explaining the injury to friends, our patient was granted a reprieve; it was the summer holiday. Somewhere, out there, is a picture in an album of the insulted face. Or at least a story that can be plied against a sibling.

Bugged

Like other healthcare providers, paramedics often extend their skills by adding patient advocates to their repertoire. Although it is not a technical skill, it requires courage, diplomacy and a thick skin when others wonder why you are going above and beyond.

Often tempted to walk away when the job is done, the line is drawn. Dedicated advocates set aside time to go the extra mile. It would be so easy to listen to the voice in your head or naysayers dismissing an act of kindness.

Back a few years, the ambulance service spent more than half its time picking up, delivering and returning patients in non-emergent situations. The moniker "horizontal cab" was well earned. It was a necessary service to the infirm.

Today, the health care system has empowered transfer services. Private providers now transport patients when there is no need for specialized care or support. A crew that can lift and provide an escort for appointments or the trip back from the ER is an essential part of our system.

One evening, Artie and I were dispatched to return an elderly gal to her nursing home bed from an earlier trip to the hospital. Waiting for hours to get an ambulance ride home, she was treated to a dry turkey sandwich in the back hall. It filled the gap, missing supper following a late afternoon fall that left her with a laceration requiring sutures.

Loading her into our ambulance, the pleasant lady issued one request; a cup of tea when she arrived at the home. The simple ask would relax her after the upsetting mishap and time lost at the hospital. There was no escort or family to accompany her this evening.

The trip home was brief. I barely learned that she taught school in the city when we backed up to the nursing home's rear entrance. Unloading was delayed, the lamp over the door was burned out or turned off, the doorway was locked. We waited inside the ambulance while Art summoned a greeter with the bell marked for deliveries.

The orderly answering the call took a couple of minutes, likely busy with the evening assignment helping elderly men into pyjamas and then bed. What a routine? People respectfully ask how we can be paramedics. We feel the same about orderlies and nurses serving in long term care institutions

Walking down the darkened halls, small opera lights just off the floor lit each side of the passageway for safety. The nursing home was in full night mode. Rooms darkened; some doors were closed to keep the hall noise from sleeping residents.

Arriving at the patient's door, a medication cart stood outside a neighbour's room. The nurse was finishing off the evening regimen. Waiting to confirm that our patient was going back to her room would save time and another move.

Some returning patients spend the night in an observation suite next to the nursing station to watch for signs of head injuries. The conversation inside ended and an older woman exited and closed the door behind her.

Receiving the nod to place the woman back in her own bed, I reached inside the darkened room and felt for the light switch. Pushing from the foot end of the stretcher, Art was in a rush to get back on the road. We were due for our first coffee. I was as interested in the doughnut as the hot drink.

Have you ever been creeped out and thought you were being watched? Your subconscious spotted someone you thought was looking at you. I got the creeps and never saw anyone. It was something. As a matter of fact, it was hundreds of somethings.

Stuck to the newly brightened walls by the overhead light were clusters of giant cockroaches. I mean, not the size of the bugs in National Geographic, but significant! The walls, ceiling and bed were spotted with the little buggers. Startled by the light or losing their footing, regular but quiet little taps sounded. The noise announcing their submission to gravity.

Brushing a couple of the unwelcome visitors off the stretcher, I attracted Artie's attention for the unplanned retreat. The nurse turned from her cart full of pills out in the hall, surprised to see the patient still on our stretcher.

Informing the nurse of the unwelcome find, she walked down to us in no hurry to see for herself. Sticking her head in the door, there was no warning, no bugs in the hall. She seemed non-plussed over our find. I wondered if the room was closed before the patient went to the ER.

Someone knew the secret. Roaches don't parachute in. They hadn't assaulted the room; they invaded the place. How long had this been their residence?

Suggesting the patient go to the wards observation room until morning received a deadpan response. An exterminator or maintenance staff could deal with the critters then. The temporary space was occupied with a "wanderer," so it was not an option. Suggesting another ward, the registered nurse looked at me like I was her supervisor.

Frustrated with our interference, the nurse suggested we lay the elderly woman on a couch in the lounge. Begrudgingly we backtracked to the lounge, transferring the recovering patient onto the uncomfortable sofa. Vinyl-covered, the surface was the first line of defence for urinary incontinence. It lacked the softer features of a mattress.

Warning the woman to lay still, I doubted she would last the night without rolling off. We placed a couple of close-by chairs backwards against the makeshift bed. Our stretcher linen became her bedding, blanket included. The only item I hated leaving was the pillow; they were in short supply. Oh well.

Still miffed by the thought of bugs in a patient's room, we did the best we could in the circumstance. Leaving disgusted, there were no other options in the middle of the night. I was still brewing a morning rant.

Checking off shift at 8 a.m., I knew the nursing supervisor would be starting her day at the nursing home. Stepping into the radio room, Ethan pushed the rolling file over to get the number. Armed with the phone number, I headed for our lounge to use an untaped line.

The nursing supervisor couldn't see the bottom of her first coffee yet as her line rung a couple of times. Recognizing the nurse's name when she answered as the mother of an old friend, I made up a happy introduction as a warm-up. It had been a long night, so I launched into the call details.

I knew her to be an old order nurse. Hearing her disgust at the patient's room description, she announced she would catch me in the hall someday for a follow-up. She cut me off, wanting to check on the resident.

Several weeks later, our paths crossed on a day shift. The nurse grabbed me by the arm and took me aside to reply to the report. It turns out the night nurse did not go behind our back, returning the patient to the infested room. She left the lady on the couch. Our move to keep the patient safe by placing the chairs against the makeshift bed was still in place when the supervisor checked.

My friend didn't reveal if the night nurse got into hot water. She stated the staff nurse did not follow through with the other wards looking for alternate accommodations. As it turns out, there was an observation bed available on another wing. By her admission, the roaches were an ongoing problem, but the contingency plan was never used.

It seems simple enough to take the lead when it comes to our patients. The credo of "patient's first" goes overlooked at times. We get caught up in the moment with deadlines and an overburdening workload, exposing crevices that the best-disciplined people can fall into. I have earned the bruises to prove it.

Mississauga

One evening in November of 1979, working the evening shift, we sat watching the six o'clock local news. Crews listened intently as reporters detailed a nasty train derailment in Mississauga two hours east of us. A couple of us commented, "cool." There were no injuries yet, but the fires looked terrible. My volunteer, firefighter side, was intrigued.

Be careful what you wish for. Our boss Donald showed up an hour later announcing that Toronto EMS called for reinforcements. Ten area ambulances were requested to respond to Square One, a Mississauga mall, for a one-time experience.

Jumping at the chance for the adventure, I called home to advise my family I was off to a disaster. Known for the overly dramatic, I probably made it sound like I was getting on Queen Elizabeth II and going off to war. Barrelling along highway 401 in a convoy of flashing lights was unique. We arrived and were poured into a sea of two hundred ambulances awaiting the worst.

Participating in what was determined to be the largest peacetime evacuation (200,000 residents) until hurricane Katrina hit New Orleans decades later, the experience was a "one-off." All in all, it was a long night. Our group assisted in a nursing home re-location and responded to a couple of garden variety ambulance calls before being cut loose for the weary ride west to London.

To this day, I cherish the signed letter from the long-standing Mayor of Mississauga, Mrs. Hazel McCallion. She dispatched thousands of documents to thank first responders for their service.

Lonely and Alone

Night shifts drag at times; a busy one can drive you crazy, testing your patience. Quiet tours make you grumpy when you are finally disturbed. Never take anything for granted, a tidbit my mentor Hugh shared early on. Get sleep between nights; your body will thank you.

Assigned to work with Alf tonight, his quiet nature made a slow night painful in the early days of my EMS career. Full of questions and still on the upside of the learning curve, he was reluctant to reply to all but the simplest of inquiries. Tonight was no exception.

A patient with slashed wrists was quite often a cry for help. Most of the cutters did not do much damage. The real message was their plea for attention, breaking the cycle. It is a cry not to be ignored. Things escalate. Our female patient was the benchmark of a scream.

Bearing half a dozen shallow cuts on each forearm, the dressings were more to protect her from infection and show concern than control the bleeding. Listening to the patient, she spelled it out. She had no means of income beyond social assistance. Living with a friend, the women pooled their resources and still struggled to survive.

The ER nurse taking the patient in the primary treatment area spoke right up when she recognized her from previous ER visits. Explaining tonight's call, the nurse ramped up her empathy and showed her concern for the injuries when she removed the dressings. Each wrist would require a few sutures.

The more critical accomplishment tonight would be the doctor's referral to the psychiatric team. The act would guarantee an assessment and, hopefully, an admission to help her out of her depression. This was in the day when there was still room at the inn. The much-reduced psych resources today are outstripped by the sheer volume of genuinely ill people.

Clearing the ER, we completed our third call. The brief drive back to the office downtown was silent. Alf was not a conversationalist. I was ready for a coffee; the time of day did not matter to me. Coffee went down the same at three am as a nine am coffee break did.

Sitting in the lounge, I grumbled at the prospect of counting dirty linen for pick up in the morning. The boss wanted an accurate count, afraid of an overcharge. It only took half an hour.

Reality sucks. Handling shitty, urine-soaked or vomit-covered sheets was something akin to walking over land mines in a pasture. You reached into the pile turning your head away, expecting one to go off. There were loads of surprises in the bags.

The reward tonight for our hazardous duty was a well-deserved lull in the call activity. Bars closed early; just the homeless could be found walking the core streets. Only the real sick called for us on nights. Others called for the less fortunate.

Our station, "the office," was about one hundred feet from the railroad tracks. One of the few outside noises to disturb you during a snooze was the occasional freight passing on a slow night shift. You could feel the vibration while reclined uncomfortably in a chair. Tonight was no exception.

The phones sat idle for a couple of hours. Alf read a book seated in the dimly lit room near the only table lamp. The gap between calls contributed to my poor posture and a sore back. The painful condition was magnified by the ringing phone, knowing we were up for the next run. Other crews slouched quietly as we stood to answer the hail.

Jimmy stuck his head out of the radio room. The one end of his handlebar moustache was bent up by the pillow on his desk. The headrest was likely spotted with drool. Sleeping, curled over face-first onto the desk, was a natural skill. Just look at him; he was the champ! "There's a body by the tracks right outside." Ok, my eyes were open.

The response took seconds. Parked at the roadside just up from our garage was a black cruiser. The one red beacon slowly whirling around on the roof looked like an electric bubble gum machine. The morning sun started to skim over the rooftops lighting the scene. There was no other traffic on the side street.

Stepping out, the lone constable stood near a body at the edge of the tracks. The fifty-foot walk gave Alf and me the chance to size up the scene. Stretcher in tow, oxygen and first aid kit on for the ride, I expected the patient to be a "leftover" from last night. Suffering from a hungover and ornery, the chief complaint.

The body was naked, save and except the grey-looking underwear on our male patient. The briefs had been the white variety in their younger days. Hands at his sides, the patient lay perpendicular to the tracks.

Close to the local homeless mission, the patient was headless. Stopping when we realized our treatment was not required would save dragging the cot one more foot through the large roadbed gravel. This was a planned, well-executed suicide.

Lying face down, head over the rails, there would be no turning back. The train was long gone. Our victim probably waited until the engine passed his location before assuming his fatal position. If the patient were visible on the approach, the train crew would have called, waking us earlier.

The fellow's shoulders were tight to the rails. Flattened to the steel ribbon, all that was left of a crushed spine and neck was a thin film of darkened flesh: the colour, the result of tons and tons of pressure from passing wheels.

It was more of a stain on the rail than skin. The remainder of the head fell between the wooden ties, severed just below the victim's ears. There was not another mark on him. There was no need to roll the torso over to examine his front. We could offer no care here other than privacy and some delayed dignity.

In a square pile next to the victim lay his clothes. Possibly his only worldly possessions, they were folded with military precision. At least that was Alf's opinion. He knew the drill; he served our country for a couple of decades in the Canadian army.

Sticking out of the treasures was a crumpled hand-written note that the officer pulled from the pile. Silently reading the personalized memorandum, the cop stopped. Reading aloud a second time, he hesitated, "Please take my clothes to Johnny at the mission behind me. We are the same size; they are no good to me anymore".

This was one of the earliest calls where I cried. We were still protected by the growing early morning sunlight. Caught mid-way between idle city streets on the railroad right of way, there was no traffic to gawk.

It was just the three of us with the victim. I turned as I teared up; my nose offered a quick sympathy drip that disappeared with the back of my hand. My secret was not so discreet. The cop also turned when our eyes met.

It took a few steps to return to our stretcher covered with a couple of sheets and a bright red wool blanket. Pulling a folded sheet off, I covered the body from head to toe. The blood was minimal with the crushing trauma. Not a drop stained the bright white hospital linen in the morning light.

Giving the responding officer our names, we could see our destination. Standing at the corner, Rob ventured out of our building to look the scene over. Missing the detail, he got the gist of it all, with the sheet spanned over the rail on the north side of the tracks. His view of the body was obscured, hidden by the steel ribbon. He later shared that he did a similar call to this scenario a couple of years prior.

How lonely was this guy? To conceive his plan and maintain the composure to write the note, undress, then fold his clothes took determination. And that was before he lay his head over the rail. I only hoped that the red tape was dispensed with, and someone delivered the belongings to Johnny, fulfilling the man's final wish.

In over my head

When thoughts of summertime activities surface, one of the first to pop up is going for a swim. Several summers as a kid were spent camping on Lake Huron at the Pinery Provincial Park. After a couple of weeks of lessons, I become a little fish.

Still comfortable in the water and a regular fan of the early 60's black and white adventure show "Sea Hunt," sport SCUBA diving piqued my curiosity. That's nostalgia for you. The course was offered through a dive club hosted by a downtown high school with a deep pool.

With the course and one dive season under my belt, I was eager for experience. Speaking up one day at the Lambeth fire hall when the city fire department could not find a partner for their lone diver, the assignment was simple. To recover a drowned youth in a pond at the city's edge.

Following a call to the fire department's alarm room, I spent the afternoon in a pond until running head-on into a kid that accidentally drowned. It was less shocking at the time than I imagined. The dive in near clear water was only an introduction.

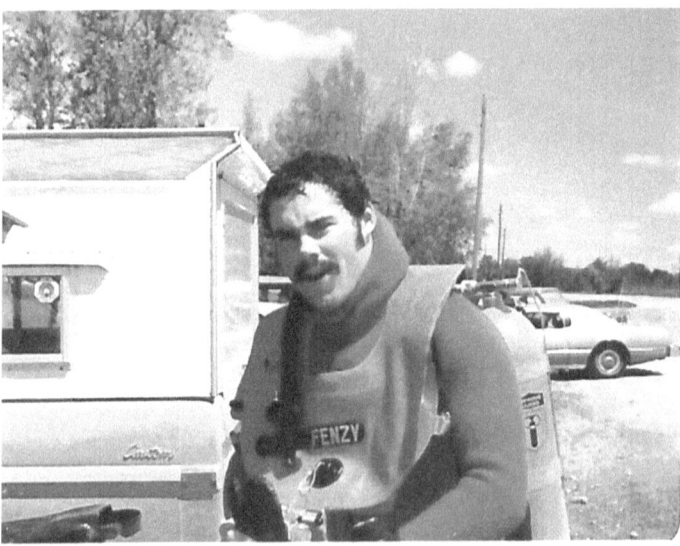

Only two months later, I started with the ambulance service. Sharing my interest in diving with the guys on the shift, two fellow medics took the course the following winter in the same school swimming pool. We travelled and dove together on several dive trips, taking in Tobermory and Key Largo in Florida. Both were hot spots for recreational diving.

Fast forward another two dive seasons; Ken and I enjoyed working as a crew. He served in our Canadian navy and told tales of his electronic specialty on ships. Ken was a diver as well. It was a sunny afternoon in August when we were called out for a swimmer drown in the Thames river.

A group of teens showing off their prowess swam several laps across the south branch of the river. The water was slow-moving, warm and inviting for some.

Darkened by algae and contaminants brought on by the summer's heat, most locals would not set foot in the rancid-smelling tributary just downstream from the city's pollution treatment plant. When the sewage facility went into overload, partially treated effluent spilled downstream into the Thames, adding to the mix.

Arriving at the water's edge, excited friends of the missing youth gathered on the bank. Pointing out the last place someone had seen the floundering swimmer, several witnesses offered their opinions. One fellow ventured the current swept the youth over the dam, carrying him west towards Delaware, miles away.

Police summoned to the scene were getting differing reports from visitors strolling by at the time. Picnickers seated on the hill above walked down with the emergency service's arrival, missing the real crisis earlier. Other parkgoers stood on the ridge, having the best vantage point for the action.

Arriving with its siren blasting, the city's rescue unit came to a halt, continuing to grind out a wail that tailed off seconds after it parked. The captain dismounted and approached us to find that we had not recovered the distressed swimmer.

He exclaimed he was out of service for diving; the fire officer described how one of the divers on his shift injured an eardrum on a recreational dive earlier in the week. He was left with a lone rescue swimmer on the unit. In his words, he was in a real "pickle."

Unsure what possessed me in the moment, I recalled to him that I replaced a diver the summer before. Dropping the rescuer's name Terry that I worked with and the recovery location, the story made its way around the campfire. Turning to Ken and me, he asked if I would be willing to use the absent diver's gear. What was that line? God hates a coward.

Returning to our ambulance, Ken laughed in my ear. "This ought to be a hoot." We were still on the drowning call, so not a word was shared with dispatch. The fire crew were on their own, so Ken became a line tender for me.

Leaving my wallet, belt and shoes in our rig, I suited up at the rear of the rescue. Still wearing my ambulance uniform, the diving equipment made me look like a fish out of water. It was hardly the time of year for a wet suit, but a swimsuit would have passed as more professional.

Sticking my head under the murky surface, a finger pressed against the glass of the diving mask was not even pink, the light erased by the sediment-filled river. With the slow-moving water, the rope around my waist was more of an encumbrance than a safety bonus. It was the captain's direction. I took his rank seriously.

I covered the first search area from the bank to a depth of about six feet in less than ten minutes. Slow going, you waved your hands back and forth in a fanning motion in the gray abyss. Looking for contact with a body lying on the bottom, the suspense had to be kept in check. Getting worked up, you would gulp air at several times the average rate shortening your bottom time.

Receiving a yank on the line was the surface signal. I was sure the seasoned diver found the missing swimmer. Ken stood on the riverbank, with the tender line, shirt open to the waist and bare belly.

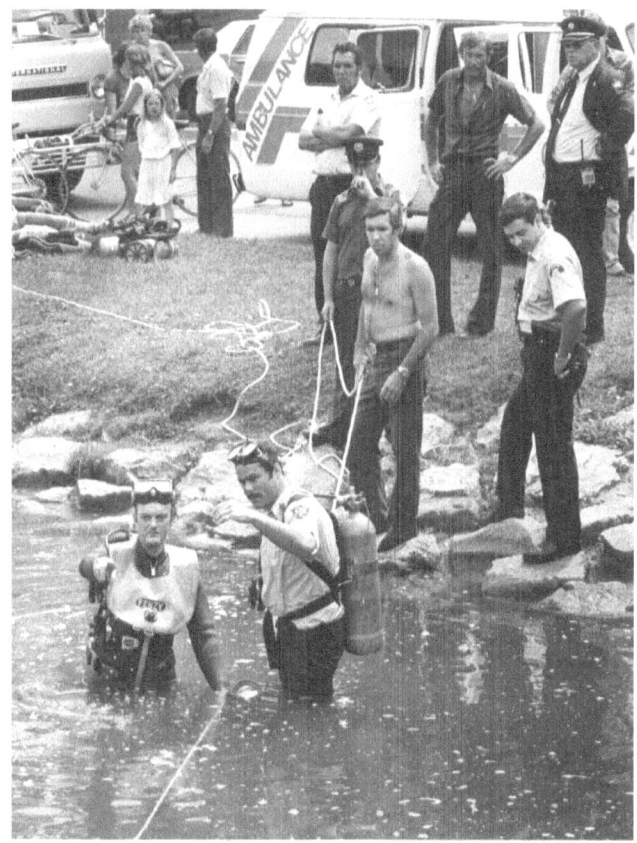

Shouting, "How are you doing? I replied, eleven hundred pounds left." I exhaled and sunk back to the soft bottom in sock feet. You did not need swim fins for this gig. It felt like you were going foot by foot in a filthy bathtub.

Bang, "shit," an "f" bomb bubbled through the mouthpiece into the regulator. You dare not drink the water; it would surely be poisonous this time of year. I swam right into an overturned picnic table, thrown or washed away in a previous season. Feeling for a divot, I had a scratch on my scalp. The damage was done; I carried on.

Playing out the rope, Ken fed out about six feet at the end of each arc. On the next sweep, I came to a grinding halt. There was a stinging feeling in my right hand as I tried to wave it for the next pass.

Reined in, I discovered a finger caught on a fishhook. The line was still attached when I pressed the digit to the glass on the mask. I always wondered what a two-hundred-pound test line looked like.

For reasons unknown, I grabbed the hook and pulled it away from the impaled finger. It wasn't too deep; the barb pulled through the wrinkled finger with a bee sting efficiency. I was free. There was no trophy fish to mount here.

Several more passes, and I reached two hundred pounds of air left on the gauge. I surfaced and returned to the shore using my best breaststroke, arriving at the muddy edge. Looking ninety exiting the water with wrinkled hands, the captain and a replacement diver called in from home met me on the shore. My shift was over.

It had been almost an hour since the disappearance. The operation passed from rescue to recovery. I was glad for the chance to squish my way back to the ambulance. Still in wet, muddy socks and stinking like a piece of garbage from the Thames, Ken and I returned to the office.

It was so close to the end of the shift that after washing my hands, head and face, I packed up and headed for home with the blessing of the shift supervisor. Calling me a keener, Neal stood and laughed as I walked away, shoes in hand still damp and smelly from the afternoon's experience.

The newspaper article the following day drew some attention. Most wondered what would compel me to voluntarily swim in the Thames in the summer. But wait, there's more. The river was like a gift that kept on giving. As if the clunk on the head was not enough.

The crease on the skull just scabbed up and quit stinging after a day or two. The finger was more of a nuisance when the cut opened or got wet; stinging lasted for days. The final insult required a trip to the doctor's office.

Arriving with more consistent symptoms of a sexually transmitted disease, the summer replacement doctor, a female, asked about recent sexual activity. Advising that I was EXTREMELY confident that that was not the cause, she asked if I had been in a hot tub or warm water.

Bingo out popped the story of the swim in the tepid contaminated river. Thank you, London. I left the docs office with the diagnosis of a urinary tract infection. Relieved it was not the other disease, I ignored the visiting doctor's smile carrying a prescription for some antibiotics. It took nearly a week before I got over the stinging.

The thinker

People still ask, "tell us about the worst thing you've ever seen." I just laugh. This story was terrible but not the worst. As a matter of fact, I would be hard-pressed to definitively select a single call. Guaranteed, there have been lots of memories vying for the award over the years.

Our service operated privately for decades. In 1969 the owner bought out the previous proprietor assuming all aspects of the business. In addition to the ambulance service, we offered oxygen rentals and operated a removal business. The oxygen part is self-explanatory.

Removals were a different cat again. Ambulance attendants were very acquainted with deceased bodies. For the right money, there was a willing workforce. The removal service supplied transportation for patient's remains from residences or a public place to the hospital morgue or funeral home. This assignment followed the official confirmation by the attending coroner that the patient was indeed dead. The process included the paperwork, making it legal to transport the remains.

As a driver/attendant, participating in removals was not mandatory. At the rate of $3.60 an hour as an attendant, the opportunity to make $8.50 for an hour's work was enough for me. There were drawbacks. A strong constitution, a.k.a stomach, helped.

In the days before private pagers and cell phones hit the market, you had to be at home or leave a number if you wanted the work. You got calls at the strangest hours. It was hit and miss, but the call-in list was short. The customers never complained when you sang to them during the ride, either.

Still living at home with my parents, I was called in one night during a bout of freezing rain. It was a pain to have the phone ring late at night. Mom and dad were understanding. They also got used to the beeping pager for the volunteer fire service.

Steves greeting during the 2 a.m. notice, "Got one on the 401 for you to shift, mate." I could only guess that it was a fatal collision due to the ice. The drive into work was treacherous; the roads were slick. Several others turned the call down with the weather. Usually requiring two for the job, I would be on my own tonight.

Picking up the black Pontiac station wagon at the office, I got the scoop from Steve in the radio room. Tommy, the shift supervisor tonight, sat next to him as the story unfolded. It was a rollover with one dead. There were body parts on the road. Great!

The trip out to the scene was chapter two of the drive. Slow going, there was no rush. Steve warned me to keep an eye out as the highway was still open and very slippery.

Nearly missing the call, I slipped on our icy parking lot, getting into the body wagon. A bruised shin from hitting the rocker panel below the car door would only be a distraction.

One break for this run, the weather and time of day; there was very little traffic to contend with. There were a handful of other drivers out there. It might be a different story on the highway.

The cloverleaf was a mess. The angle of the on-ramp usually kept you in line. With the ice tonight and the vehicle's weight, you tended to slide to the outside of your turn. Lowering my speed and keeping my two inside wheels on the gravel shoulder helped.

The scene was just beyond an overpass on the downslope. Flares warned approaching vehicles that there was a hazard ahead. I already had the scoop. Drivers that were foolish enough to travel were going thirty miles an hour.

Letting off the gas, braking began a quarter-mile short of a vehicle sitting at a sharp angle with its two rear wheels still on the gravel shoulder. You could see the right lane marked with flares was closed. An officer was cautiously replacing burnt-out safety flares at the scene. He kept watching down the road towards oncoming cars with one eye on the torch while striking it.

The safest place for me would be on the far side of the scene. I pulled over on the shoulder ahead of a second patrol car. Its lights were flashing through a glaze of ice covering their plastic lenses. Another police car blocked the right lane short of the scene. My prayer: "please hit their cars first and leave me alone."

Stepping out of the unmarked body wagon, the cop standing in the bitter cold rain didn't see the crests on my dark jacket. Ready to give me shit for wanting to rubberneck, he put off the admonition seeing the light blue uniform shirt exposed by the open parka.

Zipping up the coat, I quickly pulled a toque over my head and ears. For once, I was jealous of the constable's hat. The winter issue was four flapped and fur-lined with origins in the Hudson's Bay Company and my earliest recollection of a Northwest Mounted Police officer.

One of my best friends, Mack, nicknamed the cold weather lid a "fur-lined K-basin." A term for the plastic dish intended for vomit, he gave in and wore one a year later. I never conceded. The thought of someone puking in my hat overpowered my imaginary gag reflex.

Both constables slid over to chat in the shadow of the flares and cruiser strategically placed to protect the scene. Explaining that the driver died instantly in the car after a nasty rollover, he saved the best or the worst detail for last, depending on how you looked at it. I turned to get the inference of his gloved finger pointing out onto the right lane behind me.

Plopped upright near the middle of the right lane was a brain. Grey with the passing headlights, the organ was expelled from the driver's skull. The second constable suggested it was likely during a roll when the driver came out of his seat, trapping his head between the top of the door frame and highway.

The body part was smaller than I expected, sitting there exposed. Not rounded like the plastic training model we tossed around at college, the impact onto the road likely caused it to morph into a blob shape. This was no time to compare notes.

Returning to the wagon, I pulled the two-wheeled cart out and dragged it over to the car. Body first, parts later, the plan. Everything would be soaked before I could get back in the relative warmth of the idling Pontiac.

Sitting upright on its wheels, every side and corner of the sedan was dinged. Completing several rolls before coming to a stop, the twirling vehicle left marks in the asphalt and shoulder further back. The driver's door was easy to open; it was already ajar.

The first constable returned with some paperwork to transport to the morgue. Stuffing it in my shirt pocket, I hoped it would not fall apart with the rain. The cold water was making its way through the cheap parka.

Sitting slumped over towards the center of the front bench-style seat was a twenty-something fellow. The one side of his skull facing me was missing. Jagged edges of tissue and bone cooled off, runny streaks of blood stained his clothes. He was only clad in a shirt and jeans. Initially riding in a warm car, the abandoned coat was likely jettisoned during the crash or was in the trunk.

Clouding the door as I stood hunched over, sizing up the lift, were two odours. The first and most potent was the smell of beer. Raw brewed alcohol likely flung around during the wild ride right to the end. Then there was the stench of the regurgitated libation, also spread around the totalled vehicle's interior. Open beer cans were strewn about the car; a couple were still full.

The frigid car's second and passive smell was the undeniable flavour of body fluid and tissue further dampened by the steady rain. Etched in my memory from a few scenes now, the recall was instant. The hit on my senses stopped me cold.

Looking around the interior for the origin, the obvious was in my face. Part of the driver's collapsed skull lay on the seat. Reinforcing the primary source was the pattern of blood and tissue sprayed in a linear motion from side to side, now stuck on the cloth roof liner above the front seat.

Missing the top and side of his skull, the deceased driver was flung around and around the tumbling auto, side over-side. The violent motion scattered blood pumping from a beating heart and tissue from the open cavity once residence to the victim's brain.

The steady patter of light rain leaving its slick residue made standing next to the car challenging. Attempting to remain upright on the icy surface below became a lively jig. Lifting the man's body out of the car and sliding him onto the wheeled metal basket was hazardous. This was supposed to be a two-person call.

Head dangling over the side of the aluminum rail, blood drained for the movement onto the now wet and brittle plastic body pouch destined for the morgue. Blood-tinged water dribbled across the icy highway. An arm flopped onto the frozen road, fingers bent upward contracted from the cold, waiting for me tonight.

Almost doing the splits straddling the long aluminum basket, I grabbed the top of the driver's door to save myself. Poised over the body, moving one foot to get both on the same side of the cart was comical. A pocket full of sand would be nice now.

Finding a couple of handfuls of a cold scalp, including an eyebrow and a chunk of the skull on the driver's seat, they were tossed into the body bag barehanded. It was the icing on the cake tonight. I forgot to grab garden gloves at the base earlier. You had to steal medical examination gloves from the ER if you really wanted them.

Finally, regaining my composure, my audible laughter would have been judged as revolting at the moment if you missed the dance with no music. Strapping the body down, the competition began to get the cart back to the black wagon. The gravelled shoulder of the road crunched with ice shattering under my feet. The move went better than expected.

Loading the body up the plywood ramp was a breeze after kicking gravel around behind the black ride. There was one task left to seal the deal. It would prove to be the most gruesome.

Hidden behind the front bench seatback that tipped forward was a short-handled square shovel. Worn from gardening, the boss donated his equipment to the cause. Word was, he replaced it with a new one and submitted the receipt. I grabbed a shovel full of gravel off the shoulder of the road behind the wagon.

Making some cool curling moves, I worked my way out onto the highway. The area was ringed by flares that were sputtering their last red glow. Short of the blob, I spread the gravel. With some traction, there was at least a chance I would not wind up on my ass with a shovel full of neurons.

In a single motion, the straight edge of the shovel slid under the dormant brain. The metal was thin enough; it scraped the organ off the ice, barely leaving a trace. With the traumatically excised encephalon safely on its platform, I reversed course returning to the wagon. The tailgate was still down, making the transfer seamless.

Holding the shovel in one hand, it was time the blanket and sheet were peeled back. More than I planned for, the task of unzipping the pouch with my one free hand stalled. Setting the shovel on the tailgate, the heavy-duty vinyl bag was opened, brittle it crackled with the cold.

The tissue was placed next to its owner's head, near the other bits, also secreted away for the trip to the hospital's back hall. The shovel got an interim cleaning on the ice-crusted grass beside the road's shoulder, a less than sterile process. The leftovers unstuck from the shovel would be long gone when it warmed up. No one was the wiser.

Working against me was the warm interior in the car. The faint odour of the tissue wafted up to the front seat, making its way out of the body bag. Almost at the morgue, I counted the minutes to the destination. Helping the situation, the side and rear windows were lowered. The goosebump-producing smell trailed out the back.

Dodging the bullet

One scenario responders train for after embracing the basics of caring for one victim is the all-mighty MCI, a multi-casualty incident. Fortunately for our community, they have been few and far between. Most local occurrences have been benign despite the initial details that bystanders call in; other incidents worldwide range from life-changing to world-changing.

I know several medics that can tell you where they were when they responded to their MCI. An incident is declared whenever local resources are overwhelmed. The plan of attack changes, adapting to serving the needs of many as opposed to a few.

As a supervisor in the latter part of my career, attending routine calls was reserved for annual paramedic reviews. Paramedics are well disciplined at assessing, treating and transporting the sick and injured. The role of providing oversight on a shift is generally reserved for what I refer to as "escalated calls."

Driving between our rampantly busy emergency departments to clear ambulances from the ever-present flood of calls is a routine. Hours evaporate on a shift, meeting with nurses and paramedics to return crews to service or get them that well-earned break. Cruising along, I was returning to an ER that cleared up only an hour ago. Dispatch was busy with the morning's garden variety of medical calls. The monotony was interrupted when they assigned a call to a crew for a student choking at a school.

For a weekday, that's not so unusual. Candy stuck in a throat, congestion from a cold, maybe an allergic reaction? Cheated out of a brief pause for their coffee, paramedics responded to the "code four."

Within a minute, the communicator advised she was sending another ambulance for a second patient coughing at the same school. Unsure if the centre received two calls for the same patient, the dispatcher erred on the side of caution. A good move.

Then, there was another and another. The count jumped until the report was for six patients experiencing shortness of breath, coughing and now vomiting. Someone was thinking, call the fire department.

In addition to the Provincial ambulance radio, our supervisor's vehicles are equipped with a city services radio that works on the interdepartmental talk groups reserved for a disaster. A bonus for EMS is that the fire talk groups are also programmed into the radio to monitor. Listening can be more powerful than talking.

The closest engine company was dispatched to assist EMS. Our friends at the fire department didn't have the whole story; it was only the tip of the iceberg. The count climbed.

Speaking up, I asked for a total of six ambulances and advised I was a couple of minutes away. Looking at the crew list driving to the call, the first crew in was a bonus. Their experience would prove invaluable.

To avoid broken communications and a delay, I talked and drove at the same time. Calling the fire communications room directly, thinking they would cooperate, fell on deaf ears. Identifying myself and asking for the hazardous materials unit at our scene was not an order; it was a request. My wish went unanswered for the time being since I was not recognized in their command structure.

First in was Anna, an experienced "no BS medic." Quick to speak up to anyone, supervisors included, she was the kind of medic you wanted for this call. She is confident and vocal, both professional traits that I never questioned in the heat of the moment.

Arriving, the front lawn at the high school was littered with students. Some seated on the grass, others milling around. There wasn't much laughing and talking, the norm for teenagers. There were some concerned faces.

Passing our ambulance at the school entrance, there was no room to get off the roadway. Students blocked any chance of that. It was a walk to get to the crew standing out on the front lawn. Carrying an oxygen kit and emergency supplies to the crew surrounded by victims, we were outnumbered.

Anna stepped back from her patient; she was as cool as a cucumber. "They have breathed something in, I don't know what." Asking how many patients there were, drew the "I don't know" look. It was an honest assessment.

Calling dispatch, I offered up the initial number of thirty patients. It was an unscientific wild guess. It was the best guess, counting the patients that looked to be in distress around me. No one looked life-threatening, just upset.

Turning to Anna and her partner, I informed them, we were in MCI mode, and they were in charge of triage. Positioned perfectly, approaching crews could see them and help with the volume of victims.

Speaking to a mounting police presence, I asked everyone to announce that patients should stay on the grass and the others not affected move back. Paramedics needed to be able to identify the victims. If you counted emotions, there were over one hundred affected. It really wasn't that bad.

One female student nearby was choking then vomited on the grass. The first engine company arrived, the captain approached me, glancing around the scene. Advising I called directly asking for Haz-Mat, he carried on and sent a couple of firefighters in to check the school out. The last I saw of the two fellows, they walked into the school minus their breathing masks.

Never one to doubt another supervisor's decision, I suspected he had a plan. Arriving between several more ambulances was a full-on general fire alarm response, including a chief and lots of help. Finally, the cavalry, Haz-Mat, had landed.

Teachers knelt by their students, consoling them. Other students held friends, there was lots of crying. Asking a couple of passing teens if they knew what happened, the request drew blank stares in response.

Fire captains and their crews approached equipped for the event, hands full they too carried automated external defibrillators, first aid and oxygen kits. Asking what they could do, they could see where to go pointing out Anna in the crowd.

The principal walked up; she drew a blank on a cause. There was no more information for the moment. Our crews were confirming the obvious; no one was serious. It was time for damage control. Returning to Anna for a report on the crowd, she agreed with my observation; nearly everyone was recovering. Emotions were the slowest symptom to subside.

A police sergeant approached, followed by a fire captain. Surrounded by victims, the emergency services managers came looking for answers. Making the decision to hold, for the time being, I announced that paramedics had not examined anyone yet with severe enough symptoms to transport.

Today was an exception to the rule at significant incidents. Typically, there is a fire or criminal component, and one of the other services would be overseeing the response. Since this scene had neither element (yet), EMS drew the short straw.

The return question to the firefighter; "what have you found out?" With nothing to report, we needed a better answer than something toxic that could not be identified. The police officer made the best suggestion, "it could be OC."

Oleoresin capsicum, or "pepper spray," some call it bear, or dog spray, is not usually lethal. Used by police to control an aggressive individual, it is less dangerous than a Taser or gun. It is illegal for the public to use. The suggestion made sense since no one was in serious shape. Kids choking, red eyes, coughing, and lots of crying fit the bill.

Remove the victims' from the source; check. Place at rest and offer oxygen as required; check. The victims' symptoms were resolving quickly, pointing to a good fit. The police officer and firefighter went back to their groups. We all agreed it was the most likely culprit.

The era for cell phones had arrived. Parents began to flood the front lawn looking for their children. A handful of media folks converged on the scene. The incident attained the status of the Gong Show. It was a slow news day.

With the city street blocked off by foot traffic, paramedics were looking around for direction. Returning to Anna and several other medics, all reported kids who didn't require a trip to the hospital or refused treatment altogether. The fresh air was working.

It was time to cover our asses. As painful as it was, we needed as many kids to be identified and officially offered a trip to the ER as possible. Knowing the patients' likely answer, in a loud voice, I announced to the medics around me that we needed "no service" or refusal of service forms signed by anyone that declined treatment and transport that had not walked off. In the heat of the moment, the medics did not offer any pushback. It was a welcome response.

The one vomiting kid now recovered was still upset. Anxiety can be difficult to resolve when there is a crowd. Anna suggested to the medics with the patient that a trip to the ER was in order. Led away from prying eyes, she was eager to leave friends and gawkers behind.

Returning to our EMS crews on scene, the paper forms were flying. In the end, it would be the legacy of a non-event. Fifty-eight kids signed off, refusing service. Crews cleared, only one patient was transported to the hospital.

The media were looking for a sound bite. The scene looked dramatic. An emergency manager led me over to a small scrum of reporters for an offering to the public. They say everyone is entitled to their fifteen minutes of fame. Mine conveniently comes in fifteen-second installments.

Giving the best estimate of the culprit that the kids inhaled, it was time for a PSA (public service announcement). Always leave them with a tidbit, say the public relations pundits. A PSA aimed at closing the loop was in order.

Suggesting that anyone watching who attended the school today should seek medical attention if they continued to show symptoms filled the bill. Providing another option to anxious parents that scooped their kid up who continued to cough would cover the unexpected. A person with seasonal allergies or asthma might need some additional attention.

Someone once said terrible things happen in threes. This was no exception. A month later, another high school had an OC emergency.

A kid sprayed bear spray in through the air conditioner attached to a portable classroom. Twenty-five kids coughed and choked until fresh air provided its miracle treatment in the parking lot. That call cost me a lunch break. For the second time, the same outcome, a lot of paperwork over nothing.

The significant difference with this copycat episode was the confirmation of a culprit. One of the school's students was the recipient of some police attention following the recovery of a spray can in a nearby trash bin. There was never any mention of the outcome. Some pepper spray on his next meal might be a good lesson. I got the soap-in-the-mouth treatment as a kid for swearing.

Shortly after, someone walked through a bar downtown, spraying the noxious stuff behind him. Patrons took matters into their own hands. Hearing and seeing the offender, partiers shouted across the bar. A couple of revellers spotted buddy after he hid in plain sight for a few minutes, then walking and spraying his way out.

The roadside justice dispensed out on the street took longer to recover from than the biting vapour. I stood on Richmond Street, taking in that sight.

Middlesex-London paramedics have dodged the bullet so far. Our local MCI's have turned out to be 95% drama and 5% trauma. Sooner or later, our luck will run out. As a dedicated newshound, it seems that other countries and cities take the cake when it comes to disasters. They can keep the excitement to themselves. I avoid overtime like the plague.

No Christmas

With too many cardiac arrest calls under my belt, a single vision still evokes one of my strongest memories. Ranking highest on a paramedic's "Not Me" list must be the call for crib death. Thoughts of a lifeless baby in your arms leave most responders with an empty feeling. The reaction is brief.

Despite all the training, and that's before the newer advanced options at paramedic's fingertips, you briefly feel helpless. The sentiment passes quickly; there is work to do. The effect is compounded if you are a parent or are approaching parenthood.

Most of us settle into the Christmas spirit each year, with a light heart eager to celebrate, exchange gifts and overeat. Treats associated with special occasions never seem to give me a pass on the memory. Going to work as a paramedic, the season can go for a shit in an instant.

Tasked with a "VSA infant" call, Artie and I were the new kids on the block. Only a couple of days before Christmas eve, everyone was ready for that "special time of the year." We were scheduled to work through the season on nights.

Art had one child at the time; he was destined to be the father of two. My co-worker looked at the call from a different viewpoint than mine. I was still single and not a worry in the world. That would change.

Entering the apartment, the rest of the world faded away. Losing all sense of the reason for the season, decorations and trinkets associated with the occasion were a blur. The room smelled of fresh evergreen.

Through the preoccupation of a pulseless child, we passed a Christmas tree. Glittering lights weighed down decorated branches on the small spruce. Poking out from under the tree were several wrapped gifts, their surprises still intact. Sitting by the presents was a three-year-old child, oblivious to mom's frenzied pace.

Mom's glistening eyes and loose-fitting clothing leaned me towards a newborn. Turning back to point us into the baby's room, mom sighed, "three weeks." We both stepped past the now crying parent almost coldly as I dropped the oxygen bag on the floor. The thump startled mom: the gasp brought us to our senses. I reached into an old crib, the worn wood spindles and faded paint likely served a few babies.

Lying on his back was a tiny fellow. His lips and face reflected a dark blue by way of an underpowered bulb from the lamp on a dresser doubling as a changing table. Clothed in a small one-piece blue flannel sleeper, it was marked with stains of feedings from the past. As I scooped the infant out of the crib, thin, runny vomit ran from the corner of his cool lips.

Setting him on the changing table, Artie didn't need an order. A tiny airway appeared beside my face as I listened for a breath. I already knew there was no breathing. Two puffs of air into his mouth, and I had a small moustache from regurgitated milk and acid from his partially digested feeding.

These were the good old days. Ambulance attendants did not have small ventilation bags for infants. Art slid the airway into the baby's mouth as I started compressions. Rapidly depressing the little sternum was not going to make a difference tonight.

Compelled professionally and morally to do our best for the tiny patient, I cycled through a few rounds of compressions and ventilations before turning to mom. Announcing we were going to the hospital a mile away, she told us she would have to find a neighbour to look after the older child that we passed.

As I lifted the boy into the crook of my arm to continue CPR, she stated she would be a few minutes. She did not have a car and could not afford a cab. Hearing the plight, Artie spoke up and told her to go stand by the front door when she was ready. We would arrange a ride for her.

Walking by the older sibling, he turned as if we were regular guests and no bother. I carried his little brother out of the small flat for the last time. Breathing for the limp infant and regularly pressing on his miniature sternum was an act of compassion that would make little difference in the end.

Our patient had ceased breathing for some time. The colour did not return to his pale cheeks with artificial respiration. His mouth refilled with vomited fluid from all the movement during the resuscitation.

Turning the small boy on his side, I cradled him like a football on my forearm. Legs dangling flaccidly off each side of my arm, the palm of my hand supported his head. Fingers spread apart; they acted as support keeping his narrow airway at the right angle.

The whitish soupy mix ran out quickly onto his cheek and the dark blue sleeve on my jacket. Our suction would not have done the job. Gravity was our friend tonight.

Art jogged ahead with the oxygen kit, hitting the glass entrance door at the bottom of the stairs. Fortunately, the ground was dry tonight; snow from a couple of nights ago already melted. My recollection of the walk to the ambulance in the parking lot is an estimate.

Guided back to the ambulance by one of Art's hands on my arm, doing CPR on an infant while on the move can result in a fall, missed ventilations or both. Having my mouth poised over the infants while doing compressions, the sour milk smell would change supper plans on this shift.

The ride to the hospital was brief. Seated on a small chair just inside the passenger's side door, I missed the passing Christmas lights. I could hear Artie giving the nurse on the radio patch our report. Following the brief message, he asked the dispatcher to send the police to drive mom to the emergency room.

The ER staff were prepared for our arrival; seats just inside the waiting room door were cleared. Patients and relatives would not have their memory of Christmas dashed by the sight of a dead child.

Nurses and doctors took one look at the foot and a half-long patient on the six-foot gurney; you could read their appraisal. Their examination confirmed our primary assessment earlier in the nursery, now under the bright operating room style lights.

We had done our best but realized early on that the cards were stacked against this wee baby. The gowned staff went through the motions with a couple of advanced resuscitation procedures. The colour drained out of every face in the room.

Calling the resuscitation off after about ten minutes, the attending doctor summoned everyone out while he charted the procedures with the nurse in charge. Usually, after adult cardiac arrests, staff mill about straightening up the room and getting the patient ready so relatives could view the body.

Everyone exited with the command to take a breather. We all needed a break. Nurses with younger children talked at the end of the hall. One nurse stood wiping tears away from her eyes while looking towards the waiting room door.

The nurse in charge of the shift appeared at the door of the resuscitation room. She motioned to Art, asking where mom was, his radio patch not offering much more than the basics. Explaining that the mother had another child to care for, Art added he arranged a ride for mom with police. A clerk ran around the end of the counter to open the door to the department.

Entering with a police officer at her side, you could tell mom employed her intuition and sensed our effort's outcome. Kneeling, the constable offered to take the boy for a walk down the hall while "mommy" talked to the doctors. The innocent and silent reply from the three-year-old gave his permission. Hopefully, it would be a few years before big brother would put things together, recalling the experience.

Clearing from the emergency room couldn't come soon enough for me. Grabbing the aluminum clipboard from the counter at the nurse's station, I turned to head out. There was one last task before we departed. I ducked into the dirty utility and supply room to retrieve a small bottle of the most hideous tasting institutional mouth wash.

Tonight' was not the night to dilly dally around after a call talking to nurses. Thinking back, I am not sure who I was trying to be kinder to; mom, the nurses or me?

Calls that a paramedic can associate with a specific date tend to stick in their memory. Everything's great with my Christmas each year; our small family is close. That is until a trigger sets off a recollection of one of many calls associated with the special day. Only lasting for a moment, someone sitting across from me might miss it. That smile, blank look or sigh acknowledging the thought.

That turkey smell

Pain can crush any good memory regardless of the occasion. This Christmas experience or, more correctly, disaster was no exception. Presents opened, snacks downed, the house smelled of a turkey in its final preparation stage.

The "bird," as dad called it, would render dressing and gravy in addition to the slices of light and dark meat. Our family would sit around all afternoon as the smell of the cooking beast increased in concert with his internal temperature. The anticipation of turkey dinner for a kid on Christmas day survives as an annual rite of passage.

Mom never used a thermometer to confirm the bird's state of readiness. Instead, she wiggled a leg. The loosening appendage and darkened crackling skin were the benchmarks in our home. That was before the food handling pundits introduced their "best practice" thermometer standard. That's progress for you.

Working the evening shift this Christmas day, our family enjoyed the spoils of the season before I departed to serve the sick and injured. That was minus dinner. I would get a turkey sandwich at midnight, breaking all good rules to avoid eating after seven in the evening.

The radio room was silent during the supper hour. You had to be genuinely sick or injured to interrupt the annual feast. A couple of the fellows enjoyed a plate delivered by their wives. Sitting in the lounge, sharing the aroma of a missed meal with the other crews, the phone surprised us all. Dan and I were working the shift together tonight. Both single and no turkey dinner, we were up for the call.

Jimmy handed out the details, all too eager to dispatch both of our overactive noses away from the food-laced coffee table. The roads were silent, save a single police cruiser silently passing us in the opposite direction. The cop was likely as bored as we were.

Sent for a grease burn, I could hardly imagine someone cooking up French fried potatoes tonight. It was a wonder our friends at the fire department weren't coming along for the ride. Too often, the call for a grease burn resulted from an unsuccessful attempt to extinguish a grease fire. Other patients are burned carrying a flaming pot out to a door, tipping or dropping it on the way. Boiling grease is cruel.

Arriving at the small wartime home, a silhouette marked the front storm door. Festive lights covered a hedge lining the porch. The cold evening air was refreshing, with no new snow to contend with and dry roads. It was the singular bonus of having to work the holiday.

Walking up to the darkened entrance with our stretcher in tow, a burn kit and several bottles of sterile water were stuffed under the red wool blanket. We were greeted by a sobbing woman. Inviting us in with the cot, she warned us that the injury was severe. The smell of a cooked turkey met us at the threshold before we entered.

Opened gifts and a twinkling tree filled the small living room in the 1940's home. Led to the kitchen, we could hear our patient cursing as we passed through the short hallway. Seated on a dated vinyl chair, our patient cursed again. It was one of those hurt voices.

His wife spoke up as we entered the kitchen. She warned us about the slippery floor from spilled grease. The red-tiled floor was shiny with the by-product of a fully cooked turkey.

I can say fully cooked since the brown-skinned bird lay on the floor against a kitchen cabinet door. Lying beside the second victim was his amputated, more likely well-cooked drumstick separated by the fall and impact on the floor. Sitting beside the sink was the culprit.

Now, I was surprised by the item on the counter. Usually, only young people use tin foil roasting pans. Moms and dads were supposed to be established, cooking with enamelled roasting pans or aluminum pans with sides. The cause of tonight's incident jumped off the page.

Bent up at both ends, the thin foil pan failed from the turkey's weight, lifting it from the oven. The bright white range continued to roast along at 350 degrees. The control was not yet cancelled with the emergency.

The darkened crotch on the man's pants told the worst part of the incident. Still wearing grease-soaked trousers, the victim sipped on what looked to be a straight shot of a darkened liquor. I don't blame him; we didn't waltz through the door, pain killers in hand.

Telling everyone to leave that didn't want to see a naked man in an instant, the other couple quickly headed to the living room. Explaining to the suffering fellow that we needed to get the heat away from him as soon as possible, it was no time to scold him for not disrobing earlier. Most of the damage was already done.

Dropping his pants next to the table, his wife spoke up, adding that the "skivvies" had to go too. The grease stain began on his shirt above the beltline ending just above his knees. The failed edge of the foil roaster closest to him formed a spout pouring the boiling grease onto the victim. What we saw next took my breath away.

Ask any man to describe that sickening feeling after receiving or seeing another man get a kick, slap or physical insult to his junk. Looking at the whitened tissue on this patient's exposed genitals and his inner thighs got our undivided attention. Dan and I looked at each other, speechless.

Our burn kit would not do this fellow justice; it was only a starting point. Opening the large burn sheet in the cardboard boxed kit, the material covered the rolling cot's centre portion. Using the first bottle of sterile water, the clean sheet was soaked, the excess ran off onto the already slippery floor.

Guiding our victim over to the bed, a single linen sheet covered him. The weight of a blanket would set him off with the pain. Pouring another two bottles of the sterile solution through the improvised "burn sheet" out in the cold air, our patient shivered. It was anyone's guess if the shaking was from the pain, outside temp or both.

The ride to the hospital was brief, with the lights and sirens treatment. Dan and I agreed the shortened trip would be the least we could do for the trauma he received to his privates.

On route to the hospital, the medic's practical side in me kicked in, begging the question. Did the other couple rescue the turkey and peel the skin off, revealing the clean meal hidden below? Merry Christmas.

Home county antics

Our downtown park hosts special events every weekend during the summer. Thousands of visitors pour into the grove heading for the grassed areas and shade afforded by our "Forest City."

Seeking that fix for their love of music, specialty foods and themed merchandise on warm summer weekends, enthusiasts willingly brave the heat and the masses. The same happenings also draw partiers looking for a day away from a simpler lifestyle.

Not there for the same reason, the partiers entertain themselves with other pursuits. Drinking and drugs are the first two that come to mind. Hoping to disappear into the crowd, they are often the people that stick out. I am a people watcher.

Calls to the park have changed over the years. Today, citizens on their cell phones describe in grave detail where responders are needed. In decades past, a concerned caller had to find a phone first.

The delay often led to frustrating walks through the park to find a wandering drunk or victim, unaware they were a patient. The grounds can be like an EMS minefield on a busy afternoon. Responders have all cringed hearing calls to the venue.

Brad and I pulled up to the west side by the stage, hosting Blue Grass tunes. Unable to share the enthusiasm, we walked away from our ambulance and any connection to updates. This was before the advent of walkie-talkies for EMS.

Looking for a female "acting strangely," I commented that we were in a "target-rich area." The reply drew a grunt from Brad. We walked away from a Saturday afternoon game on our new colour television in an air-conditioned lounge for this adventure.

Strolling through a crowded park wearing uniforms towing a six-foot aluminum stretcher, oxygen and first aid kit, we stuck out. The clothes added to our non-festive demeanour. Hoping someone would run up waving wildly for us to follow them to an intoxicated woman was too much to hope for.

Arriving at a grassed area off to the side of all the noise (bluegrass is not my thing), we finally had a hit. There, sitting under a tree sipping out of a brown paper bag encased bottle, was a woman. She stopped drinking long enough to use her free hand to wave at us. Not sure if the wave was at us or for us, I pointed to my chest.

Eureka, the hand, gave a second beckoning wave. It would be a laugh if she offered a sip of her drink after making our way over. The wide-brimmed straw hat and her vintage told of flower power in her past. Reaching the lady after a near-miss with a few feet and legs along the way, I asked if she called for the ambulance.

Disappointed with the initial "no," she paused and explained her boyfriend left earlier to find a phone. Standing with a slight correction in her balance, the woman appeared to be in her thirties. Brushing the hair out of her eyes back under the brim of her hat, she looked off into the crowd.

The bottle at her side laid over slowly in the grass. White wine ran out onto the ground connecting with her bare foot. I could barely restrain myself, holding back a snicker. Pulling the brim of her hat to shield her eyes, she scanned the crowd.

Stopping to investigate the masses to our right, she pointed into the distance. "See the butt in the air?" as her index finger wiggled back and forth. Kneeling next to a family with a playpen at their side, fifty feet out, a pair of buttocks clothed in blue jeans stuck up in the air.

Music lovers around the rear end were standing up and moving away. Still, on her hands and knees, the woman gave a sidelong glance over her right shoulder. Our target was easy to spot now. Thanking our pathfinder, we rolled away. I thought the victim was drunk and had bent over to hurl onto the crunchy dry summer grass.

The proud owners of the playpen pulled the kid cage away from the proprietress of the butt. Attracting pleasing looks from the audience as we rolled up to our patient, others stood though not to greet us. The growing cluster of observers formed an unofficial perimeter around the sight.

The bum barked. Well, actually, the patient barked. Not sure what I heard, I turned to Brad for his read on the sound off. We hadn't worked a lot of shifts together, so his body language was of no help. The patient barked again then squealed.

With that, the patient turned around slowly, giving us a sidelong view. Dangling out of the side of the woman's left hip was a needle. It was buried to the barrel through the faded jeans. So, I'm thinking about a diabetic emergency. It was not usual back in the day to do the insulin thing through clothes; maybe it was a "real" crisis.

If there is one thing that startles me more than anything, it's when someone taps me when I am in a crowd. Touching my arm to get my attention is one thing; grabbing me is quite another. Not sure whether to punch as I turned, I offered a passive response to the greeting.

Looking me straight in the eye was a bedraggled-looking fellow. Several days of growth on his face, he had filthy hands and smelled like a few joints had come his way today. Asking us to help his friend, I took the medical approach first.

A non-functional pancreas is nothing to dismiss lightly. The diabetic question fell on deaf ears. "What is making your friend like this?" should have been the question right out of the gate. In a very 70s reply, our historian eagerly suggested there must be something in her "hit."

Following our informant's lead, I asked in a less than literary fashion, "What hit?" "Speed, Man, she did a hit of speed then started running around on her hands and knees!" The reply brought a laugh from a few concertgoers within hearing distance, drowning out some lively though irritating mandolin music.

With an insight into the dog-like behaviour, we had something to go on. First things first, the needle wasn't going to end up in my hand. While the patient licked the ground, I reached in for the save. The syringe offered no resistance when pulled out. It was not a surprise to see the pointy end bent from all the activity.

Wrapping the needle up in our blanket, I excluded the red wool cover from my patient care regimen for this call. Talking to the young lady, I could see she wasn't in a listening mood. It was a short struggle before realizing we would be staging a full-on animal show if one of us didn't stop.

Standing to take a rest and regroup, I could see a pair of familiar uniforms off in the distance. Without a radio to call for help, I did the only thing an ambulance attendant could do in the circumstance. Sticking a few fingers in my mouth, I whistled over the music.

A lucky break. The officers turned to find the interruption to the song coming from the bandshell. Not wanting to look helpless, I stuck a hand in the air, and with a simple wave, they turned to head our way. It would not be a direct walk. Too many bodies lay in their path.

It took a couple of minutes. The pair arrived with a game plan at the ready. It always pays to have experienced hands. The older constable addressed the barking woman by name, advising Brad and me, they had seen her earlier, he offered up that she was "stoned." Where was I during the lesson? Brad replied with the history supplied by her pal. So, it's a joint or few and some speed.

Agreeing that leaving the barking soul to her own devices would not fly, both constables each took a foot and Brad and I an arm. Walking past the end of the stretcher, the wriggling screaming woman was brought back over the stretcher from the foot end.

After a couple of "come to Jesus" moments, the police officers agreed it was time for handcuffs. So, with the cuffs and two nylon straps across her middle, the patient was stuck to our stretcher like a butterscotch Sunday to your best shirt.

You would think that the call to assist the public could not get any more ridiculous. Up comes buddy with a finger so crooked you would think he caught it in a slamming door. Sharing his current condition was a belly full of beer and the odour of more of that burnt green leafy plant responsible for an attitude adjustment.

Laughing as he wobbled on his feet, the partier related the story. It was a terrible Frisbee injury, the worst I had ever seen. Compounding the dilemma was the detail of earning the disfigurement two days earlier. The cops, Brad and I now laughed as hard as the fellow with the finger resembling a curly fry.

Not in the mood for sound medical advice like the ER is thataway, the fellow would not take the hint. Well, we were going that way anyway, so off we went to the hospital with a twofer. That's two calls for one crew.

It would just pay to take our friend to get his finger looked at. Chances were, when he sobered up, it would result in an ambulance call just the same. The second victim meant one more form to fill out and a surprised dispatcher. It all worked out in the end.

Hospital staff hearing the story of our patient's predicaments chose not to visit the festival. Sometimes it pays to leave well enough alone.

Kids

Warm and fuzzy moments in EMS are few and far between. On occasion, you come away feeling like you made a difference to someone. Opportunities crop up when you least expect them. It isn't always evident like preventing a death, appearing in a news story or returning a lost wallet.

Several medics at our land ambulance service worked a part-time gig doing medivacs on a private helicopter on our days off. I could never share this at the time, but I would have done the calls for half the price. Hello, my name is Chris; I am an air junkie.

There is nothing better than sporting a hot coffee standing at the hangar door on a day off. A call was a bonus. It could be as simple as an engine run-up and test flight after some maintenance or a full-on scene call on the side of the highway. Flying is flying.

We were dispatched earlier to a smaller city down the road for a medical patient. It was an uneventful trip late one afternoon that took us back to our University Hospital. The assignment was completed just past the supper hour. The plan; clear the hospital, pick up off the round concrete pad and fly away from the sunset, east, back to the airport.

Pilots, Nate and Bruce, returned to the machine ahead of me, carrying the folding stretcher. I took an indirect route back to the helipad to deliver the patient report to the clerk in the ER. Receiving a couple of minutes of innocent ribbing from nurses in the department over my chubby physique in a one-piece flight suit, they did not wound me.

It was apparent I was not a fighter pilot. It also took a tiny correction to inform the health care providers that I was not escaping in stolen hospital pyjamas.

Outside the hospital at the edge of the helipad, people coming and going visiting patients stopped to look out at the shiny helicopter. The warm evening air was just right for the young man to be taking in the flying machine with his parents. Commenting that we were both wearing "cool" pyjamas, the joke was on the nurses. Their wisecrack was my opening line to address the youngster.

Kneeling to talk to the budding pilot, he agreed he wanted to fly a helicopter someday. Not able to steal the glory, I admitted I worked in the back with the sick person. A split second before I could offer to walk him and dad out to look around the aircraft, the co-pilot's door closed.

The first turbine engine began to whine under pressure from a starting compressor. A second later, the fuel was added, and there was no turning back. We lost the opportunity for an impromptu tour. The second best was to leave a lasting memory.

On the corner of my collar was a small helicopter-shaped pin the company purchased for the crews and visitors to our hangar. We talked for a minute until the second engine was started. There was only a minute or two left to finish the visit without interrupting a smooth departure.

Pulling the trinket from my collar, I looked up at dad, who was smiling at the attention his son was receiving. I motioned with the badge towards his son and got the nod. Not able to really speak to the young fellow now with the whirling blades' low pitched noise, I turned the ornament, so he could see the small pewter chopper. His grin was undeniable.

Attaching the tiny present to his collar, I reached out and shook the kid's hand. Then, standing, I returned to the noisy device that repeatedly defied gravity beating the local air into submission, all the while smelling of jet fuel.

Looking back at the tyke, I believe I made his day. Little did he know he had made mine. It would be a couple of years before I became a dad.

A brief life lesson

Did you ever get up on a Saturday, no place to go and not a care in the world? Then, lazily, you pulled that Friday shirt out of the laundry basket for a second day and slacked around. Imagine that as a lifestyle beyond your control.

Very early on, there was a mentor in my career and life that taught me so many lessons. Hugh is gone now. I thanked him repeatedly over the years. He lost a battle with cancer, something most of us in the profession can relate to from arms reach.

Among the fundamental values vital to pre-hospital care, compassion ranks high. Respect for the patient and avoiding judgement are also at the top. These traits have softened with the call load, advanced procedures and equipment at paramedic's fingertips today. It is easy to get caught up in the moment of being both a practitioner and a technician. We are not nurses, though Florence Nightingale could serve as a role model.

Hugh and I would stand in the bay door at the office, exchanging stories. I had fewer life stories to share though he was eager to hear everyone's tale. Hugh could always find the good in someone's nature despite meeting people that pushed the limits. Compassion was one of Hugh's richest natural resources that he never exhausted in the thirty-seven years I knew him.

Dispatched for a bleeding peptic ulcer was not a call that brought out lots of patient care back in the day. Monitoring the patient, some oxygen, positioning feet up if the blood pressure was low, your choices were few. There were several causes for the condition, but that was beyond us. We offered the basics.

Sent to a downtown hotel, it lacked the amenities of today's lodging choices. There was no large screen colour television, bar fridge or telephone. The shingle out front of the establishment could have accurately advertised, "Hovels for rent by the month."

The rooms perched atop a local beverage room slipped from being suitable for a night's lodging decades ago in our city. Rented out now for three dollars a night, they were London's unofficial flophouses.

Arriving at the door to the hotel, Hugh, by his own admission, had crossed this threshold before. Warning me the call would be an experience, I walked in defences down like the trusting kid I was. A clerk hearing the room number admitted he called us this morning.

Leaving his post, the innkeeper reached back behind the counter. I could not see his hand for a moment, something that went over my head. Hugh said later; he thought the fellow was reaching for a bat or something to protect himself.

The innkeeper reached for a dustpan out of sight; the broom leaned against the wall a foot away. Good thing Hugh wasn't a nervous cop with his revolver at his side.

Led up an old wooden staircase, each tread creaked under our collective weight in the passageway. The resident smell occupying the building would drive most back to a safe spot somewhere out on the sidewalk. This call was an early eye-opener.

Reaching a door on the third floor, we realized our stairchair was back in the ambulance. The folding aluminum device made carrying the sick and injured easier than slogging a patient up and down stairs or an embankment. Of course, needing it would mean an extra trip back down through the scented environment.

Without tapping on the door to announce our arrival, the clerk opened the worn wooden panel to the most pungent stench yet. Lying on the bed inside was a tall elderly gentleman. Almost a foot of him hung off the single bed.

The worn-out bed collapsed on one corner from years of use, a small table and chair completed a minimalist decor. One sheet lay askew on the mattress that had not been changed in eons; its hue ranged between yellow and grey. Streaked at various angles across the wrinkled cloth were marks admitting the bleeding ulcer story.

The smell of dried blood and body fluids permeated the room. The quick diagnosis was a leaky ulcer, given the blood-streaked waste on the exposed bedding. This elderly man was beyond being down on his luck. Our patient, would likely look up with envy at someone down on their luck.

Turning to sit up and address us, the tall, lanky fellow quickly responded to our questions. He felt unwell for weeks, only leaving to use the shared washroom down the hall and find food. A friend regularly stopped by with meals from the men's mission, a resource for others in need located just down the road.

My eyes wanted to tear up now, watering from the overpowering smell; its strength went right to my taste buds. I silently yearned to run out and gargle some medicinal substance in response. Unfortunately, it was not an option yet.

A single bare light bulb emitted a pale glow from the hall through the open door. I finally noticed our patient's shirt. The cloth was discoloured from vomit and spittle that was blood-tinged and long dried. The shirt's colour and condition matched the trousers.

Standing our patient, he was eager to leave his surroundings but then turned to survey his room. It was about the time Hugh and I exchanged glances. Our fellow was clad in a one-piece pair of long Johns equipped with an old-fashioned buttoned trap door. The rear end was crusty from the repeated assault from dried blood and waste.

Senses overwhelmed, my eyes teared up in response to the smell. You couldn't hold the man back. Offering to go get our "wheelchair," he spoke right up, saying, "I ain't that sick, man." We steadied the patient up at the door to his room before leaving. He had nothing to take to the hospital, abandoning the remainder of his tattered, soiled clothes.

Rushing in behind us, broom in hand, the silent innkeeper flipped the mattress over in a single motion after pulling the one sheet onto the floor. In seconds the broom gathered a few items off the dirty wooden surface. I was hard-pressed to see a difference after the effort with the dustpan. Rolled in a ball, the sheet sat on the pan. The room was readied for the next lodger, unbelievable.

Helping our patient down the stairs, he made it under his own steam as if he was heading to the dining room for lunch. We arrived in a glass vestibule next to the stretcher we left at the bottom of the stairwell. Aided by sunlight through the grimy glass, the full extent of this fellow's condition jumped off the page.

A couple of nights in the same shirt and underwear at the cottage is one thing. Hugh pointed to the fellow's back. In disbelief, we gazed at hair growing through the waffled cotton. Matted and tangled, fine grey hair trapped the undergarment. Several buttons at the rear were missing, leaving a rough stained edge of rotted material.

I worked with the ambulance service long enough to know why Hugh reached for his bandage scissors. Nurses and orderlies at the hospital would clean up patients arriving in a dirty state with some grumbling. Having to shear off the long Johns would drive them into a state of apoplexy.

We each carried a pair of small stainless steel bandage scissors to cut dressings and remove light clothes to reveal injuries at an accident. This was a first. Telling our patient to stand still, he could hardly wait when Hugh explained what we were doing.

I have not stood that still since Mom cut gum out of my hair after falling asleep with a mouth full of pink Bazooka Joe. Afraid I would get cut in the process, I was paralyzed with fear. Getting a lecture about chewing gum in bed probably set the mood too.

Our patient stood motionless as we started. Then, cutting the material from his neck out to his shoulders, Hugh and I each took a side and began shearing the hair next to the skin, releasing the cloth. The smelly, discoloured material peeled away like the wool on a freshly shorn sheep.

Reaching the man's waist, I feared the worst. Relieved by the discovery, the patient's pubic hair was matted from the mess and not an issue. We were able to skip to his legs to finish the job. Hugh looked at me a few times; I must have had that look.

You know, "that look." The one you get doing a dirty job that just has to be done. Like the wrinkled-up face you make, picking up warm dog poop for the first time with a plastic bag covering your hand. I have never had that pleasure; I am a cat guy.

When we reached the man's ankles cutting through the stretched cuffs, it completed the humanitarian assignment. Admittedly, Hugh was to thank for the experience. I might have overlooked the option. Lying on the floor in a figure of eight, the remnants of a winter's worth of sleeping and living. Our patient was free at last!

Hugh called ahead to have an orderly meet us at the back doors to the ER near the shower. Oscar opened the ambulance door for us when we arrived, realizing we only called when we had a real mess. The worst was behind the patient and us now. It was time for the hospital to do its thing.

Thanks for the memories, Hugh.

Imagine that

Have you ever had your brain play a trick on you? Ever hear voices? The questions posed here are not to qualify or impugn your mental stability. But, surely you have listened to something at one time or another that didn't make sense or that made you stop in your tracks.

Most of us have experienced our senses picking up on an unfamiliar sight, sound, or smell before our brains could solve the mystery. Usually, the most straightforward answer is the correct one; clinicians often defer to Occam's razor theory. Try reasoning that one out when you are face to face with a dead guy.

Approaching the end of a day shift, Steve leaned out of his cubby hole, offering Ben and Rob a removal. They responded to a code 5 call earlier and left a deceased fellow at home at noontime. Both medics dismissed the incident due to its casual outcome.

It took hours some days to get a coroner to the scene, then declare the patient legally dead and release the body for transport. Weekdays were the worst when natural death calls got pushed off. Some doctors also ran family medicine practices and would finish their office visits first.

Both medics admitted that supper with family would be ready and waiting for them at home. They agreed the money was nice but would "skip it" tonight. Alf and Leon were next. Leon was single and had a beer to drink by his own admission. Alf was up for the job.

That left Tommy, the shift supervisor and me. It was a routine death; Tom would jump at an unusual call out of interest. This was your garden variety removal. Looking at me, it was a no-brainer; count me in!

Our wage was around four dollars an hour at the time. It was an opportunity to make eight and a half dollars for an hour's work. Strapping into the black Pontiac station wagon, there were only a couple of body removals in my repertoire to this point. It would also be a good experience.

Doing anything with a seasoned medic would generally offer a learning opportunity. This was Alf; he was verbally challenged. You could have renamed him "silent Sam" the moniker would have been more fitting. He was a great guy: he just didn't make small talk.

Rolling up to the ranch-style home, a police car remained on scene. Holding a death certificate and the coroner's warrant to transport the body when he opened the door, the officer inside looked relieved to see us. It was his last task before clearing the scene.

Walking us to a small bedroom, the constable stopped at a closed door. The room held the last secret in check. Was it going to be an easy removal? Hopefully, there were no goobers or big people to make us regret taking the job. Either would create more work and delay.

Lying on the bed was a fellow who looked like he would have woken up if we knocked first. Sheets pulled up under his chin, the collar on his top suggested he was wearing pyjamas, a peaceful way to depart.

The body cart, an aluminum basket with wheels at one end, would barely fit in the room alongside the small bed with the door closed. We were a bit clumsy, never having done a removal together before. At the end of the body cart, one of two tiny rubber wheels left a scuff on the wall, up by the light switch, as we turned the basket to align with the bed.

Looking at me, Alf had a puzzled look on his face. At the time, I dismissed it as his displeasure with my inexperience. The scuff mark would not disappear with the cuff of my tunic balled up, rubbing the old paint. I only gave it one try.

Opening the cover on the cart, we spread the sheet out, preparing to transfer the fellow off his bed. The bedcovers would have to sit on the floor for the moment; there was no place for Alf to put them up. We would straighten the bed linen up after transferring the fellow to our basket. It would be a respectful attempt to lessen the shock of the empty room for returning relatives.

The patient was a short but stout fellow dressed in flannel pyjamas. If you hadn't spotted the small stain at his waist, you would have missed his response when he expired. Slightly white from the lack of circulation, it was snap for a body removal assignment.

Leaning in over the man's shoulders, I was poised over his chest, preparing to quietly slide him to our stretcher. Waiting for Alf, I was ahead of myself, another telltale sign of inexperience. Still sitting at the cart's foot end were two pairs of large black rubber gloves and a body pouch.

Placed on the cart as a precaution for "stinkers," we did not need the items this afternoon. A stinker is someone who, for one reason or another, wound up decomposing before being found. That is another story. There was a voice whispering to me.

Not able to make out the spoken words, I looked up at Alf, thinking he had quietly suggested something about the lift. He would do that. Alf would often talk in hushed tones on a call, making me ask him to repeat the statement.

Looking into his eyes, they did not suggest that I missed a message. Off-balance now, I leaned back, accidentally jiggling the patient with the motion. There was that voice again. Was he complaining about the delay? Had the coroner missed a pulse on the fellow's last set of vital signs?

Sliding my hands away from the patient, I jumped up with a puzzled look. At least that's what Alf described later. Then, having started to shiver at the thought of being whispered to by a dead guy, I froze. Alf leaned in, thinking I hit the wall and was not up for the removal.

Hesitating to admit I heard voices, I leaned down to look at the patient's chest. I wanted to see for myself if there was any movement. It would be one for the history books if he was still breathing. Would we get our eight-fifty if we didn't take him to the morgue?

Looking like a first-time student of CPR, it was time for the basics. Shake and shout, well, a loud whisper would have to do. The motion rolled the man's head to the side. Eureka! Alf was likely getting ready to call in reinforcements.

Still stuck against the lifeless fellow's head was an earpiece. With the small hole turned away from his ear, you could clearly hear a voice. Unable to make out the words, I reached for the beige plastic device. A small set of twisted wires ran down and back under the pillow behind his head.

The tuning dial on the small am radio hidden under the pillow was set to a local station now broadcasting the five o'clock newscast. Mystery solved. I looked at Alf, and after a sentence and a half in a laughing tone, he waved me off to shut up. The story would have to wait.

Turning the radio off and rolling the wire around the tiny receiver, I left it on the table beside the bed. Alf looked frustrated that I took the time to pack the radio up. It was easy to slide the patient over now. Any trepidations over the mystery were long gone. Our job was a cinch from here on in.

We weren't a block away when Alf asked if I could hear the radio before finding the earpiece. Returning his snicker with my belly laugh, I admitted to being briefly scared at the prospect of hearing voices. But, as funny as it was, the moment passed. The rest of the ride to the morgue was silent. Alf and the patient returned to normal.

14

Postmortem

To close the book without acknowledging the journey would be tantamount to slamming the door in a friend's face. First, thanks to friends from Lambeth who invited me to begin the process of serving as a first responder: Warren and Mike, your early support, guidance, and training drew me in like a moth to a flame.

In the prime of my youth, how could I possibly foresee that the association with volunteer and full-time firefighters, paramedics, police, dispatchers, nurses, doctors (and the list could go on) would deliver me to retirement? What a career and fulfilling adventure. Many calls, patients, shifts, and training opportunities fueled an out-of-control enthusiasm. Witnesses often stood back as I responded in an overactive vocal display that, at times, some barely tolerated. Well, that's me.

Please accept this confession: there has always been an element of pent-up nervous energy, though I am unrepentant over the lot. To this day, I would cautiously offer support, then direction to any overzealous responder serving the public. Calm and discretion are the results of experience and association with the professionals I have enjoyed working alongside for decades. To squelch unbridled passion in a new responder would be destructive. Mentoring anyone answering a call for help should be a conscious and positive action, offered as a sharing opportunity.

My sincere thanks to friends, coworkers and professional educators that contributed to my career through the years. I hope others appreciate your dedication the way I continue to.

When the need arises, the public expects emergency responders to show up like magic, bursting with pomp and circumstance. Other times, victims wanting privacy due to their dilemma expect the "silence is golden" approach.

Regardless of the nature of the crisis or the service summoned, professionals appear as if on cue. Instantly, emergency workers are presumed to show up with a solution or cure on their belt, in their vehicle or equipment bag. Then, without hesitation, they embed themselves into the victim's emotional expectations and make everything better. The clock is running.

Life isn't always like that. In the case of EMS, it wasn't in the early days. Today, experts at the patient's side are packing more skills and resources than ever to serve the public. Literally, years of training must be sifted through in seconds to get to a working theory to understand and treat the victim's condition. It's getting to that critical inch of business to provide the care necessary to relieve suffering and stabilize a person that defines a professional paramedic and retires an "ambulance driver."

We all started out as "drivers." A term that discredited a fledgling profession. The industry went through a "technician" era inundated with new splints and devices to improve treatment...a little. Finally, with enhanced training and modern technology, the faces that come through your door today are dedicated practitioners. Medics deliver patient care based on science, technical expertise, and compassion. Despite just bruising my chest beating it, the fact remains our calling has evolved.

Through the years, paramedics shed their past baggage of medical shortcomings. Emerging as polished experts, paramedics offer pre-hospital patient management at multiple levels depending on the setting. You have only to stand back and witness the transfer of care to medical staff in the emergency room to realize they have earned respect and professional equality in medicine.

Partners, no, not wives or spouses. That individual you banged heads with learning to load the earliest of manual ambulance stretchers. Shared cold pizza with during a busy shift. The coworker handing you the correct dressing or splint as you were headfirst into a wreck at night in the rain. It has been my pleasure to have worked with several great colleagues over the years.

The list is incomplete; my admiration is endless: Bill, Peter, Chris, Fred, Larry, Ian, Charlie, Allison, Stan, Art, Nan, another Bill, Bud, Ron, another Ron, Ken, Peter, Walt, Bob, Ted, Preston, Bill, Randy, Dave and Dave and Dave, John, Bruce, Barry, Lori, Wayne, Rick, Mark, Doug, Casey, Paul, Steve, Terry. I have only scratched the surface, acknowledging medics, dispatchers, supervisors, and bosses. Without the symbiotic connection we shared, life would have differed.

To those who have served, continue to serve as responders, and to future responders, you understand or will understand that the livelihood of responding does take its toll. Shiftwork, as entertaining as it starts out to be with calls related to the time of day, day of the week, weather, day of the month, your career is wrought with stressors.

From sleep deprivation to post-traumatic stress, the pressure is tiring and can be life-altering. Listen to yourself, your family, spouse, coworkers, and practitioner. When you realize, or someone suggests it's time to seek help, it is usually overdue. Treat yourself like you are your next patient…YOU ARE!

Questions. Thinking of a new job? Looking for a professional career? All emergency services possess unique challenges and offer rewarding opportunities. If that is what you think, throw out an anchor and take a breath. Take a long and hard look before you make that first step. Ask yourself, am I that person that sticks to a plan? Can I plan? Am I a steady enough individual that I can handle challenges and stress and come back smiling? Do some research.

Find a friend, go to a college, look at some websites and seek out "information sessions." It's time to speak to professionals already in the field you are interested in. Talk to current responders, past or retired emergency workers.

If you can, attend an information session at a community college to hear instructors who have been responders explain the process for education and recruitment. Guaranteed, it will be an eye-opener. Find out early if you meet more than the educational requirements before committing to taking a course or degree.

Your personality traits, strengths and weaknesses will be tested. Getting into a responder's shoes may seem like the tricky part. Remaining upright in those shoes once in the career is the true measure of a professional.

The job can ruin relationships, marriages, and your health. Symptoms range from being that "grumpy" person that does their job but is unhappy to the extreme of mounting mental and physical health problems. If the pause and some research lead you into a career, bravo! If you have second thoughts in your honest opinion, you will probably be doing yourself a favour.

I would be laughed out of the room in an instant if I tried to pass myself off as having been the best medic. Everyone has their strengths and weaknesses. Time for reflection; there have been highs and lows related to calls, industry changes and life challenges throughout my career and life. We all face them; I paid some dues over the years; it is not the time to grumble. In the balance, I emerged the winner with few regrets.

Family. The most significant source of my strength, keeping me grounded and able, to be honest with myself. The best part: they always told me the truth, mostly when I was wrong, and that's a good thing. I missed some family events with shift work (don't all responders!); it goes with the territory. A simple rule prevailed: never forget family!

Lauren, this is for you. After patiently listening to war stories, your advice to share the experiences and wisdom amassed over the years seems a small price to pay for the gift of decades of enjoyment on the road. Your insight and help, your unwavering support along the way, are icing on the proverbial cake for your dad. Thank You. Thank You. Thank You.

To my employers, supervisors, and Chiefs over the years, I appreciate the direction you gave and deserved the sound criticism when it was issued. Your trust and confidence in me offering opportunities and promotions kept me on point. I will be forever grateful. The old adage of "work smart, not hard" isn't good enough when coming up through the ranks: "work hard and smart." Something I could have done a better job of. Despite some shortcomings, I did "ok."

Reading this collection of experiences and following the story, some might wonder if paramedics turn off their emotional sensitivity to do the job. It helps to look at the bigger picture here. We are not in the prevention business. We are not like fire inspectors that see a hazard and can be proactive and prevent a fire.

Paramedics come in hot after the fact and address the result of medical maladies and traumatic misadventures period. No one wants to hear, nor do we have the time or opportunity to offer advice on how you could or should have avoided that coronary fall or collision. Every incident is another day on the road, though some calls were more heart-wrenching than others.

If it sounds like I did not have feelings, show empathy or sympathy for the patients and victims encountered over the years, you are wrong. I have held their hands, cried with patients, watched them die, wept on a long, lonely drive home after a shift. It comes with the territory. You cope, adjust and share with friends that speak the same lingo you do. Then you get up and go out on the next call or show up for the next shift.

The incidents depicted here are true; no specifics are revealed to preserve and maintain the patients' identity and confidentiality. There is no intent to disrespect people in distress. The truth is that some events were heartbreaking, while others provided an element of humour or satire with the predicaments people find themselves in having to summon an ambulance.

To the reader, thank you. Without the possibility of someone picking this project up, perhaps the singular joy of finishing the book is the look on my daughter Lauren's face seeing her wish come true. The equally important reason for the effort is to share with the public just what responders see, do, and feel firsthand.

There will be some naysayers that will not believe the tales within. Track me down and grill me. Ask other responders about their experience; they will likely echo similar descriptions of; sights, sounds, smells, and details from the street. Stuff happens, and when it does, a paramedic or other responder will be there.

Use the question, "what's the worst thing you have ever seen?" sparingly. If you must ask that after reading Running Reds, sadly, I have failed in the attempt to share the experience. I hope you enjoyed the stories and revelations; it was a blast sharing them. I only wish paramedics could save everyone; that inclination is not possible.

ABOUT THE AUTHOR

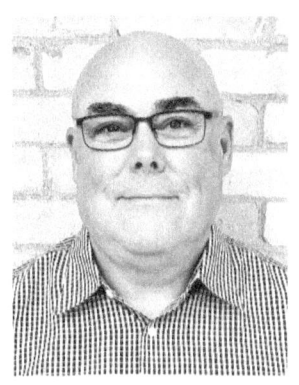

Chris Darby is a retired paramedic supervisor who served London and Middlesex County for forty-seven years.

At 18, Chris started his journey as a first responder, serving as a volunteer firefighter in Lambeth. In 1974, he joined Thames Valley Ambulance, beginning as a Casualty Care Attendant, then Primary Care Paramedic.

Driven by a lifelong interest in aviation, Chris applied and was seconded by the Province to work in Northwestern Ontario for six months as an attendant on a fixed-wing air ambulance in 1982. Chris would also spend nearly a decade working part-time on the local medivac helicopter back home in London.

Since retiring from EMS, Chris continues to follow his longstanding pursuits and share his experience, teaching part-time at Fanshawe College and volunteering with several organizations, including Airshow London. Chris enjoys golfing with his EMS friends, cooking, and travelling.

www.ingramcontent.com/pod-product-compliance
Lightning Source LLC
Chambersburg PA
CBHW031603210526

45464CB00004B/1405